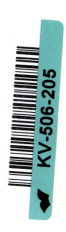
Drug Law Reform in East and Southeast Asia

Edited by Fifa Rahman and Nick Crofts

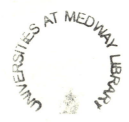
LEXINGTON BOOKS
Lanham • Boulder • New York • Toronto • Plymouth, UK

Published by Lexington Books
A wholly owned subsidiary of The Rowman & Littlefield Publishing Group, Inc.
4501 Forbes Boulevard, Suite 200, Lanham, Maryland 20706
www.rowman.com

10 Thornbury Road, Plymouth PL6 7PP, United Kingdom

British Library Cataloguing in Publication Information Available

Library of Congress Cataloging-in-Publication Data
Drug law reform in East and Southeast Asia / edited by Fifa Rahman and Nick Crofts.
p. ; cm.
Includes bibliographical references and index.
ISBN 978-0-7391-8037-2 (cloth : alk. paper)—ISBN 978-0-7391-8038-9 (electronic)
I. Rahman, Fifa, 1986– II. Crofts, Nick. [DNLM: 1. Legislation, Drug—Asia, Southeastern. 2.
Legislation, Drug—Far East. 3. Health Care Reform—Asia, Southeastern. 4. Health Care Reform—
Far East. QV 33 JA14]
HD9666.4
381'.4561510959—dc23
2013020987
978-1-7391-8492-9 (pbk: alk. paper)

♾™ The paper used in this publication meets the minimum requirements of American
National Standard for Information Sciences Permanence of Paper for Printed Library
Materials, ANSI/NISO Z39.48-1992.

Printed in the United States of America

Contents

Foreword

Drug Law Reform in Southeast Asia

Marina Mahathir

More than thirty years ago when drug use and drug trafficking became an issue of great concern in Southeast Asia, governments responded by setting up the most punitive laws possible to control it. Death penalties for drug trafficking, even for very small amounts, were instituted. Drug users were taken off to rehabilitation centers to be "cured" of their addiction. Dire warnings about the perils of drug use abounded in the media.

Despite all these, the drug issue—production, trafficking, and consumption—in Southeast Asia has not gone away and indeed has only increased. Ignoring warnings about the mandatory death penalty, traffickers continue to smuggle drugs across borders in a continuous game of cat-and-mouse with law enforcement. Millions of dollars are spent on building rehabilitation centers only to become revolving doors for an endless stream of drug user recidivists, as well as new ones. Media anti-drug campaigns wax and wane to predictably ineffective ends. Countries that initially had small numbers of drug users saw those numbers grow steadily, especially, as in the case of Indonesia, after economic and political turmoil.

Circumstances and external factors in any one society can change over time. What may have worked in one era, due to certain conditions, may not work in another time. New knowledge about the workings of the drug trade comes to light, necessitating a change in strategy and tactics. Studies about drug addiction and the social factors affecting addictive behavior bring new information and dispel past notions about what causes an individual to become addicted.

And then there's HIV. As it became clear that injecting drug users are extremely vulnerable to HIV infection, a new urgency entered the field of drug control. On the one hand, it became more imperative to solve the problem of drug use and related health consequences. On the other hand the link between HIV and drug use also led to even greater stigmatization of drug users. When human rights is even more needed in order to battle a global pandemic of stigma and prejudice, conversely many governments have done the opposite and become even harsher with drug users. The epidemic simply continues to spread and people continue to die.

Clearly something had to be done, and old ideas, practices and laws needed to be changed. New drugs became available with different issues and problems. Young people especially became more and more vulnerable to both drug addiction and all its attendant consequences, including HIV.

As always, in Southeast Asia, change needs to come from the top. Changing drug laws has become not only imperative for reasons of effectiveness but also for moral reasons. We can no longer treat drug users as sub-humans, and we can no longer deny that they live within other communities and have ties with other members of society who are also affected by these laws. To send husbands and fathers away to jail for possession of small amounts of marijuana, for example, has the effect of adding more single-mother-headed households to the community and more children brought up without a positive male role model. Making it difficult to obtain clean injecting equipment means that there will be more sharing, with a greater likelihood of spreading HIV. Refusing to provide methadone replacement therapy allows a problem to remain unsolved and insoluble.

I must thus congratulate the authors of this book, *Drug Law Reform in East and Southeast Asia*, for mapping out the issues surrounding drug use in the region and providing some solutions to its management and control. At heart, the basis for reform must be the human being involved in drug use and those nearest and dearest to him or her. I hope those in power take note of these issues covering the realities of life and move—finally—to make some changes to drug laws. After all, surely an effective solution is a better legacy than the litany of misery left by the current laws and policies.

Marina Mahathir

Preface

Mike Trace

The publication of this book on drug policy in East and Southeast Asia comes at an important time. For one hundred years, the dominant approach to the problems associated with illicit drug markets and use has been to strictly enforce their prohibition. Governments have attempted to stop the production and supply of substances as diverse as heroin, cocaine, cannabis, and amphetamines through eradication of crops, interception of shipments, and harsh punishments for those involved. On the demand side, users have been subject to criminalization and imprisonment in an effort to deter them from getting involved.

It is now increasingly clear that these strategies have not had the desired effect—the scale of the drug market and the number of users has not been reduced, and the costs of treating millions of individuals as criminals deserving of punishment, rather than citizens needing health and social services, are increasingly recognized.

We are therefore in a period where governments around the world are having to reassess their policies and programs—moving away from a reliance on law enforcement and punishment, and strengthening programs that aim to reduce particular drug related problems, such as petty crime, HIV infection or overdose deaths. Several European countries have taken this approach for many years, while the Obama administration has recently signaled a move away from the use of harsh punishment for drug possession and use. Meanwhile, the Organization of American States has commenced a regional review of future options for policy that will conclude in the summer of 2013.

So it is important that Asian governments go through a similar process of review—the regional objective, expressed through ASEAN, of creating a "drug-free Asia" by 2015 is clearly not achievable, so a new set of objectives that are more realistic and that reflect the concerns of Asian citizens need to be articulated. Specifically, the use of mass arrest and imprisonment of drug users is proving to be an expensive and counterproductive policy that can be quickly reversed through the implementation of decriminalization and diversion schemes.

There is no simple solution to the drug problem and no clear program of action that all governments should follow. But a review of options, and some sort of adjustment of course, is now clearly needed. This book gives a wide range of useful analysis and advice that policymakers across the region can make good use of as they search for drug policies and programs that are suitable for the twenty-first century.

Mike Trace
Chairman, International Drug Policy Consortium
(Former UK Government Drug Czar)

Introduction

Fifa Rahman and Nick Crofts

To counter the humanitarian and public health disaster that is the drug war, in a region where drug policy is centered around compulsory detention centers, incarceration, corporal and capital punishment, comprehensive and consistent advocacy for humane and evidence-based policy is necessary. Decades after the promulgation of laws that were intended to eradicate drug use by incarcerating, vilifying, marginalizing and traumatizing people who use drugs, the use of drugs has not at all decreased. New drugs are appearing, new populations are using drugs, and increasing seizure amounts indicate that the demand for drugs continues to increase.

And as a result of unidimensional criminalization policies, crime increases: drug producers and traders find hugely increased profits, which they use to corrupt those tasked with controlling their activities; and people who use drugs are stigmatized and brutalized, face significant obstacles to reintegrate into society, and hence are more likely to resort to crime simply to survive. Other harms also increase: in most countries in the region, HIV and hepatitis C epidemics are driven by injecting drug use because of public and governmental difficulty in dealing with drug use as a public health issue instead of a criminal justice issue.

The idea for this book arose because there is no comprehensive and authoritative source of academic material and accounts of impacts of current drug policies in East and Southeast Asia accessible to the public. There is an urgent need for information about the actual impact of current punishment-based drug policies to Asian societies, if we are to judge their success—or otherwise. Some governments call for local or regional evidence of drug policy successes and drug policy failures; others do not seek such evidence at all and revert to or retain punitive drug policies. In both cases, governments must be made aware of these successes and failures.

This book is intended for three audiences: policymakers, drug policy professionals, and the general public. Policymakers need to know that their societies are being threatened as a result of criminal punishment approaches, and that punitive drug policy is not only ineffective, it is simply not economically sound. Drug policy professionals need to know what regional policies or approaches are being considered, and whether those examples are transferable. The concerned public citizen who knows people who use drugs or are of the group that fear for private and public security would benefit from a publication that gives them the bigger picture on why drug policy professionals are advocating for change.

On the whole, the book is intended toward informing people of the harms resulting from punitive drug policy, discussing rationales for reducing harms related to drug use, illustrating effects of punitive drug policy in specific regions, providing evidence of successful drug policy and discussing possible ways forward to deal with drug use, problematic drug use, and drug trafficking.

We have attempted herein to cover the widest range of relevant issues, from the background—history, consumption patterns, associated harms; through policy and programmatic responses and their determinants; to appropriate ways to address the issues—in particular, rational, effective and humane drug treatment programs. No issue is more contentious and socially divisive than that of illicit drugs; there is no doubt that the evidence produced by our authors will arouse dissension and debate—but that is precisely the point of our constant call for evidence. Drug policy has for far too long been based on foundations other than evidence of what works, to the point where the gathering of such evidence is actually discouraged by some authorities, for fear of damaging shibboleths or vested interests.

We hope that the eventual message will be that a *unidimensional law-and-order approach* to drug policy does not reduce drug demand or drug supply, but rather multiplies and entrenches social ills, including especially corruption, and that sensible drug policy is for harm reduction measures, against criminalization of persons who use drugs and persons who are dependent on drugs, for economically sound drug policy, and for drug policy that understands that problematic drug users are to be treated as patients and not as criminals. Two lifetimes' study of people who use drugs, people who have problems with drugs, people who survive on the drug trade, and people who grow rich thereby, have convinced us of one thing—the more we look at drugs, the more we see people. And our drug policies must begin, at last, reflect this.

Chapter One

Historical Perspectives of Drug Use in Southeast Asia

Gary Reid and Nick Crofts

Drug use in Asia has a long history. Centuries of trade, migration, colonisation, ethnic movements, underdevelopment and wars have facilitated the spread of the use of different drugs throughout Asia. The introduction of manufactured psychotropic substances in the twentieth century, increasing popularity of these drugs in addition to traditional drugs, and the complexities surrounding drug use have repeatedly alarmed governments in Asia. In response to increasing drug use Asian governments have commonly adopted drastic and often harsh measures against drug use which have led to various unintended consequences with adverse health, social, economic and political impact upon drug users and the wider community. Drug control initiatives such as the Single Convention on Narcotic Drugs 1961, and follow-up treaties have for many decades focused predominantly on supply and demand reduction only. However, by the late 1980s and early 1990s the emergence of HIV epidemics among people who inject drugs (PWID) in various Asian countries facilitated the introduction and implementation of various harm reduction responses. Drug policy development has slowly shifted in Asia, taking into consideration the need for a more public health response to drug use. Yet the endorsement and traditional use of law enforcement measures by governments in Asia to tackle drug use continues to prevail. This chapter provides a historical summary of various key issues on drug use and responses in various countries of Asia pre-1900 to the present.

PRE-1900 IN INDIA, CHINA, BURMA

India

The use of cannabis has a long history in India, predating the use of raw opium.[1] Cannabis was used for medicinal purposes but also to alter consciousness, and it thus played a role in religious rituals and festivals.[2, 3] Opium was first brought to India via its western coast by Arab traders in the ninth century. Its primary use was for medicinal purposes, but by the tenth century opium use in India was widespread and included social use. The first recorded mention of opium as a product, and its cultivation, was in the early fourteenth century; the poppies were grown along the western seacoast.[4] By the early sixteenth century poppy cultivation and the sale of opium had become state monopolies, and opium was an important trade good with China and other eastern countries.[5]

In 1720 fifteen tons of Indian opium was exported to China, increasing to seventy-five tons by 1773. The British East India Company took over the opium monopoly in 1757 and attempted to popularize its use in China, to increase revenue but also to reduce consumption in Bengal among local inhabitants. In Bengal, the land designated for opium growing stretched for 500 miles with more than a million registered farmers growing opium poppy for the East India Company on 500,000 acres of prime land.[6, 7, 8] Opium produced by the British colonial government in India was the first drug to become integrated into the emerging globalization of trade and soon became entrenched in many Asian economies.[9]

In the early nineteenth century Indian exports of opium to China reached 250 tons annually, but when all restrictions on the opium trade were lifted in 1840 it increased to 2,555 tons.[10] Opium was traditionally consumed orally, but by the nineteenth century opium smoking had emerged. Despite the substantial revenue generated by the British from the opium trade, by 1893 attempts were beginning to pressure the government to suppress the trade. A Royal Commission was established which concluded it was not possible to effectively enforce prohibition.[11]

China

The word *opium* first appeared in Chinese texts in the eighth century, but it is likely that then consumption of opium was small. This changed in the sixteenth century when European merchants discovered opium's commercial appeal, and exported increasing amounts of opium from India to China. Apart from British-supplied Indian opium, after 1650, the Dutch were also exporting more than fifty tons of opium per year to China; at the time the Dutch introduced the practice of smoking opium in a pipe which expanded its popular appeal.[12, 13] In 1729, an imperial edict, the first to outlaw opium smoking and its associated activities, was introduced and lasted until 1858. However, the smuggling of opium continued as there was much revenue to be made, as did its consumption.[14]

The Opium Wars of 1839–1842 and 1856–1860, in which Britain defeated China, took place as a result of the British East India Company facing a large and growing trade imbalance as a result of Chinese control of the market. The wars, resulting in the "Unequal Treaties," were led by the British with French and American support to maintain the forced opium trade with China, against the opposition of the Chinese Emperor.[15, 16]

Britain justified the opium trade arguing that if it were to stop, the British Indian market share would immediately be absorbed by other opium producers such as Persia (now Iran) and Turkey, and China would simply increase its domestic opium production.[17, 18] At the time of the Opium Wars the use of opium and its cultivation became more widespread; an estimated ten million dependent opium consumers were spending nearly half their income on opium. By the end of the nineteenth century China was home to an estimated fifteen million dependent opium users. At the same time China was producing a large amount of its opium for domestic consumption and demand for foreign imported opium had decreased substantially.[19]

Burma

Opium was transported and consumed in Burma in the late sixteenth century. The cultivation of opium in the northeastern part of the country is believed to have been introduced by Chinese traders from Yunnan province; cultivation of the opium poppy was documented in Burma in 1736. Burmese kings discouraged the use of opium, and before colonization by the British in 1852 opium use was not widespread.[20] Following annexation of lower Burma, British administrators began importing large quantities of opium from India, establishing a government-controlled opium monopoly. In 1878, the Opium Act made it illegal for any Burmese to smoke opium, which could only be sold to registered addicts, most of whom were Chinese. Before the ban, opium use was widespread and viewed as a scourge on the country.[21]

1901–1930: THAILAND, SRI LANKA, AND CHINA

In the early twentieth century, in the Kingdom of Siam (now Thailand), opium use was widespread. In Bangkok alone there were 900 opium dens in 1905, increasing to 3,250 by 1917. By 1921 an estimated 200,000 people were dependent on opium. With the government receiving much needed tax from opium, disengagement from this commodity was extremely difficult (McCoy, 1991, 48; UNAIDS and UNDCP, 2000, 182).[22] In Sri Lanka opium use dated back to the sixteenth century, but by the early twentieth century public opinion had turned against its use, resulting in the government restricting its import. In 1907 authorities closed down sixty-five registered opium shops. However, unregistered opium shops continued trading for an estimated 60,000–68,000 opium users during the 1920s.[23, 24] In the early twentieth century China was likely home to the largest number of opium users and opium dependents in history. In 1906 an estimated 13.5 million opium users were consuming 39,000 tons of opium. It was estimated that 27 percent of adult males were dependent on opium at the time.[25]

1931–1960: INDIA, CHINA, HONG KONG, AND JAPAN

In India, the eating and smoking of opium was prohibited in 1946, unless the user was registered and able to show a medical certificate, which would allow for a personal opium supply. By 1959 sales of opium were completely banned, and the use of opium was only permitted by those registered on medical grounds.[26] The number of registered opium addicts in India was 200,000 in 1956. The fresh registration of opium users was stopped in 1959.[27]

Between 1950 and 1952 the Chinese government took draconian steps to address the ongoing widespread dependence upon opium. In 1949 an estimated 20 million people, mostly males, were dependent upon opium.[28] Those involved in cultivation, manufacture or sale of opium were subject to severe punishments, including forced labor and execution. Dependent opium users were forced to attend abstinence programs that combined psychological "rehabilitation" and vocational training programs that often involved forced labor.[29] Despite official claims of widespread success resulting from such measures, studies to measure the impact of this anti-drug campaign or of the number of lives lost as a result of the campaign do not exist.

In Hong Kong, in 1946, when opium was reclassified and placed under the Dangerous Drugs Ordinance, heroin soon became the drug of choice, and by 1955/1956 heroin offences exceeded opium offences by nearly three to one. For heroin users, offences usually resulted in the form of a custodial sentence rather than a fine as was the case with opium. Heroin offences rose substantially from 400 in 1952 to 12,000 in 1956.[30]

In Japan in 1949 the government prohibited the production of stimulants in tablet or powder form, but stimulants in liquid form, used for injection, were not covered by the prohibition. Injecting, which had been uncommon, soon became a major method of stimulant use.[31] In 1954 there were an estimated 550,000 chronic stimulant users and up to two million ex-users of stimulants in Japan.[32]

1961–1990: HONG KONG, LAOS, THAILAND, VIETNAM, CHINA, AND INDIA

The Single Convention on Narcotic Drugs 1961, a consolidation of nine multilateral drug control treaties negotiated between 1912 and 1953, was over time signed by all Asian countries. A key purpose of the Convention was to reorganize the United Nations–based drug administration and to extend the existing drug control system to include the raw materials for narcotics. The Single Convention is highly significant due to its formative role in the creation of the modern prohibitionist international drug control system. In Asian countries, and in line with other developing nations, the Single Convention led to the abolition of all non-medical and non-scientific uses of plants, such as opium and cannabis, despite the fact that their use, had for centuries, been embedded in social, cultural and religious traditions. [33, 34]

Despite the introduction of the Single Convention, drug use and availability of various new substances on the market continued to grow throughout Asia. The Single Convention and other conventions that followed (1971 Convention on Psychotropic Substances and 1988 Convention against Illicit Traffic in Narcotic Drugs and Psychotropic Substances) resulted in a range of unintended consequences, with major adverse health, social, economic and political impacts.

The enforcement of anti-opium laws in different parts of Asia was followed by a change in patterns of use from opium to heroin use: this trend was first identified in Hong Kong during the 1950s, followed by Thailand in the 1960s, and in Laos during the 1970s. These patterns of change usually took place over a ten-year span. In all three countries opium production was earlier and primarily a cottage industry, with profits largely divided between farmers and small merchants. However, the emerging heroin market saw large profits being shared between middle men, various organizations and government officials (bribes to police and customs officers became a growing necessity to ensure the expansion of national and international trade in heroin), with smaller profits received by farmers and small merchants. [35] During the mid-1970s heroin injecting was emerging and expanding in the Asian region: in the 1960s and 1970s drug users in Thailand switched from opium smoking to heroin smoking and then to heroin injection. By the 1980s administration of a drug by injecting was more common in many regions of Thailand. [36]

Drug use patterns changed again during the American war in Vietnam (1964–1973), when it was identified that opium smoking and heroin injecting were major problems among American and South Vietnamese soldiers. In Saigon in 1974 (later known as Ho Chi Minh City) it was estimated there were 150,000 drug users. After the war heroin and opium use declined considerably but reappeared during the 1980s. [37] In China, a resurgence in the use of drugs followed the free market policies and an open border policy for international trade when this was introduced in 1979. China's close proximity to the Golden Triangle (Myanmar, Thailand, and Laos) contributed to the growing number of drug users following increased accessibility and availability of heroin.[38]

By the late 1980s the transition from the smoking and ingesting of drugs to injecting was well established in many countries of Asia. At the same time explosive HIV epidemics among a growing number of PWID were identified as a result of sharing HIV-contaminated injecting equipment. In Manipur, India, on the Myanmar border, HIV infection among PWID increased from 0 percent in 1989 to 50 percent within six months.[39, 40] A rapid epidemic spread of HIV infection was also observed in 1988–1989 in Myanmar: a HIV prevalence of more than 80 percent was reported from a study of PWID in Yangon.[41] Among PWID in Bangkok, Thailand, in 1988 the HIV prevalence increased from 2 percent to 43 percent, and PWID were the first population group in the country to experience the spread of HIV.[42]

A public health approach to minimize the risk of HIV infection through various preventive measures, such as needle and syringe programs (NSP) and opioid substitution therapy (OST), as found in Australia, England, and the Netherlands, did not exist in Asia. In Asia, the traditional approaches to address drug use continued with the implementation of ongoing repressive law enforcement measures and the strengthening and increasing incarceration of drug users.

1991–2011

Throughout the 1990s the spread of HIV among PWID continued unabated in Asia, while the prevalence of illicit drug use appeared to be growing in magnitude. It was during the 1990s that addressing drug use from the perspective of law enforcement alone and the ongoing criminalizing of the drug user was for the first time seriously debated and questioned for its effectiveness and impact, including among law enforcement agencies. An emerging drug policy reform agenda surfaced in Asia closely linked to the unresolved and deepening twin epidemic of drug use and HIV. The concept of harm reduction and evidence-based public health interventions were increasingly seen as viable and relevant to the Asian context.

Commonly recognized as the most controversial of all harm reduction intervention, the first NSP in Asia was established in Kathmandu, Nepal in 1991.[43] In many countries provision of injecting equipment can be viewed as "abetment" of illicit drug consumption. The NSP in Nepal was initiated by an NGO, and by 2008, NSP were found in twenty-three sites in fourteen districts.[44] The first policy support for harm reduction in Asia occurred in the

State of Manipur, India, in 1996. The unresolved HIV epidemic among PWID in Manipur, combined with intensive national and international advocacy efforts, contributed toward the government authorities approving and implementing broad ranging harm reduction policy and programming.[45]

By the late 1990s, situation assessments on drug use and HIV in Asia undertaken by various agencies witnessed a growing recognition by the United Nations agencies, including the United Nations Office on Drugs and Crime (UNODC), that law enforcement approaches have limitations when tackling the complexity and magnitude of drug use in Asia. The option of taking up and widening harm reduction approaches in Asia was shown to be a necessity. But widespread resistance by various law enforcement agencies and drug treatment services specialists in Asia remained firm in their ongoing support for the traditional supply and demand reduction approach, with harm reduction often rejected or viewed as less a priority.

Each country in Asia has drug control legislation to address drug use issues, and in Asia the criminalization of drug users still has the capacity to overshadow the HIV-prevention efforts implemented in the majority of countries.[46] Many nations in Asia have enacted legislation on drug matters including capital punishment for drug crimes, and over the years some Asian countries, such as China, Indonesia, Malaysia, Singapore, Thailand and Vietnam, have carried out executions for drug crime convictions.[47] In 2003 the "War on Drugs Policy" introduced in Thailand saw the deaths of over 2,500 alleged drug criminals over a three-month period that created significant domestic and international condemnation.[48] In various countries of Asia emphasis on law enforcement to address the growing drug consumption has also led to mass incarceration of drug users being sent to drug treatment centres, where evidence based drug dependency treatment was seriously lacking. Mass incarceration of thousands of methamphetamine users has been most prominent in recent years in Cambodia, Laos, and Thailand where tackling the issue from a law enforcement approach, and not from a health perspective, was widespread.[49]

Nevertheless, many countries in Asia have commonly maintained a commitment and succeeded, to varying degrees, in negotiating practical compromises that seek some balance between law enforcement and public health approaches to drug use. Over the years harm reduction interventions have become increasingly viewed with better understanding and to varying degrees greater acceptance by several Asian governments. China is one such country where despite a law enforcement approach to drug use still remaining strong, and serious difficulties incorporating a health orientated or rights based approach in drug rehabilitation of drug users (see chapter 16), harm reduction interventions have gathered strength this century.

The Narcotic Control Law implemented in 2008 included significant reforms to the management of drug use in China. The new law prioritizes prevention and intervention activities in association with comprehensive drug control models that have a focus to ban the cultivation, production, trafficking, and use of drugs. But the law does state that drug users' rights are to be protected, including having the same rights to education, jobs, and social support and others in the community.[50] Acknowledging the need to reconcile the different regulatory systems and various objectives that govern drug control, China has shown its preparedness to explore alternative approaches to address drug use. This was reflected in China's endorsement of methadone maintenance therapy (MMT) clinics which are widely promoted and supported by law enforcement at state and provincial level. In 2004 there were eight pilot MMT clinics, and by 2008 there were 558 MMT clinics around the country serving more than 170,000 drug users.[51] The first NSP in China opened on a pilot basis in 1999,[52] and by 2006 there were a total of 790 NSP, around the country, of which 392 were funded by the government[53] (see chapters 15 and 16).

Until recently the approach by Malaysia toward drug use was through the criminal justice system. Mandatory treatment in a drug rehabilitation center for two years was routine for those convicted of a positive urine test for cannabis or opiates.[54] Harm reduction measures were rejected outright despite drug use being widespread and a HIV epidemic largely driven by people who inject drugs (PWID). In 2005, following increased and consistent advocacy efforts, the piloting of a methadone maintenance therapy program (MMT) and NSP were approved. These interventions were overseen and guided by a national task force on harm reduction, composed of officials from the Ministries of Health, National Anti-Drugs Agency, Royal Malaysian Police, and Prisons Department and academics and representatives of NGOs.[55] There has been quick expansion of MMT sites since their inception. In 2010 there were 94 sites increasing to 674 sites reaching 44,428 PWID in 2012. Three pilot NSP sites commenced in 2006 increasing to 297 in 2012.[56, 57] Despite government support for a harm reduction response, key challenges and barriers for sustaining and scaling up the response remain. The coexistence of harm reduction with punitive drug policies and a law enforcement approach was one area where ongoing advocacy efforts still remain critically important.

CONCLUSION

Nowhere on earth has seen a more turbulent history of drug use, of associated social conflict, corruption and war, of repressive policy, of HIV epidemics associated with injecting, than the Asian region. No other region has as many drug users, as much production or diversity of drugs, and so much incarceration of drug users and execution of those convicted of drug crimes. The roots of all these phenomena lie deep in history, particularly entwined with the history of colonialism in the region; little wonder that countries with memories of the colonial eras have identified, at least rhetorically, illicit drug use with colonization. It has taken the devastating epidemics of HIV to call attention to the often brutal responses to the use of currently illicit drugs, and the lack of humane approaches to people suffering from drug dependence.

This is changing. History shows that this region, and the character of drug use, can be volatile and is certainly dynamic. The rapidity with which, from 1997, amphetamine-type substances flooded out of Myanmar and China across the region show how quickly the drug scene can change. The speed with which China reversed its policies on methadone maintenance therapy—though certainly without resolving the policy dilemmas and leaving many reforms yet to happen—illustrates how quickly responses can change. And yet in most places in Asia the pace of drug policy reform remains very slow. HIV epidemics have opened discussion on drug policy; they are not enough to drive complete reform. There is still a long way to go before Asia as a whole can be said to have adopted humane, effective drug policies.

NOTES

1. S. Roy and S. H. Rizvi, *Nicotine Water to Heroin* (New Delhi. B. R. Publishing, 1986), 22.

2. Hasan A. Khwaya, "Social Aspects of the Use of Cannabis in India," in *Cannabis and Culture,* ed. Vera Rubin (The Hague: Mouton, 1975), 235–46.

3. Charles, Molly, David Bewley-Taylor, and Amanda Neidpath. "Drug Policy in India: Compounding Harm?" The Beckley Foundation Drug Policy Programme. Briefing Paper 10, 2005, 3. www.beckleyfoundation.org/pdf/BriefingPaper_10.pdf.

4. Tanya Machado, *Culture and Drug Abuse in Asian Settings: Research for Action* (Bangalore, India: St John's Medical College Publications, 1994), 34–37.

5. Machado, *Culture and Drug Abuse.*

6. Alfred McCoy, *The Politics of Heroin: CIA Complicity in the Global Drug Trade* (New York. Lawrence Hill Books, 1991), 224–25.

7. Machado, *Culture and Drug Abuse.*

8. A. M. B. Golding, "Two Hundred Years of Drug Abuse," *Journal of the Royal Society of Medicine* 86 (1993): 282–86.

9. Pierre-Arnaud Chouvy, "Afghanistan's Opium Production in Perspective," *China and Eurasia Forum Quarterly* 4(1) (2006): 21-24. Accessed 5 July 2012. www.silkroadstudies.org/new/docs/CEF/Quarterly/February_2006/Pierre-Arnaud_Chouvy.pdf.

10. Barbara Hodgson, *Opium: A Portrait of the Heavenly Demon* (Vancouver: Greystone Books, 1999), 68–71.

11. Machado, *Culture and Drug Abuse.*

12. Rajat Ray, S. Kattimani, and H. K. Sharma, "Opium Abuse and Its Management: Global Scenario. New Delhi." National Drug Dependence Treatment Centre All India Ray, Rajat. *South Asia: Drug Demand Reduction Report.* UNDCP Regional Office for South Asia, New Delhi, India, 1998.

13. Francis Moraes and Debra Moraes, *Opium* (Oakland: Ronin Publishing, 2003), 35.

14. Yongming Zhou, *Anti-Drug Crusades in Twentieth-Century China, Nationalism, History and State Building* (New York: Rowman & Littlefield, 1999), 13.

15. David Musto, "International Drug Control: Historical Aspects and Future Challenges." United Nations International Drug Control Programme. *World Drug Report.* (Oxford: Oxford University Press, 1997), 165–67.

16. W. Tavis Hanes and Frank Sanello. *The Opium Wars: The Addiction of One Empire and the Corruption of Another* (Naperville: Southbooks, 2002), 55–56.

17. William B. McAllister, "Conflicts of Interest in the International Drug Control System," in *Drug Control Policy: Essays in Historical and Comparative Perspective*, ed. Walker William (University Park, Pennsylvania: Pennsylvania State University Press, 1992), 143–66.

18. Musto, "International Drug Control: Historical Aspects and Future Challenges."

19. Adams, Leonard. "China: The Historical Setting of Asia's Profitable Plague," in *The Politics of Heroin in South East Asia: CIA Complicity in the Global Drug Trade*, ed. Alfred McCoy, Cathleen Read, and Leonard Adams (New York, Harper and Row, 1972), 308–10.

20. U. Khant and N. Win, "Drug Abuse in the Socialist Republic of Union of Burma," in *The International Challenge of Drug Abuse*, ed. R. C. Peterson. *NIDA Research Monograph* 19 (1978): 51–59.

21. McCoy, *The Politics of Heroin.*

22. McCoy, *The Politics of Heroin.*

23. Rajat Ray, *South Asia: Drug Demand Reduction Report* (New Delhi, India: UNDCP Regional Office for South Asia, 1998).

24. D. C. Jayasuriya, "The Drug Abuse Problem in Sri Lanka." *Medicine and Law* 14 (1995): 37–43.

25. Yi-lang Tang, Dong Zhao, Chengzheng Zhao, and Joseph Cubells, "Opiate Addiction in China: Current Situation and Treatments." *Addiction* 101, no. 5 (2006): 657–65.

26. Machado, *Culture and Drug Abuse.*

27. Ray, Kattimani, and Sharma, "Opium Abuse and Its Management."

28. Tang, Zhao, Zhao, and Cubells. "Opiate Addiction in China."

29. Tang, Zhao, Zhao, and Cubells. "Opiate Addiction in China."

30. Karen Laidler, A. J. David Hodson, and Harold Traver, "The Hong Kong Drug Market." A report for UNICRI on The UNDCP Global Study in Illicit Drug Markets (Hong Kong: University of Hong Kong, Centre for Criminology, 2000), 6–8.

31. Masayuki Tamura, "Japan: Stimulant Epidemics Past and Present." *Bulletin on Narcotics* XL1 (1 and2) (1989): 83–93.

32. Tamura, "Japan: Stimulant Epidemics Past and Present."

33. Jay Sinha, "The History and Development of the Leading International Drug Control Conventions." Report prepared for the Senate Special Committee on Illegal Drugs, Law and Government Division Parliamentary Research Branch, Library of Parliament, Parliament of Canada, Ottawa, Canada, 2001; 1. www.parl.gc.ca/Content/SEN/Committee/371/ille/library/history-e.htm.

34. David Bewley-Taylor and Martin Jelsma, "Fifty Years of the 1961 Single Convention on Narcotic Drugs: A Reinterpretation." Series on Legislative Reform of Drug Policies Number 1, Transnational Institute, 2011, 1.

35. Joseph Westermeyer, "The Pro-Heroin Effects of Anti-Opium Laws in Asia," *Archives of General Psychiatry* 33 (1976): 1135–39.

36. Gerry Stimson, "The Global Diffusion of Injecting Drug Use: Implications for Human Immunodeficiency Virus Infection," *Bulletin on Narcotics* 1 (1993): 3–17.

37. Tran Hien Nguyen, "Drug Use and HIV Infection in Vietnam." Global Research Network Meeting on HIV Prevention in Drug-Using Populations, Inaugural Meeting Report, Geneva, June 25–26, 1998.

38. Alex Wodak, "A Guide for HIV/AIDS Control among and from Injecting Drug Users in China." Report for the Western Pacific Regional Office World Health Organization, Manila, 1999, 6.

39. T. N. Naik, S Sarkar, H. L. Singh, S. C. Bhunia, Y. I. Singh, P. K. Singh, and S. C. Pal. "Intravenous Drug Users: A New High-Risk Group for HIV Infection in India," *AIDS* 5, no. 1 (1991): 117–18.

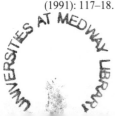

40. S. Sarkar, N. Das, Panda Samiran, T Naik, Kamalesh Sarkar, B. C. Singh, J. M. Ralte, S. M. Aier., and S. P. Tripathy. "Rapid Spread of HIV among Injecting Drug Users in North-Eastern States of India," *Bulletin on Narcotics* 45, no. 1 (1993): 91–104.

41. Vichai Poshyachinda, "Drugs and AIDS in Southeast-Asia," *Forensic Science International* 62, nos. 1–2 (1993): 15–28.

42. David D. Celentano, Jaroon Jittiwutikorn, Matthew J. Hodge, Chris Beyrer, and Kenrad E. Nelson, "Epidemiology of HIV-1 Infection in Opiate Users in Northern Thailand." *Journal of Acquired Immune Deficiency Syndromes and Human Retrovirology* 17 (1998): 73–78.

43. Aaron Peake, Sujata Rana, Shiba Hari Maharjan, Damien Jolley, and Nick Crofts, "Declining Risk for HIV among Injecting Drug Users in Kathmandu, Nepal: The Impact of a Harm-Reduction Programme," *AIDS* 9 (1995): 1067–70.

44. WHO (World Health Organization). *Report on People Who Inject Drugs in the South-East Asia Region* (New Delhi: WHO-SEARO, 2010), 118.

45. Morung Makunga, "Best Practices: Facing the Policy Challenges in HIV/AIDS: Manipur Experience." Paper presented the United Nations General Assembly Special Session on Drugs, Panel on Drug Abuse and HIV/AIDS, New York, June 9, 1998.

46. WHO, *Report on People Who Inject Drugs.*

47. Rick Lines, "The Death Penalty for Drug Offences: A Violation of International Human Rights Law." International Harm Reduction Association, London, 2007. www.ihra.net/files/2010/07/01/DeathPenaltyReport2007.pdf .

48. HRW (Human Rights Watch). *Thailand Not Enough Graves: The War on Drugs, HIV/AIDS, and Violations of Human Rights* (New York: BSI, 2004), 2–3.

49. Nick Thomson, "Detention as Treatment: Detention of Methamphetamine Users in Cambodia, Laos and Thailand." Nossal Institute for Global Health, University of Melbourne, Open Society Institute, Public Health Program, 2010. www.unhcr.org/refworld/docid/4cbd342f2.html.

50. Li Jianhua, H. Ha. Toan, Cunmin Zhang, and Hongjie Liu. "The Chinese Government's Response to Drug Use and HIV/AIDS: A Review of Policies and Programs," *Harm Reduction Journal* 7 (2010): 4–5. Accessed 29 July 2012. www.harmreductionjournal.com/content/7/1/4/.

51. Jianhua, Toan, Zhang, and Liu, "The Chinese Government's Response to Drug Use and HIV/AIDS."

52. Sheena G. Sullivan and Zunyou Wu, "Rapid Scale Up of Harm Reduction in China," *International Journal of Drug Policy* 18 (2007): 118–28.

53. Jianhua, Toan, Zhang, and Liu, "The Chinese Government's Response to Drug Use and HIV/AIDS."

54. Adeeba Kamarulzaman, "Impact of HIV Prevention Programs on Drug Users in Malaysia," *Journal of Acquired Immune Deficiency Syndrome* 52 (2009): S17–S19.

55. Kamarulzaman, "Impact of HIV Prevention Programs on Drug Users in Malaysia."

56. HRI (Harm Reduction International), *The Global State of Harm Reduction 2012: Towards an Integrated Response* (London: HRI, 2012).

57. Kamarulzaman, "Impact of HIV Prevention Programs on Drug Users in Malaysia."

BIBLIOGRAPHY

Adams, Leonard. "China: The Historical Setting of Asia's Profitable Plague." In *The Politics of Heroin in South East Asia: CIA Complicity in the Global Drug Trade*, edited by Alfred McCoy, Cathleen Read, and Leonard Adams, 308–10. New York: Harper and Row, 1972.

Bewley-Taylor, David and Jelsma, Martin. "Fifty Years of the 1961 Single Convention on Narcotic Drugs: A Reinterpretation." Series on Legislative Reform of Drug Policies Number 1, Transnational Institute, 2011, 1.

Celentano, David D., Jaroon Jittiwutikorn, Matthew J. Hodge, Chris Beyrer, and Kenrad E. Nelson. "Epidemiology of HIV-1 Infection in Opiate Users in Northern Thailand." *Journal of Acquired Immune Deficiency Syndromes and Human Retrovirology* 17 (1998): 73–78.

Charles, Molly, David Bewley-Taylor, and Amanda Neidpath. "Drug Policy in India: Compounding Harm?" The Beckley Foundation Drug Policy Programme. Briefing Paper 10, 2005, 3. www.beckleyfoundation.org/pdf/BriefingPaper_10.pdf.

Chouvy, Pierre-Arnaud. "Afghanistan's Opium Production in Perspective." *China and Eurasia Forum Quarterly* 4, no. 1 (2006): 21–24. Accessed 5 July 2012. www.silkroadstudies.org/new/docs/CEF/Quarterly/February_2006/Pierre-Arnaud_Chouvy.pdf.

Golding, A. M. B. "Two Hundred Years of Drug Abuse." *Journal of the Royal Society of Medicine* 86 (1993): 282–86.

Hanes, W. Tavis and Frank Sanello. *The Opium Wars: The Addiction of One Empire and the Corruption of Another.* Naperville: Southbooks, 2002.

Hodgson, Barbara. *Opium: A Portrait of the Heavenly Demon.* Vancouver: Greystone Books, 1999.

HRI (Harm Reduction International). *The Global State of Harm Reduction 2012: Towards an Integrated Response.* London: HRI, 2012.

HRW (Human Rights Watch). *Thailand Not Enough Graves: The War on Drugs, HIV/AIDS, and Violations of Human Rights.* New York: BSI, 2004.

Jayasuriya, D. C. "The Drug Abuse Problem in Sri Lanka." *Medicine and Law* 14 (1995): 37–43.

Jianhua, Li, Toan H. Ha, Cunmin Zhang, and Hongjie Liu. "The Chinese Government's Response to Drug Use and HIV/AIDS: A Review of Policies and Programs." *Harm Reduction Journal* 7 (2010): 4–5 Accessed 29 July 2012. www.harmreductionjournal.com/content/7/1/4/.

Kamarulzaman, Adeeba. "Impact of HIV Prevention Programs on Drug Users in Malaysia." *Journal of Acquired Immune Deficiency Syndrome* 52 (2009): S17–S19.

Khant, U. and Win, N. "Drug Abuse in the Socialist Republic of Union of Burma." In *The International Challenge of Drug Abuse*, edited by R. C. Peterson, 51–59. *NIDA Research Monograph* 19 (1978).

Khwaya, Hasan A. "Social Aspects of the Use of Cannabis in India." In *Cannabis and Culture,* edited by Vera Rubin, 235–46. The Hague: Mouton Publishers, 1975.

Laidler, Karen A. J., David Hodson, and Harold Traver. "The Hong Kong Drug Market." A Report for UNICRI on The UNDCP Global Study in Illicit Drug markets. Hong Kong: Centre for Criminology, University of Hong Kong, 2000, 6–8.

Lines, Rick. "The Death Penalty for Drug Offences: a Violation of International Human Rights Law." International Harm Reduction Association, London, 2007. www.ihra.net/files/2010/07/01/DeathPenaltyReport2007.pdf.

Machado, Tanya. *Culture and Drug Abuse in Asian Settings: Research for Action.* Bangalore: St. John's Medical College Publications. India, 1994.

Makunga, Morung. "Best Practices: Facing the Policy Challenges in HIV/AIDS: Manipur Experience." Paper presented the United Nations General Assembly Special Session on Drugs, Panel on Drug Abuse and HIV/AIDS, New York, June 9, 1998.

McAllister, William B. "Conflicts of Interest in the International Drug Control System." In *Drug Control Policy: Essays in Historical and Comparative Perspective,* edited by Walker William, 145–66. University Park: Pennsylvania State University Press, 1992.

McCoy, Alfred. *The Politics of Heroin: CIA Complicity in the Global Drug Trade.* New York. Lawrence Hill Books, 1991.

Moraes, Francis and Moraes Debra. *Opium.* Oakland: Ronin Publishing, 2003.

Musto, David. "International Drug Control: Historical Aspects and Future Challenges." United Nations International Drug Control Programme. *World Drug Report.* Oxford: Oxford University Press, 1997.

Naik, T. N., S. Sarkar, H. L. Singh, S. C. Bhunia, Y. I. Singh, P. K. Singh, and S. C. Pal. "Intravenous Drug Users: A New High-Risk Group for HIV Infection in India." *AIDS* 5, no. 1 (1991): 117–18.

Nguyen, Tran Hien. "Drug use and HIV infection in Vietnam." Global Research Network Meeting on HIV Prevention in Drug-Using Populations, Inaugural Meeting Report, Geneva, June 25–26, 1998.

Peake, Aaron, Sujata Rana, Shiba Hari Maharjan, Damien Jolley, and Nick Crofts. "Declining Risk for HIV among Injecting Drug Users in Kathmandu, Nepal: The Impact of Harm-Reduction Programme." *AIDS* 9 (1995): 1067–70.

Poshyachinda, Vichai. "Drugs and AIDS in Southeast-Asia." *Forensic Science International.* 62, nos. 1–2 (1993): 15–28.

Ray, Rajat. *South Asia: Drug Demand Reduction Report.* UNDCP Regional Office for South Asia, New Delhi, India, 1998.

Ray, Rajat, S. Kattimani, and H. K. Sharma. "Opium Abuse and Its Management: Global Scenario. New Delhi." National Drug Dependence Treatment Centre All India Ray, Rajat. *South Asia: Drug Demand Reduction Report.* UNDCP Regional Office for South Asia, New Delhi, India, 1998.

Roy, S. and S. H. Rizvi. *Nicotine Water to Heroin.* New Delhi: B. R. Publishing Corporation, 1986.

Sarkar, S., N. Das, Samiran Panda, T. Naik, Kamalesh Sarkar, B. C. Singh, J. M. Ralte, S. M. Aier, and S. P. Tripathy. "Rapid Spread of HIV among Injecting Drug Users in North-Eastern States of India." *Bulletin on Narcotics* 45, no. 1 (1993): 91–104.

Sinha, Jay. "The History and Development of the Leading International Drug Control Conventions." Report prepared for the Senate Special Committee on Illegal Drugs, Law and Government Division Parliamentary Research Branch, Library of Parliament, Parliament of Canada, Ottawa, Canada, 2001, 1. www.parl.gc.ca/Content/SEN/Committee/371/ille/library/history-e.htm.

Stimson, Gerry. "The Global Diffusion of Injecting Drug Use: Implications for Human Immunodeficiency Virus Infection." *Bulletin on Narcotics* 1 (1993): 3–17.

Sullivan, Sheena G., and Zunyou Wu. "Rapid Scale Up of Harm Reduction in China." *International Journal of Drug Policy* 18 (2007): 118–28.

Tamura, Masayuki. "Japan: Stimulant Epidemics Past and Present." *Bulletin on Narcotics* 41, nos. 1–2 (1989): 83–93.

Tang, Yi-lang, Dong Zhao, Chengzheng Zhao, and Joseph Cubells. "Opiate Addiction in China: Current Situation and Treatments." *Addiction* 101, no. 5 (2006): 657–65.

Thomson, Nick. "Detention as Treatment: Detention of Methamphetamine Users in Cambodia, Laos and Thailand." Nossal Institute for Global Health, University of Melbourne, Open Society Institute, Public Health Program, 2010. www.unhcr.org/refworld/docid/4cbd342f2.html.

Westermeyer, Joseph. "The Pro-Heroin Effects of Anti-Opium Laws in Asia." *Archives of General Psychiatry* 33 (1976): 1135–39.

WHO (World Health Organization). *Report on People Who Inject Drugs in the South-East Asia Region.* New Delhi: WHO-SEARO, 2010.

Wodak, Alex. "A Guide for HIV/AIDS Control among and from Injecting Drug Users in China." Report for the Western Pacific Regional Office World Health Organization, Manila, 1999.

Zhou, Yongming. *Anti-Drug Crusades in Twentieth-Cntury China: Nationalism, History and State Building.* New York: Rowman & Littlefield, 1999.

Chapter Two

Harm Reduction Is Good Public Health

S. S. Lee, David Jacka, and Nick Crofts

Harm reduction is a simple generic concept, literally meaning the continuing attempt to minimize the adverse consequences of a phenomenon—without necessarily reducing the occurrence of the phenomenon itself. The concept is most easily understandable if it is applied to health issues, which is routinely the case in the practice of modern medicine. For example, harm reduction for a sedentary, overweight person, who has, as a result, high blood pressure, would refer to exercise and a healthier diet to treat the underlying cause and treatment with medication to reduce the occurrence of complications resulting from poorly controlled blood pressure. There is little controversy when the idea of harm reduction is used in combating a chronic medical condition with potentially serious adverse consequences. Few would argue that antihypertensive medication is inappropriate until the ideal target weight has been achieved.

But perhaps a clearer example of both community and personal benefits from harm reduction interventions is seen in the use of helmets and seat belts by motorcyclists and car drivers, respectively. Neither has been shown to increase dangerous driving or the incidence of untoward occurrences, and the benefit for society goes clearly well beyond that of personal injury reduction should a crash occur. Despite the harm reducing "safety" hardware, we mostly accept that these interventions have little impact on the background behavior of the rider or driver, yet the interventions have worldwide accepted merit in their own right.

The US Institute of Medicine (IoM), in its 1988 report on the Future of Public Health, proposed the influential definition: "Public health is what we, as a society, do collectively to assure the conditions for people to be healthy."[1]

The IoM report makes it clear that society cannot guarantee complete physical and mental well-being and that there will always be a certain amount of injury or disease that is beyond the reach of individuals or government; the role of public health is then just to "assure the conditions for people to be healthy."

With harm reduction, the public provision of these conditions to "be healthy" accepts the reality of less-than-healthy personal behavior (including self-administration of illicit drugs) and attempts to assure conditions for people to optimally moderate their behaviors and avoid substantial ill health.

In reality, harm reduction remains a contentious approach because of its specific association with illicit drug (commonly heroin) use and dependence. For approximately a century, zero tolerance of many drugs by broader society, enshrined in the strategy of promoting and enforcing abstinence, has been the common goal of the approach to drug use, despite this appearing ever less achievable. The complexities of drug-related harm, of which blood-borne infection with human immunodeficiency virus (HIV) is the most visible prototype, have led to the evolution of a harm reduction approach as a companion and alternative to abstinence. Harm reduction in this specific context focuses on the reduction of negative health impacts of injecting drug use, the core component of which has so far been invariably associated with HIV prevention. The rationale is that if people who inject drugs (PWID) can be protected from HIV infection, their long-term health outcomes will be improved, along with the critical reduction of virus transmission onward to non-injecting members of the society.

Over the years, harm reduction has grown from a concept to a concrete suite of interventions, including methadone substitution for heroin dependence and widespread access to sterile needles and syringes. The social movements of harm reductionists, locally and internationally, have seen the definition of harm reduction expanded to incorporate state policies, programs, and services; its scope extended to health, social and economic perspectives; and the components of drug-use related "harm" broadened from that of individuals to communities and whole of society.[2]

Understandably, good coverage of interventions is essential if harm reduction is to achieve measurable health outcomes. Policy support for harm reduction is crucial, but such advocacy from social movements and health professionals is often perceived as a threat to policies of zero tolerance, as the success of either approach hinges similarly on the adequacy of coverage. Not surprisingly, it is often at policy level that the principles of harm reduction clash with those of zero tolerance. In the last two decades, HIV has silently permeated almost all communities of PWID in Asia. Despite the urgency for controlling HIV transmission, the development of harm reduction to scale has continued to confront an uphill battle. Why is it so hard to formulate and promulgate harm reduction policy and practice when the public health good is so evident and so well documented? Are there lessons that we can learn from harm reduction policy development?

THE TRIGGER

Policy does not evolve on its own.

In the era of evidence-based policy formulation, scientific research is expected to deliver evidence, providing the rationale for a respective policy which can then be developed and nurtured through the country's policy pathway. For harm reduction, this would mean that either local research is in place or that adequate and relevant evidence generated in other countries is available for reference. There must also be knowledgeable professionals to bring forward the available evidence for deliberation in a policy framework. Very rarely have things happened in such a systematic manner for harm reduction, except perhaps in Australia with their formulation of a national drug strategy, in 1985, shortly after HIV was discovered and its transmission associated with heroin injection delineated by the scientific community.[3, 4] It has taken most Asian countries as many as twenty years to have in place a policy that encompasses this principle of harm reduction. For most of those years there were only scant pilot studies in countries like Vietnam, Malaysia,

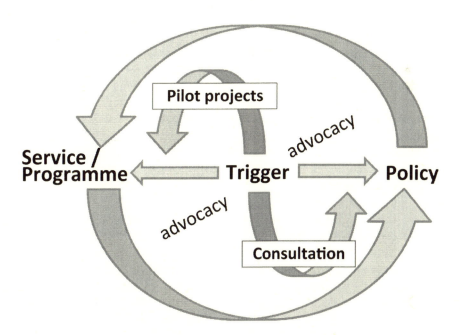

Figure 2.1.   The Policy-Action Cycle in Harm Reduction

and China, without provision for countrywide services nor a strategy for addressing drug-related harm.

What was missing? Apparently, an appreciation of HIV epidemiology and the association with heroin injection in the home country or internationally was insufficient to drive policy forward. The high HIV prevalence in PWID in Asian countries was already well known in the late 1980s,[5] yet this scientific evidence did not in most create a trigger for action. In some countries, however, the actual numbers did count if they were high enough. In Taiwan, reported HIV cases in PWID doubled in 2003 and culminated in a seven-fold increase by 2004, an observation that caught public health authorities by surprise. In 2005, a harm reduction strategy was developed alongside a pilot project, which was followed by rapid scaling up of methadone substitution treatment. A similar situation occurred in 2004 in Macao when alarmingly PWID accounted for 60 percent of all reported HIV cases in that year, followed by the discovery of an unusual genetic cluster of the virus in injectors. Methadone treatment was rolled out as a result. In Malaysia, the trigger was the discovery that the country was unlikely to achieve the Millennium Development Goal of halting HIV spread in 2005.[6] Pilot harm reduction services were introduced, beginning with methadone treatment that year and needle exchange scheme in the following year. By the end of 2007, around 5,000 heroin users were on methadone with a target to reach 75,000 by 2015. The stimulus for the harm reduction movement in mainland China was less conspicuous. The high HIV prevalence in PWID had been known since the 1980s. With the support of foreign aid, pilot projects had been introduced in high prevalence provinces including Yunnan, Guangxi and Xinjiang, but it was not until the country was awarded large grants by the Global Fund[7] that a longer-term, sustainable program began. The turning point was the promulgation of the AIDS Prevention and Control Regulations in 2006 and the accompanying five-year Action Plan describing the use of harm reduction strategies, including methadone treatment and needle exchange programs. By late 2011, there were over 700 methadone clinics serving 330,000 heroin users.[8] Instead of a single major trigger, it appears to have been an accumulation of triggers which potentiated one another to change the policy response to heroin use in the country.

Must there be an HIV epidemic to trigger the policy response? Perhaps not necessarily. . . . Hong Kong was an example where methadone clinics were established before the AIDS era. Methadone treatment was run as a trial in 1972, almost ten years before the HIV epidemic was first reported in the United States. On completion of the trial phase, a consultant invited by the Hong Kong Government evaluated the program and provided advice on which methadone treatment was formally established in 1976. Within two years, enrollment rapidly reached 10,000 and daily attendance 7,500, through a network of over twenty clinics. That program was started because of the presence of a high number of dependent heroin users and the worsening situation with public security. To this day, the HIV prevalence in PWID in Hong Kong has remained low at less than 1 percent of that population.

POLICY AND THE ROADMAPS

For PWID and the community at large, having methadone treatment available and sterile needles and syringes readily accessible are the ultimate goals of harm reduction. Rapid actions in response to new epidemics are crucial to save lives. When HIV swept through the region in the late 1980s and early 1990s, there was hardly a country that hastened to establish harm reduction services. The controversy surrounding harm reduction as perceived by abstinence-based drug rehabilitation workers and the dominance of zero-tolerance public policy were probably the main reasons for the inertia. Some countries looked for more evidence on the effectiveness of harm reduction interventions. Despite research reports since the 1970s on the positive health outcomes of methadone treatment and sterile needle and syringe access, there have always been remarks that these interventions were insufficiently convincing, or that because of perceptions of local cultural difference, locally generated evidence was needed.

Instead of emergency response to scale, the setting up of pilot projects or going on innumerable study tours were the norm, especially in countries where harm reduction was a new concept and an unfamiliar new term. Exposure to methadone treatment and needle and syringe program activities was gradually, incrementally translated into experiences, confidence, expertise and advocacy, and which definitely assisted the institutionalization of harm reduction. Unfortunately in some countries, pilots remained as pilots for years, perhaps reflecting the lack public health push for a breakthrough in policy support.

For many young countries in Asia and the Pacific, public health "policy" is taken to be identical to "law." While all countries go by "rule of law," the procedure adopted for policy development varies not just by the subject confronted but also the legal system in place. In this region, it is the civil law system that is more commonly enforced, which unlike common law that is weighed heavily by legal precedents, civil law traditions are guided by the ruling of an empowered state in accordance with constitutional law. As the term "harm reduction" was not listed in any constitutional or legal dictionary, the policy support demanded by professionals meant enactment of new designated ordinances or legal instruments specifically defining and incorporating harm reduction.

In common law countries, reference to related legislation, for example principles embodied in drug addiction laws or health service regulations, could be made without resorting to the passage of new laws. In Hong Kong, for example, despite there never having been any laws on harm reduction, this did not mean that methadone treatment could not be implemented. Policies and practices could be realized through means not disallowed by law. Policies can be "those laws, regulations, formal and informal rules and understandings that are adopted on a collective basis to guide individual and collective behaviour."[9] For harm reduction, policy is assumed to be in place if there is an agreed mechanism through which specific steps, either written or not written, are available to achieve the set purposes, as long as these go in line with principles and cases allowed in existing laws which serve as precedent.

The policy environment at country level has also often been influenced by international forces. Many countries in Asia and the Pacific have naturally looked to the United Nations (UN) for policy support. Like ministries within a national government, policies are "owned" by an UN equivalent for state ministry. The United Nations International Drug Control Programme (UNDCP), predecessor of United Nations Office on Drugs and Crime (UN-ODC), was the *de facto* UN equivalent for an international policy ministry on issues relating to illicit drug abuse. When the HIV epidemic hit the world, harm reduction was not a policy advised by UNDCP until it joined the Joint United Nations Programme on HIV/AIDS (UNAIDS) family in 1999, five years after the latter came into being. The global policy environment was extremely confused between the 1980s and the turn of the century, when the spread of HIV among PWID gained momentum in Asia and around the world, with the divergence of policy responses of developed nations impairing the pace of expansion of the harm reduction movement into public health.

THE PEOPLE

At the community level, harm reduction is a pragmatic practice for people in need. To dependent PWID, the crucial elements of a harm reduction response are that it be sufficiently operationalized, available, and accessible. An epidemiological trigger can remind the health authorities and public of an issue demanding attention, but policy does not evolve naturally and passively without somebody to push for it. The "people" is the notable key behind policy development. For many minority health issues, advocacy comes from patients suffering from the condition, health professionals knowledgeable about the issues from research or clinical practice, or both. Unlike many other minority health issues however, harm reduction is linked with a community sector that is stigmatized, marginalized, and composed of people who rarely have bargaining power or positive public visibility. In Asian countries, there were very few people in the community of PWID who are willing to come forward and advocate for policy reform. Admitting to the personal use of illicit drugs, particularly by injection, may potentially lead to prosecution for a criminal offense. This vulnerability factor stands between the usual potent personal or family advocacy and the development of humane, responsive policy. On the other hand, while drug dependence is a recognized international disease diagnosis and health problem, there are rarely advocates from within the medical specialist profession in the Asian region pushing for a harm reduction approach to heroin use. This is hardly surprising with drug dependence conventionally compartmentalized as a part of mental health and abstinence rather than harm reduction being the traditional specialist mental health approach to any substance abuse. The association of illicit drug injection with HIV transmission has only incidentally brought a fresh approach and a public health portfolio to the arena of illicit drug use and dependence.

Who then were the people who started the policy wheel rolling in favor of harm reduction? Widespread HIV transmission at the global level has exposed and internationalized the policy development process and response in Asian countries in a number of ways. International consultants have brought the issues to national governments and, likewise, international NGOs have brought the issues to their national counterparts. Until a critical mass of people committed to the cause has accumulated at country level to support change, harm reduction as a policy is not in sight. The legal environment, if facilitative, can hasten the process, irrespective of whether civil or common law system is in place.

The "coming out" of people living with HIV/AIDS serves as an example as to how harm reduction policy might be advocated for. Conscientious medical professionals in the public health or HIV fields also play a key role as opinion leaders and community catalysts. People learn from others in neighboring countries when it comes to the development and operationalization of harm reduction policy and practice.

In Hong Kong, the then Commissioner for Narcotics, a public security official rather than public health professional, fought for the creation of twenty methadone clinics to be immediately set up when he was convinced by a medical consultant that such should be the way ahead. Knowledge is necessary but insufficient to move policy ahead. The visibility of passion for people and people with passion can be seen in every country where harm reduction interventions have been implemented the ground.

Country	High HIV prevalence or report in IDU	Harm reduction start date: methadone / needle access	Latest HIV prevalence in IDU[1]	Harm reduction law	Legal structure[2]
Hong Kong	No	1976 / nil	0.5% [2010]	No	Common law
China	Yes	2004 / 2002	6.4% [2011][3]	No	Civil Law
Taiwan	Yes	2006 / 2006	11.0% [2010][4]	Yes	Civil Law
Indonesia	Yes	2003 / 1999	36.4% [2011][5]	Yes	Civil Law
Malaysia	Yes	2004 / 2005	8.7% [2011][6]	Yes	Common Law
Singapore	Yes[7]	Nil / Nil	unknown	No	Common Law
Vietnam	Yes	2008 / 2002	13.4% [2011][8]	Yes	Civil Law
Australia	Yes	1972 / 1982	1.0% [2010][9]	No	Common Law
Country	High HIV prevalence or report in IDU	Harm reduction start date: methadone / needle access	Latest HIV prevalence in IDU[1]	Harm reduction law	Legal structure[2]
Cambodia	Yes	2010 / 2003	24% [2010]	No	Civil Law
China	Yes	2004 / 2002	6.4% [2011]	No	Civil Law
Hong Kong SAR	No	1976 / nil	0.5% [2010]	No	Common law
Taiwan	Yes	2006 / 2006	11.0% [2010][3]	Yes	Civil Law
Indonesia	Yes	2003 / 1999	36.4% [2011]	Yes	Civil Law
Malaysia	Yes	2004 / 2005	8.7% [2011]	Yes	Common Law
Myanmar	Yes	2005 / 2004	21.9% [2011]	No	Common Law
Singapore	Yes[4]	Nil / Nil	unknown	No	Common Law
Vietnam	Yes	2008 / 2002	13.4% [2011]	Yes	Civil Law
Australia	Yes	1972 / 1982	1.0% [2010]	No	Common Law

Table 2.1

PUBLIC HEALTH GOOD

How much health good has harm reduction achieved? To the scientific community, reduction of HIV transmission is probably the most important health outcome, with implications that are far-reaching. By reducing HIV transmission, fewer PWID are exposed to the lifelong burden of HIV treatment and the severe medical illnesses arising from immune deficiency caused by HIV. Beyond that individual, their sexual and injecting partners are not placed at risk of HIV infection nor their unborn children. The transmission of HIV from the person at high risk through drug injection to those of lower risk through casual or spousal sexual transmission or through maternal to child transmission can be prevented.

With substitution treatment for heroin dependence, withdrawal symptoms and craving fade, and the desperation of dependence leading to criminality and high risk behaviors are likewise, gone. The majority of PWID slowly recover their way back to a "normal" life and become, once again, productive members of their family, community and the workforce. Under the harm reduction umbrella, the provision of community-based HIV prevention and drug dependence treatment reduce the need for more expensive, institutionalized treatment. It has not been uncommon to find residential drug rehabilitation centers closing down through reduced demand. In Hong Kong in the 1970s, when methadone treatment was initiated, the health benefits were not conspicuous; however, the treatment led to a sharp reduction in the crime. With rapid expansion of methadone clinics, the city simply became safer; measurably fewer drug users were sufficiently desperate and willing to commit offenses to get money to buy heroin. At that time, public security benefit was more evident than public health good. That safer environment came at the right moment as Hong Kong moved through the 1980s and emerged as a leading economy in the region. Economic assessments have repeatedly identified that every dollar spent on harm reduction measures saved multiple dollars on law enforcement, medical care and institutionalized treatment.

Upon finally receiving policy support, harm reduction programs have normally been implemented as rapidly scaled, public health services, rather than research projects. This is rightly so, though the downside is that evaluation has rarely been accorded sufficient priority.

The complexity of the lives of chaotic illicit drug users amplifies the lack of an efficient, parallel, service monitoring system to track health, psychosocial, community and security outcomes. Time and again, policymakers have looked back at (relatively) expensive harm reduction programs, questioned their effectiveness and seemingly forgotten why the substitution treatment and needle syringe programs were implemented in the first place. Many of the emerging economies have seen the HIV prevalence in PWID peak and fall away under donor supported harm reduction programs. The challenge for public health in Asia in the twenty-first century will be to maintain government health investment in harm reduction for these marginalized and stigmatized PWID, when the HIV epidemic seems to have responded so readily and other non-communicable disease epidemic demands emerge.

While the benefits and cost-effectiveness of harm reduction appear obvious, the debates and re-examinations continue to recur in almost every city implementing harm reduction. The common criticism that some PWID engaged in harm reduction services continue to use illicit drugs is taken as an indication that the strategy has "failed," even though the health and social harms have reduced significantly.

Comparison has often been made unfavorably between harm reduction services and abstinence programs. The latter are usually praised for achieving the goal of total abstinence in a small number of highly selected PWID, while ignoring their failure with the majority of participants and the alternative effectiveness of substitution treatment and needle syringe programs in allowing every drug user to remain with their family and to re-integrate in their society. In fact, a significant proportion of PWID eventually enter treatment and abstain from drug use if they are well supported through harm reduction services over an unrestricted number of years. The invisibility of the slow recovering drug user in treatment and those quietly but successfully leaving treatment, is often not eye-catching enough for sustained policy support.

It has taken decades for harm reduction policy to be successfully established in most Asian countries; without ongoing public health support, proactive documentation of impact and support to give a voice to its beneficiaries, its foundation will be shaken and efforts to maintain the policies undermined.

NOTES

1. IOM (Institute of Medicine). *The Future of Public Health* (National Academy Press Washington, DC: Committee for the Study of the Future of Public Health, 1988).
2. UKHRA (UK Harm Reduction Alliance). "Definition of Harm Reduction." Accessed July 24, 2012. www.ukhra.org/harm_reduction_definition.html .
3. Commonwealth of Australia. Australian Government: Ministerial Council on Drug Strategy National Drug Strategy, 2010–2015. Accessed August 27, 2012. www.nationaldrugstrategy.gov.au/internet/drugstrategy/publishing.nsf/Content/ DB4076D49F13309FCA257854007BAF30/$File/nds2015.pdf.
4. Adeeba Kamarulzaman, "Impact of HIV Prevention Programs on Drug Users in Malaysia," *Journal of Acquired Immune Deficiency Syndrome* 52, no. 1 (2009): S17–9.
5. Bruce G. Weniger, Khanchit Limpakarnjanarat, Kumnuan Ungchusak, Sombat Thanprasertsuk, Kachit Choopanya, Suphak Vanichseni, Thongchai Uneklabh, Prasert Thongcharoen, and Chantapong Wasi. "The Epidemiology of HIV Infection and AIDS in Thailand," *AIDS* 5, no. 2 (1991): S71–85.
6. Kamarulzaman, "Impact of HIV Prevention Programs on Drug Users in Malaysia," S17–9.
7. Global Fund to Fight AIDS, Tuberculosis and Malaria, established in 2002.
8. Li, Li, Zunyou Wu, Li-Jung Liang, Chunqing Lin, Linglin Zhang, Sam Guo, Keming Rou, and Jianhua Li. "An Intervention Targeting Service Providers and Clients for Methadone Maintenance Treatment in China: A Cluster-randomized Trial," *Addiction* 2012 [Epub ahead of print 13 July 2012] DOI: 10.1111/j.1360-0443.2012.04020.x.
9. Lawrence Wallack, "Media Advocacy: Promoting Health through Mass Communication," in *Health Behaviour and Health Education: Theory Research and Practice*, edited by Karen Glanz., Frances M. Lewis, and Barbara K. Rimer, 370–86 (San Francisco, CA: Jossey-Bass, 1990).

BIBLIOGRAPHY

Commonwealth of Australia. Australian Government: Ministerial Council on Drug Strategy National Drug Strategy 2010–2015. Accessed August 27, 2012. www.nationaldrugstrategy. gov.au/internet/drugstrategy/publishing.nsf/Content/DB4076D49F13309FCA257854007 BAF30/$File/nds2015.pdf.

IOM (Institute of Medicine). *The Future of Public Health.* National Academy Press Washington, DC: Committee for the Study of the Future of Public Health, 1988.

Kamarulzaman, Adeeba. "Impact of HIV Prevention Programs on Drug Users in Malaysia." *Journal of Acquired Immune Deficiency Syndrome* 52, no. 1 (2009): S17–S19.

Li, Li, Zunyou Wu, Li-Jung Liang, Chunqing Lin, Linglin Zhang, Sam Guo, Keming Rou, and Jianhua Li. "An Intervention Targeting Service Providers and Clients for Methadone Maintenance Treatment in China: A Cluster-Randomized Trial." *Addiction* 2012 (Epub ahead of print 13 July 2012) DOI: 10.1111/j.1360-0443.2012.04020.x.

UKHRA (UK Harm Reduction Alliance). "Definition of Harm Reduction." Accessed July 24, 2012. www.ukhra.org/harm_reduction_definition.html.

Wallack, Lawrence. "Media Advocacy: Promoting Health through Mass Communication." In *Health Behaviour and Health Education: Theory Research and Practice*, edited by Karen Glanz, Frances M. Lewis, and Barbara K. Rimer, 370–86. San Francisco, CA: Jossey-Bass, 1990.

Weniger, Bruce G., Khanchit Limpakarnjanarat, Kumnuan Ungchusak, Sombat Thanprasertsuk, Kachit Choopanya, Suphak Vanichseni, Thongchai Uneklabh, Prasert Thongcharoen, and Chantapong Wasi. "The Epidemiology of HIV Infection and AIDS in Thailand." *AIDS* 5, no. 2 (1991): S71–S85.

Chapter Three

Turning a Page

*Human Rights and Drug Policy in
East and Southeast Asia*

Joanne Csete and Fifa Rahman

> [In Singapore,] the police . . . are empowered . . . to test the urine for drugs of any person who behaves in a suspicious manner. If the result is positive, rehabilitation treatment is compulsory. Such a law will be considered unconstitutional in some countries, and such urine tests will lead to lawsuits for damages for battery and assault. . . . As a result, the community's interests are sacrificed because of the human rights of drug consumers and traffickers.
>
> —Wong Kan Seng, minister for Foreign Affairs, Singapore, at
> World Conference on Human Rights, Vienna, 16 June 1993

Lee Kuan Yew was prime minister of Singapore from the founding of the city-state in 1965 until 1990. Singapore's economic "miracle" occurred under his leadership. Looking back on his life in politics, Lee was quoted at age eighty-seven in 2010 as reflecting that "I had to do some nasty things, locking fellows up without trial," but that these things were necessary to unite an otherwise ethnically and religiously fragmented society and to facilitate economic growth.[1]

In 2012, South Korean presidential candidate Park Geun-hye, in the heat of the electoral campaign, stopped to apologize for human rights abuses committed by her father, Park Chung-hee, who was president of the Republic of Korea from 1962 to 1979, a period in which South Korea emerged as an economic power.[2] "Behind the stellar growth were sacrifices by workers who suffered under a repressive labor environment; behind the efforts for national security to protect [ourselves] from North Korea were human rights abuses committed by state power," she said.[3] Media reports suggested that Ms.

Park's campaign viewed this statement as necessary to appeal to voters who regard her father's human rights record as a stain on the country's history.

Ms. Park, as do many accounts of the story of the East Asian "tiger" economies, adopts a common narrative of human rights violations as part of the cost of "stellar" economic growth in the region. The fact that Ms. Park felt it necessary to address this point in her campaign perhaps signals something of a shift in the importance of human rights norms in the public mind in some parts of East and Southeast Asia. If so, there is still a long way to go. Human Rights Watch's 2012 global survey highlights continuing repression of opposition voices, crackdowns on human rights activists and lawyers, and undermining of workers' rights to organize and assemble in virtually all countries of the region.[4]

Africa, the Americas, and Europe all have regional human rights bodies that are intended to complement global human rights norms and have served, at least at times, to offer some form of justice where national remedies were not possible. No such bodies exist on a regional level in Asia. A debate continues more in Asia than in other parts of the world about whether traditional values, especially respect for the family and for the culture of the community, do or should trump individual rights as defined in human rights instruments.[5] Indeed, as the quote opening this chapter illustrates, Singapore, for example, has brought to United Nations human rights discussions its strong views on Asian values, the inherent imperialism and Western nature of human rights, and the need for social order at all costs to advance development.[6, 7]

A full appreciation of human rights thinking in East and Southeast Asia is beyond the scope of this chapter. Few countries anywhere in the world probably can be said to be imbued with a true human rights culture in mainstream society. And it is obvious that in many countries in all regions, societies make damaging moral judgments against people whose behavior challenges mainstream norms, including people who use illicit drugs or who live with addiction. For the purposes of this chapter, we wish simply to note that in East and Southeast Asia social disdain for people involved with illicit drugs, powerful states easily able to crack down on those outside the social mainstream, and the absence or weakness of civil society institutions able to assert the rights of people who use drugs constitute, together, a recipe for drug policy that is anything but just.

SUSCEPTIBILITY OF PEOPLE WHO USE DRUGS TO HUMAN RIGHTS ABUSE

Awareness of the link between HIV and drug use, especially drug injection, has occasioned re-examination of approaches to policy on illicit drugs in many countries and among multinational institutions (see des Jarlais et al. in this book). In 2001, the unanimous declaration from the first UN General Assembly high-level meeting on HIV/AIDS committed member states to "harm reduction efforts related to drug use" and to "expanded access to essential commodities, including . . . sterile injecting equipment."[8] This declaration alone, if taken seriously, would have ensured that countries revisit drug policies and law enforcement practices that stand in the way of ensuring life-saving health services for people who use drugs.

As has by now been well documented, crackdowns and other repressive policing directed at people who inject drugs frequently cause them to go into hiding and be separated from HIV and health services, and often a singular focus on drug users as criminals results in policy-level neglect of health and social services for them.[9] A study in Ukraine estimated for example that almost 20 percent of new HIV infection could be prevented in a five-year period if police brutality were eliminated.[10]

As other accounts in this book have shown, it is not just the right to life-saving health services that is violated in repressive policing of drug users. It is clear that people who live with addiction are especially vulnerable to police abuse. They are the low-hanging fruit when police need to fill arrest quotas.[11] If interrogated when in drug withdrawal, they are susceptible to being coerced to confess to the crime for which they are charged or to other unsolved crimes in exchange for drugs, which a UN special expert has defined as a form of torture particular to people with addictions.[12]

In a study conducted in Indonesia with local participants, it was found that 60 percent of interviewees reported physical abuse by police, which included beatings with fists, hands, and boots, beatings with objects such as folded chairs, pistol butts, and wrenches, burning with cigarettes, and inappropriate sexual touching during street searches.[13] When drug users are beaten or otherwise mistreated by police, unlawfully searched or forced to undergo drug testing, as has been documented in East and Southeast Asia, there is often no public outcry, limited access to legal counsel, and no independent police complaints commission.

Police also perpetrate various other human rights abuses that limit and circumvent the positive effects of harm reduction. In a survey conducted among 53 police officers in Malaysia, slightly more than half of the respondents said that they would seize needles and syringes provided by government-endorsed NSEP, whether or not an arrest was made.[14] There continue to be numerous incidents of police waiting outside methadone clinics and drug drop-in centers to make arrests to fulfill their yearly key performance indicators.[15] Actions such as these result in individuals being afraid to attend harm reduction services, and are clear violations of the right to health.

Individuals are also deprived of the right to health while in police station lockups in Malaysia, where they are not given access to medical practitioners, despite the existence of protocols requiring the same. Despite a 2011 decision by Judge Lee Swee Seng in the Malaysian High Court deeming the actions of police in depriving the plaintiff (a thirty-one-year-old male arrested for drugs) of medical attention constituted "oppressive, arbitrary or unconstitutional action by the servants of the government,"[16] deaths in police custody among individuals who use drugs continue to occur. The Honorable Judge opined, "something is not quite right in the institution represented by the men in blue."[17] In Thailand, the "men in blue" upon instruction of the government conducted mass assassinations of individuals who use drugs, described further by Kaplan et al. in this book.

As noted by Baldwin et al. and Biddulph et al. in this book, in East and Southeast Asia, people convicted of consuming illicit drugs in much of the region may find themselves detained for compulsory "treatment" in facilities that often offer no health services whatsoever and resemble prisons or forced labor camps more than treatment centers.[18, 19] A fundamental principle of the right to health is that coerced use of health services is a human rights violation. The right to health services is also clearly understood to be the right to services that are voluntary and "of good quality and scientifically sound."[20]

There is nothing about compulsory "treatment" centers that could remotely be characterized as scientifically sound as treatment for drug dependence.[21] Many countries in East and Southeast Asia have quite good policies guaranteeing people's access to a minimum core of basic health services.[22] One must then suppose that some other factor—moral judgment and social disdain directed to drug users perhaps—impedes lack of access to basic care and support for this population. In addition, people with opiate dependency in the region who may be among the few who have access to methadone or buprenorphine maintenance therapy may also find that if detained for a drug offense, access to their medications may be refused or interrupted.[23]

In short, people who use drugs are particularly vulnerable to violations of their right to due process; their right to bodily security, which is violated when they are mistreated by the police or forced to undergo urinalysis; their right not to be subjected to cruel, inhuman and degrading treatment or torture; and their right to health services.

RIGHTS-CENTERED POLICY ON ILLICIT DRUGS

In a number of countries outside Asia, notably in Europe, experience has shown that it is possible to control drugs and HIV related to drugs while also protecting the rights of people who use drugs, including their right to health. These countries—including Portugal, Switzerland, the Czech Republic and the Netherlands, among others—reject the usual practice of seeing policing as the principal response to drug consumption.[24] They make it an explicit policy priority to ensure easy access to health and social services for people who use drugs. In these countries, drug use itself and possession of quantities of illicit drugs deemed to be for individual use are not criminal offenses but rather administrative offenses subject to a fine or, in the case of Portugal, not offenses at all. Policy priorities of this kind enable the police to keep their focus on major trafficking and related crimes. All of the countries that have adopted policies that balance policing with readily accessible health and social services have enjoyed good success in controlling HIV among people who inject drugs.[25]

Though there is no single formula to define "rights-based drug policy," the work of the high-profile Global Commission on Drug Policy,[26] whose members include numerous former heads of state and business and social leaders from around the world, suggests several essential elements:

- Empowered national drug policy authorities that include not just police and prosecutors but health, education and social sector officials.
- Law, policy, and law enforcement practices that distinguish individual use and possession from major drug offenses (e.g., trafficking), with non-criminal sanctions for individual-level infractions.
- The state ensures provision of humane, affordable, voluntary, scientifically sound treatment for drug dependence.
- The states ensures access to HIV and hepatitis prevention and care for people who use drugs, including harm reduction services, drug policy, and law provide a solid grounding for these services.

The United Nations has not always clearly favored all of these elements. UN bodies have still not called for decriminalization of individual drug use and possession, for example, even though both the Global Commission on Drug Policy and the similarly high-level Global Commission on HIV and the Law (2012) have issued that call. The Joint United Nations Programme on HIV/AIDS (UNAIDS) and the UN secretary-general have called for revisiting punitive drug laws that impede HIV responses and are associated with human rights violations.[27, 28] The UN Office on Drugs and Crime has been somewhat slower than other UN bodies to embrace human rights ideas in its work. However, in 2010, outgoing UNODC executive director Antonio Maria Costa issued a statement recognizing an urgent need for drug control policies to be "better synchronized with the need to protect human rights."[29] In contrast with the statement that introduced this chapter, for example, Costa noted:

> Effective drug control cannot exist without fair criminal justice and successful crime prevention. Human rights offer guidance on the delicate balance between the protection of fundamental freedoms and the protection of public

health, morals and security. It [*sic*] sets out the broad responsibilities of the state to respect, protect and fulfill the health and well-being of its peoples and specific due process guarantees, such as for those suspected or accused of a criminal offense. (para 3)

This was a departure from UNODC's previous strong focus on drug supply reduction at all costs. This statement was followed by a UNODC (2012) guideline on respecting human rights norms in its own work across the world. That guideline recognizes that state actions in drug control may cause human rights violations, and UNODC as an organization needs to be prepared to adjust its support accordingly.

The three UN drug conventions of 1961, 1971, and 1988 are widely ratified in Asia and across the world.[30] They are of a prohibitionist character, and the 1988 convention specifically enjoins countries to apply criminal law to "the possession, purchase, or cultivation of narcotic drugs or psychotropic substances for person consumption" (Art. 3.2). Nonetheless, many countries have marshaled legal arguments and established alternatives to criminalization of minor offenses without being considered in violation of the treaties.[31] In addition, it is frequently overlooked that all three of the conventions commit state parties to providing essential services for people who live with drug dependence, including "early identification, treatment, education, aftercare, rehabilitation, and social reintegration" (1961 convention, Art. 38.1). Taking the conventions seriously should mean dramatically scaled up access to such services compared to what is available in many countries.

For East and Southeast Asia in particular, the United Nations in 2012 turned its attention in an important way to the heinous human rights abuses committed in compulsory "treatment" centers across the region. The joint statement on this subject, which resulted from a long period of advocacy on the part of civil society in the region and internationally, condemns the "deprivation of liberty without due process" associated with many of these centers.[32] It echoes the findings of human rights groups that the centers in several countries are "reported to involve physical and sexual violence, forced labor, sub-standard conditions, denial of health care and other measures that violate human rights."[33] The UN bodies call for the closure of these centers in all countries with a guarantee of appropriate health and social support for those detained in them.

Advocacy for human rights-based drug policy is difficult in several countries in Asia due to government aversion to human rights terminology, and the inapplicability of human rights arguments in courts. In addition to this, the political fear of seeming "weak" toward drug users is omnipresent.

Asian leaders often speak about their intentions to improve human rights records. In 2011, the Malaysian Prime Minister Najib Razak abolished the preventive detention law and stated that he wanted Malaysia to become the "best democracy,"[34] and in 2012 Thai Prime Minister Yingluck Shinawatra said that she wanted to "ensure that the rule of law prevails and the basic rights of the people guaranteed, in particular vulnerable groups."[35]

At time of writing it seems that this is mere rhetoric; especially in relation to changing drug policy. Cohen and Csete comment: "Protecting the rights of vulnerable groups is consistent with the highest ideals of democracy and public welfare . . . governments must accept that there is nothing divisive about respecting people's rights, and that applying the rule of law to police and drug users alike benefits society as a whole."[36]

At this writing, there is a seemingly important movement in many Latin American countries promoting drug laws and policies that will loosen the grip of violent drug gangs on the region and reduce the repression application of criminal law to minor drug offenses.[37] While this movement has been advanced partly by public statements by sitting presidents, it is sustained in many countries by a strong and very human rights-centered civil society. East and Southeast Asia for the most part do not yet enjoy a similarly strong and rights-oriented civil society, but the young groups that do have a focus on drug policy reform will undoubtedly grow stronger.

A few Asian states have shown signs of modifying to some degree their drug policies. As noted in Baldwin's chapter in this book, in 2010, the Malaysian government announced a plan to close all of its compulsory treatment facilities and replace them with voluntary treatment centers called "Cure & Care" centers, which provide services such as methadone maintenance, HIV treatment and peer support groups, in clear contrast to the compulsory centers, which focused solely on counseling and religious education. Government support for harm reduction services in Indonesia, Vietnam, and China have been seen as positive developments by many observers.[38] The fortress of repressive drug policy in the region will not be toppled any time soon. But it is possible that with increasing global acceptance of the value of drug policy that is consistent with human rights protection, Asian governments will increasingly find themselves out of step with global trends if they ignore the human rights link to drug policy.

NOTES

1. Seth Mydans, "Days of Reflection for Man Who Defined Singapore," *New York Times*, September 10, 2010. Accessed September 25, 2012. www.nytimes.com/2010/09/11/world/asia/11lee.html?pagewanted=all&_moc.semityn.www.

2. APF News Agency, "South Korea Presidential Runner Park Apologises for Father." *Bangkok Post*, September 24, 2012. Accessed September 25, 2012. www.bangkokpost.com/news/asia/313765/s-korean-dictator-daughter-apologises-for-abuses.

3. APF News Agency, "South Korea Presidential Runner Park Apologises for Father."

4. HRW (Human Rights Watch). *World Report 2012* (New York: HRW, 2012). Accessed September 25, 2012. www.hrw.org/world-report-2012.

5. Amartya Sen, "Human Rights and Asian Values," *The New Republic* 33 (1997): 33–40.

6. Wong Kan Seng, "The Real World of Human Rights." Speech to UN World Conference on Human Rights, Vienna, June 16, 1993.

7. Christina M. Cerna, "Universality of Human Rights and Cultural Diversity: Implementation of Human Rights in Different Socio-Cultural Contexts." *Human Rights Quarterly* 16 (1994): 740–52.

8. UN General Assembly. "Declaration of Commitment on HIV/AIDS." 2001. New York: United Nations (UN doc. A/RES/S-26/2), para 52. Accessed September 25, 2012. www.un.org/ga/aids/docs/aress262.pdf.

9. Ralf Jürgens, Joanne Csete, Joseph J. Amon, Stefan Baral, and Chris Beyrer, "People Who Use Drugs, HIV and Human Rights," *Lancet* 376 (2010): 475–85.

10. Steffanie A. Strathdee, Timothy B. Hallett, Natalia Bobrova, Tim Rhodes, Robert Booth, R. Abdool, and Catherine A. Hankins. "HIV and Risk Environment for Injecting Drug Users: the Past, Present and Future." *Lancet* 376 (2010): 268–84.

11. Jürgens, Csete, Amon, Baral, and Beyrer, "People Who Use Drugs, HIV and Human Rights," 475–85.

12. Roxanne Saucier, Daniel Wolfe, Kathleen Kingsbury, and Paul Silva, eds. "Treated with Cruelty: Abuses in the Name of Drug Rehabilitation." New York: Open Society Foundations, 2012. Accessed September 24, 2012. www.soros.org/sites/default/files/treatedwithcruelty.pdf.

13. Sara Davis, Agus Triwahyuono, and Risa Alexander. "Survey of Abuses against Injecting Drug Users in Indonesia," *Harm Reduction Journal* 6 (2009): 28–29.

14. Fifa Rahman and Guganesan Parasuraman, "Police Knowledge of Needle-and-Syringe Programs and Harm Reduction in Malaysia." Paper presented at the 6th International Society for the Study of Drug Policy (ISSDP) Conference, Canterbury Cathedral Lodge, Canterbury, Kent, United Kingdom, May 30–31, 2012.

15. Azahari Said (Manager, NSEP, Malaysian AIDS Council), in discussion with author, October 2012.

16. Suzana bt Md Aris (claiming as administrator of the estate and a dependent of Mohd Anuar bin Sharip, deceased) v DSP Ishak bin Hussain & Ors (2011) 1 MLJ 107, *Malayan Law Journal*, para 2, per Lee Swee Seng JC.

17. Suzana bt Md Aris (claiming as administrator of the estate and a dependant of Mohd Anuar bin Sharip, deceased) v DSP Ishak bin Hussain & Ors (2011) 1 MLJ 107, *Malayan Law Journal*, para 5.

18. Daniel Wolfe, M. Patrizia Carrieri, and Donald Shepard. "Treatment and Care for Injecting Drug Users with HIV Infection: a review of Barriers and Ways Forward," *Lancet* 376 (2010): 355–66.

19. ILO/OHCHR/UNDP/UNESCO/UNPF/UNHCR/UNICEF/UNODC/UNWOMEN/WFP/WHP/ UNAIDS (International Labour Organisation, Office of the High Commissioner for Human Rights, United Nations Development Programme, United Nations Educational Scientific and Cultural Organisation, United Nations population Fund, United Nations High Commissioner for Refugees, United Nations Childrens Fund, United Nations Office on Drugs and Crime, United Nations Entity for Gender Equality and Empowerment of Women, World Food Programme, World Health Organisation and Joint United Nations Programme on HIV/AIDS). 2012. "Joint Statement: Compulsory Drug Detention and Rehabilitation Centers." Accessed October 17, 2012. www.ilo.org/aids/Whatsnew/WCMS_175377/lang--en/index.htm.

20. UN Committee on Economic, Social and Cultural Rights, "General Comment no. 14: The Right to the Highest Attainable Standard of Health." 2000. Geneva: United Nations (UN doc. no. D/C.12/2000/4).

21. UNAIDS, Office of the United Nations High Commissioner for Human Rights, UN Development Programme, UNESCO, UNFPA, UNHCR, UNICEF, UN Office on Drugs and Crime, UN Women, World Food Programme, World Health Organization and International Labour Organization. 2012. "Joint Statement: Compulsory Drug Detention and Rehabilitation Centres." Geneva: United Nations. Accessed September 24, 2012. www.ohchr.org/en/NewsEvents/Pages/DisplayNews.aspx?NewsID=11941&LangID=E.

22. Sven Olsson Hort and Stein Kuhnle, "The Coming of East and South-East Asian Welfare States," *European Journal of Social Policy* 10 (2000): 162–84.

23. Wolfe, Carrieri, and Shepard, "Treatment and Care for Injecting Drug Users with HIV Infection."

24. Global Commission on Drug Policy, "War on Drugs: Report of the Global Commission on Drug Policy" (Rio de Janeiro: GCDP, 2011). Accessed September 25, 2012. www.globalcommissionondrugs.org/wp-content/themes/gcdp_v1/pdf/Global_Commission_Report_English.pdf.

25. Global Commission on Drug Policy, "War on Drugs."

26. Global Commission on Drug Policy, "War on Drugs."

27. UNAIDS (Joint United Nations Programme on HIV/AIDS), "Joint Action for Results: UNAIDS Outcome Framework 2009–2011." Geneva: United Nations, 2009. Accessed September 25, 2012. http://data.unaids.org/pub/BaseDocument/2010/jc1713_joint_action_en.pdf.

28. Ban Ki-moon, "The Protection of Human Rights in the Context of Human Immunodeficiency Virus (HIV) and Acquired Immune Deficiency Syndrome (AIDS): Report of the Secretary-General, " (New York: United Nations, 2010; UN doc. no. A/HRC/16/69).

29. Antonio Maria Costa, "Drug Control Crime Prevention and Criminal Justice: A Human Rights Perspective—Note by the Executive Director" (Vienna: UN Commission on Narcotic Drugs, 2010; UN doc. no. E/CN.7/2010/CRP.6 – E/CN.15/2010/CRP.1).

30. The texts of the UN drug conventions and the ratification status of the three treaties are available from the web site of the International Narcotics Control Board, www.incb.org.

31. Robin Room and Peter Reuter, "How Well Do International Drug Conventions Protect Public Health?" *Lancet* 379 (2012): 84–91.

32. UNAIDS, Office of the United Nations High Commissioner for Human Rights, UN Development Programme, UNESCO, UNFPA, UNHCR, UNICEF, UN Office on Drugs and Crime, UN Women, World Food Programme, World Health Organization and International Labour Organization, "Joint Statement: Compulsory Drug Detention and Rehabilitation Centre," (Geneva: United Nations, 2012). Accessed September 24, 2012. www.ohchr.org/en/NewsEvents/Pages/DisplayNews.aspx?NewsID=11941&LangID=E.

33. UNAIDS, "Joint Statement."

34. 1Malaysia: The Personal Website of Dato' Sri Najib Razak, "ISA Repealed to Make Malaysia Best Democracy, Says Najib." Accessed October 19, 2010. http://1malaysia.com.my/zh/news_archive/isa-repealed-to-make-malaysia-best-democracy-says-najib/.

35. Ministry of Foreign Affairs of the Kingdom of Thailand, "Statement by Her Excellency Ms. Yingluck Shinawatra, Prime Minister of the Kingdom of Thailand at the General Debate of the 67th Session of the United Nations General Assembly, New York, September 27, 2012." Accessed October 19, 2012. www.mfa.go.th/main/en/media-center/14/28027-Statement--by-Her-Excellency-Ms.-Yingluck-Shinawat.html.

36. Jonathan Cohen and Joanne Csete, "As Strong as the Weakest Pillar: Harm Reduction, Law Enforcement and Human Rights," *International Journal of Drug Policy* 17 (2006): 101.

37. Juan Forero, "Latin Countries Pursue Alternatives to US Drug War," *Washington Post*, April 10, 2012. Accessed September 24, 2012. www.washingtonpost.com/world/the_americas/latin-american-countries-pursue-alternatives-to-us-drug-war/2012/04/10/gIQAFPEe7S_story.html.

38. HRI (Harm Reduction International), "Global State of Harm Reduction 2012" (London: HRI, 2012). Accessed September 25, 2012. www.ihra.net/files/2012/07/24/GlobalState2012_Web.pdf.

BIBLIOGRAPHY

1Malaysia: The Personal Website of Dato' Sri Najib Razak. "ISA Repealed to Make Malaysia Best Democracy, Says Najib." Accessed October 19, 2010. http://1malaysia.com.my/zh/news_archive/isa-repealed-to-make-malaysia-best-democracy-says-najib/.

APF News Agency. "South Korea Presidential Runner Park Apologises for Father." *Bangkok Post*, September 24, 2012. Accessed September 25, 2012. www.bangkokpost.com/news/asia/313765/s-korean-dictator-daughter-apologises-for-abuses.

Ban Ki-moon. "The Protection of Human Rights in the Context of Human Immunodeficiency Virus (HIV) and Acquired Immune Deficiency Syndrome (AIDS): Report of the Secretary-General." New York: United Nations, 2010 (UN doc. no. A/HRC/16/69).

Cerna, Christina M. "Universality of Human Rights and Cultural Diversity: Implementation of Human Rights in Different Socio-Cultural Contexts." *Human Rights Quarterly* 16 (1994): 740–52.

Cohen, Jonathan and Joanne Csete. "As Strong as the Weakest Pillar: Harm Reduction, Law Enforcement and Human Rights." *International Journal of Drug Policy* 17 (2006): 101.

Costa, Antonio Maria. "Drug Control Crime Prevention and Criminal Justice: A Human Rights Perspective—Note by the Executive Director." Vienna: UN Commission on Narcotic Drugs, 2010 (UN doc. no. E/CN.7/2010/CRP.6–E/CN.15/2010/CRP.1).

Davis, Sara L. M., Agus Triwahyuono, and Risa Alexander. "Survey of Abuses Against Injecting Drug Users in Indonesia." *Harm Reduction Journal* 6 (2009): 28–29.

Forero, Juan. "Latin Countries Pursue Alternatives to US Drug War." *Washington Post*, April 10, 2012. Accessed September 24, 2012. www.washingtonpost.com/world/the_americas/latin-american-countries-pursue-alternatives-to-us-drug-war/2012/04/10/gIQAFPEe7S_story.html.

Global Commission on Drug Policy. "War on Drugs: Report of the Global Commission on Drug Policy." Rio de Janeiro: GCDP, 2011. Accessed September 25, 2012. www.globalcommissionondrugs.org/wp-content/themes/gcdp_v1/pdf/Global_Commission_Report_English.pdf.

Hort, Sven Olsson and Stein Kuhnle. "The Coming of East and South-East Asian Welfare States." *European Journal of Social Policy* 10 (2000): 162–84.

HRI (Harm Reduction International). " Global State of Harm Reduction 2012. " London: HRI, 2012. Accessed September 25, 2012. www.ihra.net/files/2012/07/24/GlobalState2012_Web.pdf.

HRW (Human Rights Watch). *World Report 2012*. New York: HRW, 2012. Accessed September 25, 2012. www.hrw.org/world-report-2012.

ILO/OHCHR/UNDP/UNESCO/UNPF/UNHCR/UNICEF/UNODC/UNWOMEN/WFP/WHP/UNAIDS (International Labour Organisation, Office of the High Commissioner for Human Rights, United Nations Development Programme, United Nations Educational Scientific and Cultural Organisation, United Nations population Fund, United Nations High Commissioner for Refugees, United Nations Childrens Fund, United Nations Office on Drugs and Crime, United Nations Entity for Gender Equality and Empowerment of Women, World Food Programme, World Health Organisation and Joint United Nations Programme on HIV/AIDS). 2012. "Joint Statement: Compulsory Drug Detention and Rehabilitation Centers." Accessed October 17, 2012. www.ilo.org/aids/Whatsnew/WCMS_175377/lang--en/index.htm.

Jürgens, Ralf, Joanne Csete, Joseph J. Amon, Stefan Baral, and Chris Beyrer. "People Who Use Drugs, HIV and Human Rights." *Lancet* 376 (2010): 475–85.

Ministry of Foreign Affairs of the Kingdom of Thailand. "Statement by Her Excellency Ms. Yingluck Shinawatra, Prime Minister of the Kingdom of Thailand at the General Debate of the 67th Session of the United Nations General Assembly, New York, September 27, 2012." Accessed October 19, 2012. www.mfa.go.th/main/en/media-center/14/28027-Statement--by-Her-Excellency-Ms.-Yingluck-Shinawat.html.

Mydans, Seth. "Days of Reflection for Man Who Defined Singapore." *New York Times*, September 10, 2010. Accessed September 25, 2012. www.nytimes.com/2010/09/11/world/asia/11lee.html?pagewanted=all&_moc.semityn.www.

Rahman, Fifa and Guganesan Parasuraman, "Police Knowledge of Needle-and-Syringe Programs and Harm Reduction in Malaysia." Paper presented at the 6th International Society for the Study of Drug Policy (ISSDP) Conference, Canterbury Cathedral Lodge, Canterbury, Kent, United Kingdom, May 30–31, 2012.

Room, Robin and Peter Reuter. "How Well Do International Drug Conventions Protect Public Health?" *Lancet* 379 (2012): 84–91.

Said, Azahari (manager, NSEP, Malaysian AIDS Council), in discussion with author, October 2012.

Saucier, Roxanne, Daniel Wolfe, Kathleen Kingsbury, and Paul Silva, eds. "Treated with Cruelty: Abuses in the Name of Drug Rehabilitation." New York: Open Society Foundations, 2011. Accessed September 24, 2012. www.soros.org/sites/default/files/treatedwithcruelty.pdf.

Sen, Amartya. "Human Rights and Asian Values." *The New Republic* 33 (1997): 33–40.

Seng, Wong Kan. "The Real World of Human Rights." Speech to UN World Conference on Human Rights, Vienna, June 16, 1993.

Strathdee, Steffanie A., Timothy B. Hallett, Natalia Bobrova, Tim Rhodes, Robert Booth, R. Abdool, and Catherine A. Hankins. "HIV and Risk Environment for Injecting Drug Users: the Past, Present and Future." *Lancet* 376 (2010): 268–84.

Suzana bt Md Aris (claiming as administrator of the estate and a dependant of Mohd Anuar bin Sharip, deceased) v DSP Ishak bin Hussain & Ors (2011) 1 MLJ 107, *Malayan Law Journal*, para 5.

UNAIDS (Joint United Nations Programme on HIV/AIDS). "Joint Action for Results: UN-AIDS Outcome Framework 2009–2011." Geneva: United Nations, 2009. Accessed September 25, 2012. http://data.unaids.org/pub/BaseDocument/2010/jc1713_joint_action_en.pdf.

UNAIDS, Office of the United Nations High Commissioner for Human Rights, UN Development Programme, UNESCO, UNFPA, UNHCR, UNICEF, UN Office on Drugs and Crime, UN Women, World Food Programme, World Health Organization, and International Labour Organization. "Joint Statement: Compulsory Drug Detention and Rehabilitation Centres." Geneva: United Nations, 2012. Accessed September 24, 2012. www.ohchr.org/en/NewsEvents/Pages/DisplayNews.aspx?NewsID=11941&LangID=E.

UN Committee on Economic, Social and Cultural Rights. "General Comment no. 14: The Right to the Highest Attainable Standard of Health." Geneva: United Nations, 2000. (UN doc. no. D/C.12/2000/4).

UN General Assembly. "Declaration of Commitment on HIV/AIDS." 2001. New York: United Nations (UN doc. A/RES/S-26/2), para 52. Accessed September 25, 2012. www.un.org/ga/aids/docs/aress262.pdf.

Wolfe, Daniel, M. Patrizia Carrieri, and Donald Shepard. "Treatment and Care for Injecting Drug Users with HIV Infection: a review of Barriers and Ways Forward." *Lancet* 376 (2010): 355–66.

Chapter Four

Drug Users and Imprisonment

Kate Dolan and Ana Rodas

The imprisonment of drug users is a typical approach to problems of drug use in most countries. The vast numbers of drug users who are detained in prison means that prisons have an important role in drug policy. Therefore, the prison setting should be an ideal one for the provision of treatment of drug dependence, given the vast numbers of drug users they hold. This chapter examines drug users and imprisonment, the continuation of drug use while imprisoned, and harms resulting from that use and post release from prison. In terms of response to drug users in prison, the chapter also examines judicial corporal punishment for drugs, abuse by prison officials, and the death penalty. Finally we examine approaches that are effective in treating drug users and in particular methadone maintenance treatment for prisoners. We conclude with a brief look at decriminalization and recommendations.

INTRODUCTION

According to the UNODC, globally, the prevalence of HIV, sexually transmitted infections, hepatitis B, hepatitis C, and tuberculosis in prison populations is two to ten times as high as in the general population. [1] While the global prison census is about ten million people, [2] a staggering thirty million individuals enter and leave prison systems each year. Approximately one third of prison inmates are pre-trial detainees, awaiting court. Virtually all prisoners will return to their communities, many within a few months to a year. An additional half a million drug users are held in closed settings, or compulsory centers for drug users (and sex workers in Vietnam) found across Asia. Many drug users are held in these compulsory centers without due legal process, often without a predetermined release date, and subjected to corporal punishment. Relapse to drug use post-release can result in longer stays in these centers.

DRUG USERS AND IMPRISONMENT

People who inject drugs (PWID) are vastly over-represented in prison. Globally, PWID account for more than 30 percent of prisoners but less than 2 or 3 percent of the general population.[3] PWID have a very high chance of being imprisoned at some time in their life, and usually on multiple occasions. One study that sampled PWIDs from twelve cities found that over 60 percent reported a history of imprisonment.[4] A cross-sectional survey in ten European cities found that over half of the heroin and cocaine users had been in prison.[5] One-third of all heroin-dependent individuals in the United States pass through a correctional center annually.[6] Australian PWID reported a similar level of incarceration and an average of five imprisonments.[7]

A review of recidivism in fifteen US states found that one-quarter of individuals released from prison returned within three years.[8] These figures show that the approach of imprisoning vast numbers of drug users does not rehabilitate drug users. Another aspect to the repeated re-incarceration of PWID is the creation of a very dynamic population. The prison population is not a static one that people enter and stay in for long periods of time. Rather, legal systems generate an incredible number of movements into, out of, and through the system, that can catalyze the spread of a range of infections such as TB, HIV, and HCV. The high proportion of PWID coupled with the dynamic nature of prison populations contributes to HIV transmission among prisoners and to the broader community once inmates are released. As we will cover in the next sections, not only do inmates go untreated for their drug dependence, they are rarely provided with the means to reduce their risk of acquiring blood-borne viral infections such as HIV and hepatitis C in prison.

PRISONERS AND DRUG USE

In the United Kingdom, 80 percent of prisoners reported having used illicit drugs.[9] Of sentenced prisoners, 32 percent of men and 34 percent of women reported severe drug dependence on at least one illicit drug.[10] Many prisoners continue to using drugs while they are in prison,[11, 12] this is in spite of various measures to stop drugs from entering prison and punishment for those caught using drugs. In Britain, about 40 percent of prisoners reported using drugs inside prison.[13] According to Stöver (2001),[14] the percentage of heroin-dependent prisoners who continue to inject in prisons ranges between 16 percent and 60 percent across European studies. An even higher level was reported from a German study where 75 percent of imprisoned injectors continued to inject in prison.[15]

HARMS IN PRISON

Inmates face a range of harms from being incarcerated. These include switching the type of drug they use, initiation into drug use or into injecting, blood-borne viral infections from sharing syringes, and loss of tolerance to drugs leading to an increase risk of fatal overdose on release. In some cases drug users are sentenced to death for their drug use.

Switching Drugs Used and Initiation into Drug Use and Injecting

Some studies suggest that prisoners switch between drugs when they enter prison. The length of the prison sentence, mandatory drug testing, and psychosocial characteristics of prisoners have been reported as the most important influences on such switching from one drug to another.[16] When prisoners are subjected to drug testing,[17] some prisoners may switch from one with a long period for detection (e.g., cannabis) to a drug with a brief period for detection (e.g., heroin) to minimise detection and punishment, although the numbers who reported doing this in an English survey of prisoners was small.[18]

Prisons can be a place where individuals will commence their drug use. A study of three thousand prisoners in the United Kingdom found that over one-quarter of the heroin users reported that they had began using heroin in prison.[19] An estimated 10 percent of Australian inmates commenced injecting while in prison.[20]

HIV and Hepatitis C in Prison

HIV prevalence is universally higher in prison than in the surrounding community, with levels of infection reaching 50 percent among prisoners in some countries.[21, 22] The dynamic nature of prison populations facilitates HIV transmission. In 2011, over ten million people were in prison (International Centre for Prison Studies, 2011), but an estimated thirty million people were imprisoned and released to the community that year. Studies of prisoners document a high prevalence of injecting and an extremely high prevalence of syringe sharing in prison. In Thailand, Thaisri (2003)[23] reported that 25 percent of 689 inmates injected and of them 78 percent shared syringes. Studies of prisoners with a history of injecting find even higher rates of injecting in prison. In Pakistan, 80 percent of PWIDs had been to jail, where reports of injecting ranged from 22 percent to 70 percent in two cities and syringe sharing was 56 percent.[24] In Pakistan, 4 percent of prisoners were injecting drug users.[25] An Afghan study found that 17 percent and 11 percent of PWIDs reported having injected drugs in prison in Kabul and Herat, respectively.[26]

HIV transmission in prison is difficult to document owing to uncertainties regarding precise date of infection, the rapid turnover of inmates, low levels of HIV testing, and inmates' reluctance to report risk behaviors to prison authorities (Dolan, 1997; 1999). Nevertheless, a growing number of reports of HIV transmission in prison, including outbreaks, have been made.[27, 28, 29, 30, 31, 32]

In Thailand, the first outbreak of HIV began among PWIDs in a Bangkok prison in 1988.[33] Incarceration and the sharing of needles in prison were the only two independent risk factors for HIV transmission in a cohort of injectors in the community. HIV incidence in Thai prisons was very high, at thirty-five per one hundred persons per year.[34] An outbreak of HIV in one Lithuanian prison resulted in almost 300 inmates being infected within a six-month period. This outbreak doubled the number of HIV cases in Lithuania.[35] Meanwhile an outbreak in Russian prisons resulted in over 400 inmates acquiring HIV in a brief period.[36] Iran reported two large outbreaks of HIV in prisons with hundreds infected.[37] These outbreaks were the impetus for the introduction of needle and syringe and methadone programs in Iranian prisons.[38] HIV outbreaks in prison have been reported even where prevalence is very low such as Scotland[39] and Australia.[40] These findings indicate the need for HIV prevention in prisons is not just for inmates but also for the wider community once inmates are released.

Imprisonment has been found to be an independent factor for acquiring hepatitis C virus.[41, 42] Disruption of methadone treatment, especially due to brief periods of imprisonment, was associated with a significant increase in HCV incidence.[43]

Overdose

Although some inmates will continue to use drugs in prison, they rarely use at a level which maintains their tolerance to drugs.[44] Once released, ex-inmates seek drugs and commence using at levels they used pre-incarceration. This level of use places them at an increased risk of fatal overdose on release from prison. The crucial period is the first two to four weeks after release from prison.[45]

In Vietnam, ex-residents of drug rehabilitation centers were significantly more likely to have overdosed in the previous twelve months than users who had not been in such centers (45 percent vs. 27 percent, p = 0.001).[46] PWIDs in the developing world appear to have a higher rate of mortality than their counterparts in the developed world. Vietnamese PWIDs all-cause mortality rate (6.3 percent per year) was thirteen-fold higher than the rate in the general population after standardization for age and sex.[47] This rate was higher than rates reported from studies of PWID in India (4.3 percent per year)[48] and Thailand (3.8 percent per year)[49] and is much higher than rates in the United States (0.7 percent per year)[50] and Australia (0.8 percent per year).[51] In Thailand, 252 PWIDs were surveyed about their experience of non-fatal overdoses. A history of non-fatal overdose was reported by 30 percent of participants and was independently associated with a history of incarceration.[52]

Methadone Treatment for Heroin Users in Prison

Methadone maintenance treatment (MMT) is an effective and cost-effective treatment for heroin dependence.[53] Clients in MMT are retained in treatment, reduce their heroin use[54] and risk behavior[55] and experience improvements in health, social, and criminal justice outcomes.[56, 57, 58, 59, 60] In order for treatment to be optimized, clients need adequate dosages,[61] ongoing treatment[62] and ancillary services.[63]

Prison-based methadone programs reduce drug use in prison,[64] criminality,[65, 66] re-incarceration and mortality among recently released prisoners.[67, 68, 69, 70] And pre-release prison methadone was associated significantly with increased treatment entry and retention after release if treatment continued.[71]

According to the World Health Organization, methadone is an essential medicine in all countries with problem opioid-user populations.[72] The United Nations Office on Drugs and Crime[73] recommend MMT in prisons as a strategy to reduce drug injection and HIV transmission. While MMT is implemented in the community setting in seventy countries,[74] it is implemented in prison in about twenty-nine countries.[75] However coverage within prisons is poor with less than 1 percent to 14 percent of all inmates being treated. Further some thirty-seven countries offer MMT to PWIDs in community settings, but not prisons. India and Malaysia provide methadone to prisoners.

Treatment for ATS Users in Prison

Japan has introduced the Matrix Model for stimulant abusers in prison.[76] It consists of six major treatment components: individual/conjoint counseling, early recovery group, relapse prevention group, social support group, family education group, and urine testing.[77]

Needle and Syringe Programs for Prisoners

While eighty-two countries operate NSPs in the community, only ten countries do so for prison inmates.[78] Results from studies of NSP in prison are very favourable,[79] but no Asian country offers this program.

The Impact of Incarceration

Drucker (2011) highlights the flow-on effects of incarceration.[80] Imprisonment does not impact on drug users only but their families, communities and the overall economy are also affected. According to Drucker (2011) an even larger population, the family members of those who have been incarcerated, is adversely affected in ways that help to sustain an epidemic of mass incarceration. These innocent victims, especially children, are psychologically and socially wounded. Children with incarcerated parents are significantly more likely to become incarcerated themselves. These children experience disadvantages such as school failure, increased health and psychological problems and homelessness. Imprisonment strains already shaky marriages as the main breadwinner is removed and often held hundreds of miles away from home making visits exceedingly difficult. Chances are that the ex-offender will re-enter society significantly worse than when he left in terms of being employable.

COST EFFECTIVENESS OF DRUG TREATMENT

One dollar spent on drug courts is estimated to save approximately $4 in avoided costs of incarceration and health care,[81] and prison-based treatment saves between $2 to $6.[82] The US National Institutes on Drug Abuse (NIDA) estimated that the United States spends $9 billion incarcerating drug offenders each year, whereas treating these people would cost a third as much. Spending money to provide treatment for heavy cocaine users would reduce drug consumption by nearly four times as much as spending the same amount on law enforcement.[83]

JUDICIAL CORPORAL PUNISHMENT FOR DRUGS

Judicial corporal punishment is state-sanctioned beating, caning, or whipping of a person for drug use, purchase, or possession. According to Harm Reduction International,[84] these human rights abuses against people who use drugs and excessively punitive approaches to drug control are not only wrong in themselves but are also counterproductive for individuals, communities and public health.

Thousands of drug users and alcohol consumers are subjected to judicially sanctioned caning, flogging, lashing, or whipping each year.[85] Judicial corporal punishment is practiced in over forty countries including Singapore, Malaysia, Iran, Yemen, Saudi Arabia, Qatar, United Arab Emirates, Libya, Brunei, Darussalam, Maldives, Indonesia (Aceh), and Nigeria (northern states). The use of caning, flogging, lashing, and whipping is in direct violation of international law that prohibits the use of corporal punishment. UN human rights monitors have expressed their concern a number of times about the legislation in various countries that allow law enforcement to inflict these types of cruel, inhumane, and degrading punishments. The reports states that state-sanctioned violence such as this is in clear violation of international law. In Singapore, relapse to drug use is harshly punished: "Those who relapse upon their release . . . would be sentenced to a minimum of seven years' and a maximum of thirteen years' imprisonment, as well as a minimum of six and a maximum of twelve strokes of the cane." Relapse, it should be noted, is a common, expected, and manageable element of drug treatment. There is no evidence that this approach reduces drug use or any other harms resulting from drug use.

CLOSED SETTINGS

Recently, attention has focused on how drug users are treated by the criminal justice system. Advocates of drug use as a victimless crime argue for the diversion of drug users away from penal institutions and into treatment programs. In 2009, the Indonesian Supreme Court encouraged judges to send drug users to drug rehabilitation centers instead of prison.[86] However, "treatment centers" or "rehabilitation centers" in some Asian countries lack health care, treatment programs where due process and human rights are violated (see Baldwin and Thomson in this book). These centers consist of prison-like confinement with little empirical data on treatment outcomes. Reports suggest that persons undergoing this punitive "treatment" suffer physical and psychological harms and high rates of relapse to drug use.[87, 88]

In Malaysia, the drug treatment system does not make a distinction between occasional drug users and dependent drug users.[89] Detainees in Malaysian government "treatment centers" have reported being beaten with bricks, punched, caned by religious teachers, made to crawl through animal excrement, and made to drink dirty water as part of their induction to the center.[90] In Malaysia, there is an estimated 70 percent to 90 percent relapse rate after incarceration.[91]

In Cambodia, drug users are often arrested during police raids and confined in treatment centers that are managed by military staff as opposed to health staff with appropriate addiction and counselling skills.[92] In 2009, the International Harm Reduction Development Program reported that detainees endured food shortages, custodial deaths, and sexual abuse.

Approximately fifty thousand to one hundred thousand drug users are detained in Vietnamese compulsory treatment centers where HIV antiviral treatment is unavailable in spite of a reported HIV prevalence of 75 percent.[93] Individuals tested for HIV are rarely informed of the result.[94] Vietnam's law stipulates a mandatory detention of drug users for a period of one to two years for rehabilitation. In addition, there is a further two years of "post rehabilitation management" which can be extended to six years.[95, 96] Up to 28 percent of PWIDs have reported sharing needles. Evidence shows an association between drug rehabilitation and HIV transmission in Vietnam where HIV prevalence in six centers ranged from 30 percent to 65 percent.[97] Residents work for private companies with little or no pay and are required to meet production quotas or face severe punishment.[98] In Vietnam, 95 percent of those who leave compulsory drug treatment centers relapse to drug use.[99] This has resulted in further punitive policy responses that have seen an increase in periods of detention for up to six years.[100]

For China's three to four million PWIDs[101] the most common forms of drug treatment are detoxification and re-education through labor (see Biddulph in this book). In 2005 the Chinese government introduced a "National People's War on Illicit Drugs" intended to increase the number of drug users detained in compulsory detoxification centers.[102] In that same year a total of 350,000 drug users were detained in detoxification or RTL centers.[103, 104] Conditions in detox and RTL centers have been reported by detainees as consisting of repeated mandatory HIV testing but without being told the results, inadequate access to health care, disruption of antivretroviral therapy, enhanced risk of HIV infection, and poor living conditions.[105] Evaluations of compulsory drug detention in China estimate them to have relapse rates of about 95 percent.[106] In China, there is no after care or follow-up provided (WHO, 2009), and a 79 percent relapse rate.[107] There are a number of human rights issues in compulsory detention in China, including a lack of due legal process and forced labor, exercise, and "moral education."[108, 109]

In Thailand, most drug users end up in "forced treatment."[110] From October 2008 to June 2009, there were an estimated 39,287 people in compulsory drug detention centers in Thailand.[111] Empirical data on the experiences of drug users in compulsory drug treatment in Thailand is scant. However, a study conducted by Csete and Dube[112] of 252 community-recruited PWIDs found that having undergone compulsory drug detention was associated with having had drugs planted on one's person by the police, reported greater spending on illicit drugs, and poly drug use. Beyrer et al. (2003)[113] found that 27 percent of 1,865 drug users in the study reported a history of imprisonment. Of those women who reported a history of imprisonment 22.7 percent were HIV positive compared to 5 percent of those reporting no period of imprisonment. Among the male sample with IDU history (n = 485) it was found that 56 percent had a history of incarceration. Among this group, 38.2 percent of those who had been incarcerated were HIV positive compared to 20.2 percent of those reporting no history of imprisonment. And of those with incarceration history 16 percent reported using drugs in prison and 36 percent shared needles.

WHO has produced clinical guidelines for withdrawal management and treatment of drug dependence in closed settings.[114] These guidelines detail how to management inmates experiencing withdrawals from drugs and alcohol and how to treat their drug dependency.

DEATH PENALTY

In 2011, thirty-two countries or territories had laws prescribing the death penalty for drug offences, a practice that is in violation of international law. [115] Mandatory capital punishment for certain drug offences exists in twelve countries.[116] These countries are Brunei-Darussalam, Egypt, Iran, Kuwait, Lao PDR, Malaysia, Oman, Singapore, Sudan, Syria, United Arab Emirates, and Yemen. Drug offenders make up the majority of those who are condemned to die. Although exact numbers are difficult to obtain, it is clear that hundreds of people are executed every year for a drug-related offence. The vast majority of executions occur in just a few countries. The Global Overview estimated that executions for drugs happened in twelve countries over the last five years. The use of the death penalty for drug offences has declined over the recent past. Recently Singapore's Law Minister K. Shanmugam introduced legal changes before parliament that would end mandatory death sentences in drug trafficking cases[117] (see Rahman's chapter on the death penalty in this book).

DECRIMINALIZATION

Over twenty countries have adopted some form of decriminalization of drug possession without any increase in drug use.[118] These authors concluded that "the law enforcement model adopted has little impact on the levels of drug use within a country and yet the criminalization of people who use drugs causes significant harms to the individual and society."

The report from the Global Commission on HIV and the Law argues that regulation of illicit drugs may have a positive effect on HIV prevention.[119] Thus it advocates that decriminalization, as opposed to legalization, may be a viable option to allow the legal arm of the law to still function in a protective way that does not increase harms for drug users and the community. Adopting a decriminalization framework means that drug use and possession of small amounts can still remain illegal, but instead of being dealt with through the criminal justice system, such cases would be dealt with through civil law. Brazil, Mexico, and Portugal have all experimented with the decriminalization of drug use for personal use and no significant increase in drug use has been reported. The call for decriminalization by the Commission is that by removing the fear of arrest and draconian punishment, drug users would be less stigmatized and more willing to be tested for HIV and access treatment for their drug use.

CONCLUSION AND RECOMMENDATIONS

The criminalization of drug users with attendant imprisonment causes numerous harms. It is counterproductive in that it does not treat offenders' drug problems, but rather some inmates start using drugs or injecting when they are imprisoned. Other inmates are infected with HIV or hepatitis C when in prison. *But perhaps the most absurd aspect is that the imprisonment of drug offenders is more costly than the provision of treatment.* The approach of using compulsory drug treatment appears to be worse than imprisonment as human right abuses and no due legal process are common place. Many drug users are held in the compulsory centers often without a predetermined release date, and subjected to corporal punishment. Relapse to drug use post-release can result in longer stays in these centers. Severe punishment is meted out to detainees who attempt escape.[120] Many countries imprison drug offenders while on remand when this is not required.

The vast number of prisoners with a drug problem is astounding. One-third of men and women in UK prisons reported severe drug dependence on at least one illicit drug. Yet treatment is scarce or not based on evidence. Countries need to examine the WHO-produced Clinical Guidelines for withdrawal management and treatment of drug dependence in closed settings.[121] These guidelines detail how to manage inmates experiencing withdrawals from drugs and alcohol and how to treat their drug dependency.

The benefits of prison methadone treatment are similar to those in community settings. If countries were serious about treatment, reducing crime, re-incarceration and overdose deaths then prison methadone program would be the norm rather than the rare thing they are today.

NOTES

1. UNODC (United Nations Office of Drugs and Crime), *HIV Prevention, Treatment and Care in Prisons and Other Closed Settings: A Comprehensive Package of Interventions* (Vienna: UNODC, 2012).

2. International Centre for Prison Studies. "World Prison Briefs 2011." Accessed August 14, 2012.www.prisonstudies.org/info/worldbrief/.

3. Bradley Mathers, Louisa Degenhardt, Benjamin Phillips, Lucas Weissing, Matthew Hickman, Steffanie Strathdee, Alex Wodak, Samiran Panda, Mark Tyndall, Abdalla Toufik, and Richard Mattick, "Global Epidemiology of Injecting Drug Use and HIV among People who Inject Drugs: a Systematic Review," *Lancet* 372, no. 9651 (2008): 1733–45.

4. Andrew Ball, Don des Jarlais, Martin Donohoe, Samual Friedman, David Goldberg, Gillian Hunter, Gerry Stimson, and Alex Wodak. "Multi-City Study on Drug Injecting and Risk of HIV Infection" (Geneva: World Health Organisation, 1994).

5. Joan March, Eugenia Oviedo-Joekes, and Manuel Romero, "Drugs and Social Exclusion in Ten European Cities," *European Addiction Research* 12, no. 1 (2006): 33–41.

6. Amy Boutwell, Ank Nijhawan, Nichol Zaller, and Josiah Rich, "Arrested on Heroin: A National Opportunity." *Journal of Opioid Management* 3 (2007): 328–32.

7. Kate Dolan, Alex Wodak, and Wayne Hall, "HIV Risk Behaviour and Prevention in Prison: A Bleach Programme for Inmates in NSW." *Drug Alcohol Review* 18, no. 2 (1999): 139–43.

8. Redonna Chandler, Bennet Fletcher, and Nora Volkow, "Treating Drug Abuse and Addiction in the Criminal Justice System: improving Public Health and Safety." *The Journal of the American Medical Association* 301, no. 2 (2009): 183–90.

9. Annabel Boys, Michael Farrell, Glyn Bebbington, Traolach Brugha, Jeremy Coid, Paul Jenkins, Nicola Lewis, John Marsden, Rachel Meltzer, Nicola Singleton, and Colin Taylor, "Drug Use and Initiation in Prison: Results from a National Prison Survey in England and Wales," *Addiction* 97, no. 12 (2002): 1551–60.

10. Nicola Singleton, Michael Farrell, and Howard Meltzer, "Substance Misuse among Prisoners in England and Wales," *International Review of Psychiatry* 15 (2003): 150–52.

11. Kate Dolan, Wayne Hall, and Alex Wodak. "Methadone Maintenance Reduces Injecting in Prison," *British Medical Journal* 312 (1996): 1162.

12. Seena Fazel, Parveen Bains, and Helen Doll, "Substance Abuse and Dependence in Prisoners: A Systematic Review," *Addiction* 101 (2006): 181–91

13. Nicola Singleton, Elizabeth Pendry, Tracy Simpson, Eileen Goddard, Michael Farrell, John Marsden, and Colin Taylor, "The Impact of Mandatory Drug Testing in Prisons," Home Office Online Report 03/05, Home Office, London, 2005.

14. Heino Stöver, ed. *Overview Study. Assistance to Drug Users in European Prisons* (Lisbon: EMCDDA, 2001).

15. Klaus Stark, Ute Herrmann, Stephan Ehrhardt, and Ulrich Bienzle, "A Syringe Exchange Programme in Prison as Prevention Strategy against HIV Infection and Hepatitis B and C in Berlin, Germany," *Epidemiology and Infection* 134, no. 4 (2006): 814–19.

16. Boys et al., *Drug Use and Initiation in Prisons*, 1551–60.

17. Kate Dolan, David Rouen, and Jo Kimber, "An Overview of the Use of Urine, Hair, Sweat and Saliva to detect Drug Use," *Drug and Alcohol Review* 23, no. 2 (2004): 213–17.

18. Singleton et al., *The Impact of Mandatory Drug Testing in Prisons.*

19. Boys et al., *Drug Use and Initiation in Prisons*, 1551–60.

20. Scott Rutter, Kate Dolan, and Alex Wodak, "Sex, Drugs and Viruses in Sin City Sydney. Report on Australian Study of HIV and Injecting Drug Use." National Drug and Alcohol Research Center Technical Report No. 37 (Sydney: University of New South Wales [UNSW], 1996).

21. Kate Dolan, Ben Kite, Emma Black, Carmen Aceijas, and Gerry Stimson, "HIV in Prison in Low-Income and Middle-Income Countries," *Lancet Infectious Diseases* 7, no. 1 (2007): 32–41.

22. UNAIDS (Joint United Nations Programme on HIV/AIDS). *Global Report: UNAIDS Report on The Global AIDS Epidemic.* Geneva: UNAIDS, 2010.

23. Hansa Thaisri,John Lerwitworapong, Suthon Vongsheree, Pathom Sawanpanyalert, Chanchai Chadbanchachai, Archawin Rojanawiwat, Wichuda Kongpromsook, Wiroj Paungtubtim, Pongnuwat Sri-ngam, and Rachaneekorn Jaisue, "HIV Infection and Risk Factors among Bangkok Prisoners, Thailand: A Prospective Cohort Study," *BMC Infectious Diseases* 3, no. 25 (2003), DOI:10.1186/1471-2334-3-25.

24. Nai Zindagi. "Rapid Situation Assessments of HIV Prevalence and Risk Factors among People Injecting Drugs in Four Cities of the Punjab." Islamabad, 2009, accessed January 10, 2013.

25. Shehla Baqi, Naheed Nabi, Syed Hasan, Amir Khan, Omrana Pasha, Naila Kayani, Rehan Haque, Inaam-ul Haq, Mohammad Khurshid, Susan Fisher-Hoch, Stephen Luby, and Joseph McCormick, "HIV Antibody Seroprevalence and Associated Risk Factors in Sex Workers, Drug Users, and Prisoners in Sindh, Pakistan," *Journal of Acquired Immune Deficiency Syndromes & Human Retrovirology* 18, no. 1 (1998): 73–79.

26. World Bank, *Afghanistan HIV/AIDS Prevention Project:* June 2008.

27. T. Brewer Fordham, David Vlahov, Ellen Taylor, Drusilla Hall, Alvaro Munoz, and Frank Polk, "Transmission of HIV-1 within a Statewide Prison System," *AIDS* 2, no. 5 (1988): 363–67.

28. CDC, "Acquired Immunodeficiency Syndrome in Correctional Facilities: A Report of the National Institute of Justice and the American Correctional Association," *MMWR. Morbidity and Mortality Weekly Report 35*, no. 12 (1986): 195–99.

29. Kate Dolan and Alex Wodak, "HIV Transmission in a Prison System in an Australian State," *Medical Journal of Australia* 171, no. 1 (1999): 14–17.

30. Robert Horsburgh, Joseph Jarvis, Trudy McArthur, Terri Ignacio, and Patricia Stock, "Seroconversion to HIV in Prison Inmates," *American Journal of Public Health* 80, no. 2 (1990): 209–10.

31. Randal Mutter, Richard Grimes, and Darwin Labarthe, "Evidence of Intraprison Spread of HIV Infection," *Archives of Internal Medicine* 154, no. 7 (1994): 793–95.

32. T. Fordham Brewer, David Vlahov, Ellen Taylor, Drusilla Hall, Alvaro Munoz, and Frank Polk, "Transmission of HIV-1 within a Statewide Prison System," *AIDS* 2, no. 5 (1988): 363–67.

33. Kachit Choopanya, Suphak Vanichseni, Don Des Jarlais, Kanokporn Plangsringarm, Wandee Sonchai, Manuel Carballo, Patricia Friedman, and Samuel Friedman, "Risk Factors and HIV Seropositivity among Injecting Drug Users in Bangkok," *AIDS* 5, no. 12 (1991): 1509–13.

34. Kachit Choopanya, Don Des Jarlais, Suphak Vanichseni, Dwip Kitayaporn, Phillip Mock, Suwanee Raktham, Krit Hireanras, William Heyward, Sathit Sujarita, and Timothy Mastro, "Incarceration and Risk for HIV Infection among Injecting Drug Users in Bangkok," *Journal of Acquired Immune Deficiency Syndromes & Human Retrovirology* 29, no. 1 (2002): 86–94.

35. Dolan et al., *HIV in Prison*, 32–41.

36. Dolan et al., *HIV in Prison*, 32–41.

37. Dolan et al., *HIV in Prison*, 32–41.

38. Marziyeh Farnia, Bahman Ebrahimi, Ali Shams, and Saman Zamani, "Scaling up Methadone Maintenance Treatment for Opioid-Dependent Prisoners in Iran," *International Journal of Drug Policy* 21, no. 5 (2010): 422–24.

39. Avril Taylor, David Goldberg, John Emslie, Laurence Gruer, Sheila Cameron, James Black, Barbara Davis, James McGregor, Edward Follet, Janina Harvey, John Basson, and James McGavigan, "Outbreak of HIV Infection in a Scottish prison," *British Medical Journal* 310, no. 289 (1995): 289.

40. Dolan and Wodak, *HIV Transmission in a Prison System*, 14–17.

41. Markus Backmund, Kirsten Meyer, MartinWächtler, and Dieter Eichenlaub, "Hepatitis C Virus Infection in Injection Drug Users in Bavaria: Risk Factors for Seropositivity," *European Journal of Epidemiology* 18 (2003): 563–68.

42. Markus Backmund, Jens Reimer, Kirsten Meyer, Tilman Gerlach, and Reinhart Zachoval, "Hepatitis C Virus Infection and Injection Drug Users: Prevention, Risk Factors, and Treatment," *Clinical Infectious Diseases* 40, no. 5 (2005): S330–S335.

43. Kate Dolan, James Shearer, Bethany White, Jialun Zhou, and Alex Wodak, "Four-Year Follow-up of Imprisoned Male Heroin Users and Methadone Treatment: Mortality, Re-incarceration and Hepatitis C Infection," *Addiction* 100, no. 6 (2005): 820–28.

44. Kate Dolan, Alex Wodak, Wayne Hall, Matt Gaughwin, and Fiona Rae, "HIV Risk Behaviour of IDUs before, during, and after Imprisonment in NSW," *Addiction Research* 4, no. 2 (1996): 151–60.

45. Michael Farrell and John Marsden, "Acute Risk of Drug-Related Death among Newly Released Prisoners in England and Wales," *Addiction* 103, no. 2 (2008): 251–55.

46. Anne Bergenstrom, Vu Minh Quan, Le Van Nam, Kristen McClausland, Nguyen Phuong Thuoc, David Celentano, and Vivian Go, "Cross-Sectional Study on Prevalence of Non-Fatal Drug Overdose and Associated Risk Characteristics among Out-of-Treatment Injecting Drug Users in North Vietnam," *Substance Use & Misuse* 43, no. 1 (2008): 73–84.

47. Vu Quan, Apinun Aramrattana, Tasanai Vongchak, Carl Latkin, Deborah Donnell, Ting-Yuang Liu, Kanokporn Wiboonnatakul, and David Celentano, "Mortality among Injec-

tion Drug Users in Northern Thailand: A Prospective Cohort Study," *Journal of Addiction Medicine* 4, no. 4 (2010): 217–22. DOI: 10.1097/ADM.0b013e3181c78bf4.

48. Quan et al., *Mortality among Injection Drug Users*, 217–22.

49. Sunil Solomon, David Celentano, Aylur Srikrishnan, Conjeevaram Vasudevan, Santha-nam Anand, Muniratnam Kumar, Suniti Solomon, Gregory Lucas, and Shruti Mehta, "Mortal-ity among Injection Drug Users in Chennai, India (2005–2008)," *AIDS* 23 (2009): 997–1004.

50. David Vlahov, Cunlin Wang, Danielle Ompad, Crystal M. Fuller, Wendy Caceres, Law-rence Ouellet, Peter Kerndt, Don Des Jarlais, and Richard Garfein, "Mortality Risk among Recent-Onset Injection Drug Users in Five U.S. Cities," *Substance Use and Misuse* 43 (2008): 413–28.

51. Mark Stoove, Paul Dietze, Campbell Aitken, and Damien Jolley, "Mortality among Injecting Drug Users in Melbourne: A 16-year Follow-up of the Victorian Injecting Cohort Study (VICS)," *Drug and Alcohol Dependence* 96 (2008): 281–85.

52. M-J. Milloy, Nadia Fairbairn, Kanna Hayashi, Paisan Suwannawong, Karyn Kaplan, Evan Wood, and Thomas Kerr, "Research Overdose Experiences among Injection Drug Users in Bangkok, Thailand," *Harm Reduction Journal* 7, no. 1 (2010): DOI: 10.1186/1477-7517-7-9.

53. Dagmar Hedrich, Paula Alves, Michael Farrell, Heino Stöver, Lars Møller, and Soraya Maye, "The Effectiveness of Opioid Maintenance Treatment in Prison Settings: a Systematic Review," *Addiction* 107, no. 3 (2012): 501–17.

54. Kate Dolan, Alex Wodak, and Wayne Hall, "Methadone Maintenance Treatment Re-duces Heroin Injection in NSW Prisons," *Drug and Alcohol Review* 17, no. 2 (1998): 153–58.

55. Kate Dolan, James Shearer, Margaret MacDonald, Richard Mattick, Wayne Hall, and Alex Wodak. "A Randomized Controlled Trial of Methadone Maintenance Treatment vs. Wait List Control in an Australian Prison," *Drug and Alcohol Dependence* 72, no. 1 (2003): 59–65.

56. Hugh Tilson, Apinun Aramrattana, Samuel Bozzette, David Celentano, Mathea Falco, Theodore Hammett, Andrei Kozlov, Shenghan Lai, Ajay Mahal, Richard Schottenfeld, and S. Solomon. (Committee on the Prevention of HIV Infection among Injecting Drug Users in High-Risk Countries). "Preventing HIV Infection among Injecting Drug Users in High-Risk Countries. An Assessment of the Evidence," (Washington, DC: Global Board of Health, Insti-tute of Medicine of the National Academies, 2006).

57. Linda Gowing, Michael Farrell, Reinhart Bornemann, Lynn Sullivan, and Robert Ali, (2008). "Substitution Treatment of Injecting Opioid Users for Prevention of HIV Infection," *Cochrane Database of Systematic Reviews* 2, no. CD004145 (2008): DOI:10.1002/14651858.CD004145.pub3.

58. Richard Mattick, Courtney Breen, Jo Kimber, and Marina Davoli, "Methadone Mainte-nance Therapy versus no Opioid Replacement Therapy for Opioid Dependence," *Cochrane Database of Systematic Reviews* 3, no. CD002209 (2009): DOI: 10.1002/14651858.CD002209.pub2.

59. Anna Bargagli, Marina Davoli, Silvia Minozzi, Simona Vecchi, and Carlo Perucci, "A Systematic Review of Observational Studies on Treatment of Opioid Dependence," Back-ground Document Prepared for 3rd meeting of Technical Development Group (TDG) for the WHO Guidelines for Psychosocially Assisted Pharmacotherapy of Opioid Dependence, WHO, Geneva, Switzerland, September 17–21, 2007.

60. Kate Dolan, Heather Worth, Ousman Badjie, and J'Belle Foster, "Review of Compulso-ry and Voluntary Treatment for Drug Users in Asia" (Sydney: University of New South Wales [UNSW], 2012).

61. Dolan, Hall, and Wodak, *Methadone Maintenance Reduces Injecting in Prison*, 1162.

62. Dolan et al., *Four-Year Follow-Up*, 820–28.

63. Laura Amato, Marina Davoli, Silvia Minozzi, Robert Ali, and Marica Ferri, "Methadone at Tapered Doses for the Management of Opioid Withdrawal," *Cochrane Database Systematic Reviews* 3, no. CD003409 (2005). www.ncbi.nlm.nih.gov/pubmed/12804464. Accessed Sep-tember 13, 2012. DOI: 10.1002/14651858.CD003409.pub3.

64. Dolan et al., "A Randomized Controlled Trial," 59–65.

65. Timothy Kinlock, Michael Gordon, Robert Schwartz, and Kevin O'Grady, "A Study of Methadone Maintenance for Male Prisoners: 3-month Post Release Outcomes," *Criminal Justice Behavior* 35 (2008): 34–47.

66. Michael Gordon, Timothy Kinlock, Robert Schwartz, and Kevin O'Grady, "A Randomized Clinical Trial of Methadone Maintenance for Prisoners: Findings at 6 Months Post-Release," *Addiction* 103 (2008): 1333–42.

67. Dolan et al., *Four-Year Follow-Up*, 820–28.

68. Sarah Larney, Barbara Toson, Lucy Burns, and Kate Dolan, "Opioid Substitution Treatment in Prison and post-release: Effects on Criminal Recidivism and Mortality," *Monograph Series* No. 37, NDLERF, Canberra, 2011.

69. Gordon et al., *A Randomized Clinical*, 1333–42.

70. Eran Bellin, Jennifer Wesson, Vincent Tomasino, James Nolan, Alvin Glick, and Sonia Oquendo, "High Dose Methadone reduces Criminal Recidivism in Opiate Addicts," *Addiction Research and Theory* 7 (1999): 19–29.

71. Sarah Larney, Barbara Toson, Lucy Burns, and Kate Dolan, "Effect of Prison-based Opioid Substitution Treatment and Post-release Retention in Treatment on Risk of Re-incarceration," *Addiction* 107, no. 2 (2012): 372–80.

72. WHO (World Health Organization), *Model List of Essential Medicines, 2011* (Geneva: WHO, 2011). Accessed August 2012. http://whqlibdoc.who.int/hq/2011/a95053_eng.pdf.

73. UNODC, *HIV Prevention, Treatment and Care in Prisons*.

74. HRI (Harm Reduction International), *Global State of Harm Reduction 2012: Towards an Integrated Response* (London: HRI, 2012).

75. Sarah Larney and Kate Dolan, "A Literature Review of International Implementation of Opioid Substitution Treatment in Prisons: Equivalence of Care?" *European Addiction Research* 15 (2009): 107–12.

76. Takayuki Harada and Hiroyuki Shinkai, "New Initiatives for Drug Abuse Treatment in Japanese Prisons," *International Journal of Comparative and Applied Criminal Justice* 34, no. 2 (2010): 391–404.

77. Jeanne Obert, Michael McCann, Patricia Marinelli-Casey, Ahndrea Weiner, Sam Minsky, Paul Brethen, and Richard Rawson, "The Matrix Model of Outpatient Stimulant Abuse Treatment: History and Description," *Journal of Psychoactive Drugs* 32, no. 2 (2000): 157–64.

78. HRI, *Global State of Harm Reduction 2012*.

79. Ralf Jürgens, Andrew Ball, and Annette Verster, "Interventions to Reduce HIV Transmission related to Injecting Drug Use in Prison," *Lancet Infectious Diseases* 9, no. 1 (2009): 57–66.

80. Ernest Drucker, *A Plague of Prisons. The Epidemiology of Mass Incarceration in America* (New York: The New Press, 2011).

81. T. K. Logan, William Hoyt, Kathryn McCollister, Michael French, Carl Leukefeld, and Lisa Minton, "Economic Evaluation of Drug Courts: Methodology, Results, and Policy Implications," *Evaluation and Program Planning* 27, no. 4 (2004): 381–96.

82. Marilyn Daley, Craig Love, Donal Shepherd, Cheryl Petersen, Karen White, and Wayne Hall. "Cost-Effectiveness of Connecticut's in-Prison Substance Abuse Treatment," *Journal of Offender Rehabilitation* 39, no. 3 (2004): 69–92.

83. Peter C. Rydell and Susan S. Everingham, "Controlling Cocaine: Supply Versus Demand Programs" (Santa Monica, CA: RAND Monograph Report, RAND Corporation, 1994). www.rand.org/pubs/monograph_reports/MR331.

84. HRI (Harm Reduction International), *Judicial Corporal Punishment for Drug and Alcohol Offences in Selected Countries* (London: HRI, 2012).

85. Patrick Gallahue, "The Death Penalty for Drug Offences Global Overview 2011: Shared Responsibility and Shared Consequences" (London: Harm Reduction International, 2011).

86. Ketua Mahkamah Agung Republik Indonesia (Head of the Supreme Court of the Republic of Indonesia). *Surat Edaran Nomor: 07 Tahun 2009. Tentang Menempatkan Pemakai Narkoba Ke Dalam Panti Terapi Dan Rehabilitasi (Circular Number: 07 Year 2009. About Placing Drug Users into Therapy and Rehabilitation Centres)*. Jakarta, Indonesia, 2009.

87. Elizabeth Cohen and Joseph Amon, "Health and Human Rights Concerns of Drug Users in Detention in Guangxi Providence, China," *PLoS Med* 5, no. 12 (2008): e234. DOI: 10.1371/journal.pmed.0050234.

88. HRW (Human Rights Watch). *Skin on the Cable: The Illegal Arrest, Arbitrary Detention and Torture of People Who Use Drugs in Cambodia* (New York: Human Rights Watch, 2010).

89. WHO-WPRO (World Health Organization-Western Pacific Regional Office), *Assessment of Compulsory Treatment of People who use Drugs in Cambodia, China, Malaysia and Viet Nam: An Application of Selected Human Rights Principles* (Manila: WHO-WPRO, 2009). Accessed December 8, 2011.www.wpro.who.int/publications /PUB_9789290614173.htm.

90. WHO-WPRO (World Health Organization-Western Pacific Regional Office), *Assessment of Compulsory Treatment of People who use Drugs in Cambodia, China, Malaysia and Viet Nam.*

91. Gary Reid, Adeeba Kamarulzaman, and Sangeeta Sran, "Malaysia and Harm Reduction: the Challenges and Responses," *International Journal of Drug Policy* 18, no. 2 (2007): 136–40.

92. HRW, *Skin on the Cable.*

93. Theodore Hammett, Wu Zunyou, Tran Duc, David Stephens, Sheena Sullivan, Wei Liu, Yi Chen, Doan Ngu, and Don Des Jarlais, "'Social Evils' and Harm Reduction: The Evolving Policy Environment for Human Immunodeficiency Virus Prevention among Injecting Drug Users in China and Vietnam," *Addiction* 103 (2007): 137–45.

94. IHRDP (International Harm Reduction Development Program), *Human Rights Abuses in the Name of Drug Treatment: Reports from the Field* (New York: Open Society Institute, 2009).

95. Roxanne Saucier, Nancy Berlinger, Nicholas Thomson, Michael Gusmano, and Daniel Wolfe, "The Limits of Equivalence: Ethical Dilemmas in Providing Care in Drug Detention Centers," *International Journal of Prisoner Health* 6, no. 2 (2010): 37–43.

96. WHO-WPRO, *Assessment of Compulsory Treatment of People Who Use Drugs.*

97. Gayle Martin, David Stephens, David Burrows, Uyen N. Vu, Lam T. Nguyen, Sac X. Tran, and Duc T. Tran, "Does Drug Rehabilitation in Closed Setting Work in Vietnam?" Presentation, International Harm Reduction Conference, Accessed January 13, 2012.www.unodc.org/documents/eastasiaandpacific/presentation/2009/hiv-aids/ihra-conference/Does_drug_rehabilitation_in_closed_settings_work_in_Viet_nam_Duc.pdf.

98. Jane Parry, "Vietnam is Urged to Close Drug Detention Centers after Widespread Abuse is Discovered," *BMJ* 8, no. 343 (2011): DOI: 10.1136/bmj.d5739.

99. WHO-WPRO, *Assessment of Compulsory Treatment of People Who Use Drugs.*

100. Hammett et al., *"Social Evils" and Harm Reduction*, 137–45.

101. Cohen, and Amon, *Health and Human Rights Concerns*, e234.

102. Cohen, and Amon, *Health and Human Rights Concerns*, e234.

103. Niklas Swanstrom and Yin He, *China's War on Narcotics: Two Perspectives* (Washington, DC: Central Asia—Caucasus Institute and Silk Road Studies Program, 2006).

104. Cohen, and Amon, *Health and Human Rights Concerns*, e234.

105. Cohen, and Amon, *Health and Human Rights Concerns*, e234.

106. Cohen, and Amon, *Health and Human Rights Concerns*, e234.

107. Ingo Michels, Min Zhao, and Lin Lu, "Drug Abuse and its Treatment in China," *Journal of Addiction and Research Practice* 53, no. 4 (2007): 228–37.

108. Larney and Dolan, *A Literature Review*, 107–12.

109. WHO-WPRO, *Assessment of Compulsory Treatment of People Who Use Drugs.*

110. Joanne Csete and Siddharth Dube, "An Inappropriate Tool: Criminal Law and HIV in Asia," *AIDS* 24, no. 3 (2010): S80–S85.

111. MOFA (Ministry of Foreign Affairs, Kingdom of Thailand). (undated) Questionnaires for the Secretariat of the Working Group on Arbitrary Detention on the issue of Detention of Drug Users. Accessed October 19, 2012. www.mfa.go.th/humanrights/implementation-of-un-resolutions/66-answers-to-questionnaire-for-the-secretariat-of-the-working-group-on-arbitrary-detention-on-the-issue-of-detention-of-drug-users-.

112. Csete and Dube, *An Inappropriate Tool*, S80–S85.

113. Chris Beyrer, Jaroon Jittiwutikarn, Waranya Teokul, Myat Htoo Razak, Vinai Suriyanon, Namptip Srirak, Tasani Vongchuk, Sodsai Tovanabutra, Teera Sripaipan, and David Celentano, "Drug Use, Increasing Incarceration Rates, and Prison-Associated HIV Risks in Thailand," *AIDS and Behaviour* 7, no. 2 (2003): 155–61.
114. Larney and Dolan, *A Literature Review*, 107–12.
115. Gallahue, *The Death Penalty for Drug Offences*.
116. Gallahue, *The Death Penalty for Drug Offences*.
117. AAP, "Australian Woman faces Death in Malaysia," *Sydney Morning Herald*, July 31, 2012. Accessed October 19, 2012.http://m.smh.com.au/national/australian-woman-faces-death-in-malaysia-20120730-23a87.html.
118. Ari Rosmarinand Niamh Eastwood.,"Quiet Revolution: Drug Decriminalisation Policies in Practice across the Globe," Release, London, 2012. Accessed October 19, 2012. www.release.org.uk/downloads/publications/release-quiet-revolution-drug-decriminalisation-policies.pdf.
119. UNDP (United Nations Development Programme), *Global Commission on HIV and the Law: Risks, Rights and Health* (New York: UNDP, 2012).
120. IHRDP, *Human rights Abuses*.
121. Larney and Dolan, *A Literature Review*, 107–12.

BIBLIOGRAPHY

AAP. "Australian Woman faces Death in Malaysia." *Sydney Morning Herald*, July 31, 2012. Accessed October 19, 2012. http://m.smh.com.au/national/australian-woman-faces-death-in-malaysia-20120730-23a87.html.

Amato, Laura, Marina Davoli, Silvia Minozzi, Robert Ali, and Marica Ferri. "Methadone at Tapered Doses for the Management of Opioid Withdrawal." *Cochrane Database Systematic Reviews* 3, no. CD003409 (2005). Accessed September 13, 2012. DOI: 10.1002/14651858.CD003409.pub3.

Backmund, Markus, Kirsten Meyer, Martin Wächtler, and Dieter Eichenlaub. "Hepatitis C Virus Infection in Injection Drug Users in Bavaria: Risk Factors for Seropositivity." *European Journal of Epidemiology* 18 (2003): 563–68.

Backmund, Markus, Jens Reimer, Kirsten Meyer, Tilman Gerlach, and Reinhart Zachoval. "Hepatitis C Virus Infection and Injection Drug Users: Prevention, Risk Factors, and Treatment." *Clinical Infectious Diseases* 40, no. 5 (2005): S330–S335.

Ball, Andrew, Don des Jarlais, Martin Donohoe, Samual Friedman, David Goldberg, Gillian Hunter, Gerry Stimson, and Alex Wodak. "Multi-City Study on Drug Injecting and Risk of HIV Infection." Geneva: World Health Organisation, 1994.

Baqi, Shehla, Naheed Nabi, Syed Hasan, Amir Khan, Omrana Pasha, Naila Kayani, Rehan Haque, Inaam-ul Haq, Mohammad Khurshid, Susan Fisher-Hoch, Stephen Luby, and Joseph McCormick. "HIV Antibody Seroprevalence and Associated Risk Factors in Sex Workers, Drug Users and Prisoners in Sindh, Pakistan." *Journal of Acquired Immune Deficiency Syndromes & Human Retrovirology* 18, no. 1 (1998): 73–79.

Bargagli, Anna, Marina Davoli, Silvia Minozzi, Simona Vecchi, and Carlo Perucci. "A Systematic Review of Observational Studies on Treatment of Opioid Dependence." Background Document Prepared for 3rd meeting of Technical Development Group (TDG) for the WHO Guidelines for Psychosocially Assisted Pharmacotherapy of Opioid Dependence, WHO, Geneva, Switzerland, September 17–21, 2007.

Bellin, Eran, Jennifer Wesson, Vincent Tomasino, James Nolan, Alvin Glick, and Sonia Oquendo. "High Dose Methadone reduces Criminal Recidivism in Opiate Addicts." *Addiction Research and Theory* 7 (1999): 19–29.

Bergenstrom, Anne, Vu Minh Quan, Le Van Nam, Kristen McClausland, Nguyen Phuong Thuoc, David Celentano, and Vivian Go. "Cross-Sectional Study on Prevalence of Non-Fatal Drug Overdose and Associated Risk Characteristics among Out-of-Treatment Injecting Drug Users in North Vietnam." *Substance Use & Misuse* 43, no. 1 (2008): 73–84.

Beyrer, Chris, Jaroon Jittiwutikarn, Waranya Teokul, Myat Htoo Razak, Vinai Suriyanon, Namptip Srirak, Tasani Vongchuk, Sodsai Tovanabutra, Teera Sripaipan, and David Celentano, "Drug Use, Increasing Incarceration Rates, and Prison-Associated HIV risks in Thailand." *AIDS and Behaviour* 7, no. 2 (2003): 155–61.

Boutwell, Amy, Ank Nijhawan, Nichol Zaller, and Josiah Rich. "Arrested on Heroin: a National Opportunity." *Journal of Opioid Management* 3 (2007): 328–32.

Boys, Annabel, Michael Farrell, Glyn Bebbington, Traolach Brugha, Jeremy Coid, Paul Jenkins, Nicola Lewis, John Marsden, Rachel Meltzer, Nicola Singleton, and Colin Taylor. "Drug Use and Initiation in Prison: Results from a National Prison Survey in England and Wales." *Addiction* 97, no. 12 (2002): 1551–60.

Brewer, T. Fordham, David Vlahov, Ellen Taylor, Drusilla Hall, Alvaro Munoz, and Frank Polk. "Transmission of HIV-1 within a Statewide Prison System." *AIDS* 2, no. 5 (1988): 363–67.

CDC. "Acquired Immunodeficiency Syndrome in Correctional Facilities: A Report of the National Institute of Justice and the American Correctional Association." *MMWR. Morbidity and Mortality Weekly Report 35*, no. 12 (1986): 195–99.

Chandler, Redonna, Bennet Fletcher, and Nora Volkow. "Treating Drug Abuse and Addiction in the Criminal Justice System: improving Public Health and Safety." *The Journal of the American Medical Association* 301, no. 2 (2009): 183–90.

Choopanya, Kachit, Suphak Vanichseni, Don Des Jarlais, Kanokporn Plangsringarm, Wandee Sonchai, Manuel Carballo, Patricia Friedman, and Samuel Friedman. "Risk Factors and HIV Seropositivity among Injecting Drug Users in Bangkok." *AIDS* 5, no. 12 (1991): 1509–13.

Choopanya, Kachit, Don Des Jarlais, Suphak Vanichseni, Dwip Kitayaporn, Phillip Mock, Suwanee Raktham, Krit Hireanras, William Heyward, Sathit Sujarita, and Timothy Mastro. "Incarceration and Risk for HIV Infection among Injecting Drug Users in Bangkok." *Journal of Acquired Immune Deficiency Syndromes & Human Retrovirology* 29, no. 1 (2002): 86–94.

Cohen, Elizabeth and Joseph Amon. "Health and Human Rights Concerns of Drug Users in Detention in Guangxi Providence, China." *PLoS Med* 5, no. 12 (2008): e234. DOI:10.1371/journal.pmed.0050234.

Csete, Joanne and Siddharth Dube. "An Inappropriate Tool: Criminal Law and HIV in Asia." *AIDS* 24, no. 3 (2010): S80–S85.

Daley, Marilyn, Craig Love, Donal Shepherd, Cheryl Petersen, Karen White, and Wayne Hall. "Cost-Effectiveness of Connecticut's in-Prison Substance Abuse Treatment." *Journal of Offender Rehabilitation* 39, no. 3 (2004): 69–92.

Dolan, Kate, Wayne Hall, and Alex Wodak "Methadone Maintenance Reduces Injecting in Prison." *British Medical Journal* 312 (1996): 1162.

Dolan, Kate and Alex Wodak. "HIV Transmission in a Prison System in an Australian State." *The Medical Journal of Australia* 171, no. 1 (1999): 14–17.

Dolan, Kate, James Shearer, Margaret MacDonald, Richard Mattick, Wayne Hall, and Alex Wodak. "A Randomized Controlled Trial of Methadone Maintenance Treatment vs. Wait List Control in an Australian Prison." *Drug and Alcohol Dependence* 72, no. 1 (2003): 59–65.

Dolan, Kate, David Rouen, and Jo Kimber. "An Overview of the Use of Urine, Hair, Sweat and Saliva to detect Drug Use." *Drug and Alcohol Review* 23, no. 2 (2004): 213–17.

Dolan, Kate, James Shearer, Bethany White, Jialun Zhou, and Alex Wodak. "Four-year Follow-up of Imprisoned Male Heroin Users and Methadone Treatment: Mortality, Re-Incarceration and Hepatitis C Infection." *Addiction* 100, no. 6 (2005): 820–28.

Dolan, Kate, Ben Kite, Emma Black, Carmen Aceijas, and Gerry Stimson. "HIV in Prison in Low-income and Middle-income Countries." *Lancet Infectious Diseases* 7, no. 1 (2007): 32–41.

Dolan, Kate, Heather Worth, Ousman Badjie, and J'Belle Foster. "Review of Compulsory and Voluntary Treatment for Drug Users in Asia." Sydney: University of New South Wales (UNSW), 2012.

Drucker, Ernest. *A Plague of Prisons. The Epidemiology of Mass Incarceration in America.* New York: The New Press, 2011.

Farnia, Marziyeh, Bahman Ebrahimi, Ali Shams, and Saman Zamani. "Scaling up Methadone Maintenance Treatment for Opioid-Dependent Prisoners in Iran." *International Journal of Drug Policy* 21, no. 5 (2010): 422–24.

Farrell, Michael and John Marsden. "Acute Risk of Drug-related Death among Newly Released Prisoners in England and Wales." *Addiction* 103, no. 2 (2008): 251–55.

Fazel, Seena, Parveen Bains, and Helen Doll. "Substance Abuse and Dependence in Prisoners: A Systematic Review." *Addiction* 101 (2006): 181–91.

Gallahue, Patrick. "The Death Penalty for Drug Offences Global Overview 2011: Shared Responsibility and Shared Consequences." London: Harm Reduction International, 2011.

Gordon, Michael, Timothy Kinlock, Robert Schwartz, and Kevin O'Grady. "A Randomized Clinical Trial of Methadone Maintenance for Prisoners: Findings at 6 Months Post-Release." *Addiction* 103 (2008): 1333–42.

Gowing, Linda, Michael Farrell, Reinhart Bornemann, Lynn Sullivan, and Robert Ali. "Substitution Treatment of Injecting Opioid Users for Prevention of HIV Infection." *Cochrane Database of Systematic Reviews* 2, no. CD004145 (2008): DOI:10.1002/146-51858.CD004145.pub3.

Hammett, Theodore, Wu Zunyou, Tran Duc, David Stephens, Sheena Sullivan, Wei Liu., Yi Chen, Doan Ngu, and Don Des Jarlais. "'Social Evils' and Harm Reduction: The Evolving Policy Environment for Human Immunodeficiency Virus Prevention among Injecting Drug Users in China and Vietnam." *Addiction* 103 (2007): 137–45.

Harada, Takayuki and Hiroyuki Shinkai. "New Initiatives for Drug Abuse Treatment in Japanese Prisons." *International Journal of Comparative and Applied Criminal Justice* 34, no. 2 (2010): 391–404.

Hedrich, Dagmar, Paula Alves, Michael Farrell, Heino Stöver, Lars Møller, and Soraya Maye. "The Effectiveness of Opioid Maintenance Treatment in Prison Settings: a Systematic Review." *Addiction* 107, no. 3 (2012): 501–17.

Horsburgh, Robert, Joseph Jarvis, Trudy McArthur, Terri Ignacio, and Patricia Stock. "Seroconversion to HIV in Prison Inmates." *American Journal of Public Health* 80, no. 2 (1990): 209–10.

HRI (Harm Reduction International). *Global State of Harm Reduction 2012: Towards an Integrated Response.* London: HRI, 2012.

———. *Judicial Corporal Punishment for Drug and Alcohol Offences in Selected Countries.* London: HRI, 2012.

HRW (Human Rights Watch). *Skin on the Cable: The Illegal Arrest, Arbitrary Detention and Torture of People Who Use Drugs in Cambodia.* New York: Human Rights Watch, 2010.

IHRDP (International Harm Reduction Development Program). *Human Rights Abuses in the Name of Drug Treatment: Reports from the Field.* New York: Open Society Institute, 2009.

International Centre for Prison Studies. "World Prison Briefs 2011." Accessed August 14, 2012. www.prisonstudies.org/info/worldbrief/.

Jürgens, Ralf, Andrew Ball, and Annette Verster. "Interventions to Reduce HIV Transmission Related to Injecting Drug Use in Prison." *Lancet Infectious Diseases* 9, no. 1 (2009): 57–66.

Ketua Mahkamah Agung Republik Indonesia (Head of the Supreme Court of the Republic of Indonesia). *Surat Edaran Nomor: 07 Tahun 2009. Tentang Menempatkan Pemakai Narkoba Ke Dalam Panti Terapi Dan Rehabilitasi (Circular Number: 07 Year 2009. About Placing Drug Users into Therapy and Rehabilitation Centres).* Jakarta, Indonesia, 2009.

Kinlock, Timothy, Michael Gordon, Robert Schwartz, and Kevin O'Grady. "A Study of Methadone Maintenance for Male Prisoners: 3-Month Post Release Outcomes." *Criminal Justice Behavior* 35 (2008): 34–47.

Larney, Sarah and Kate Dolan. "A Literature Review of International Implementation of Opioid Substitution Treatment in Prisons: Equivalence of Care?" *European Addiction Research* 15 (2009): 107–12.

Larney, Sarah, Barbara Toson, Lucy Burns, and Kate Dolan. "Effect of Prison-based Opioid Substitution Treatment and Post-release Retention in Treatment on Risk of Re-incarceration." *Addiction* 107, no. 2 (2012): 372–80.

Logan, T. K., William Hoyt, Kathryn McCollister, Michael French, Carl Leukefeld, and Lisa Minton. "Economic Evaluation of Drug Courts: Methodology, Results, and Policy Implications." *Evaluation and Program Planning* 27, no. 4 (2004): 381–96.

March, Joan, Eugenia Oviedo-Joekes, and Manuel Romero. "Drugs and Social Exclusion in Ten European Cities." *European Addiction Research* 12, no. 1 (2006): 33–41.

Martin, Gayle, David Stephens, David Burrows, Uyen N. Vu, Lam T. Nguyen, Sac X. Tran, and Duc T. Tran. "Does Drug Rehabilitation in Closed Setting Work in Vietnam?" Presentation, International Harm Reduction Conference, 2010. Accessed January 13, 2012. www.unodc.org/documents/eastasiaandpacific/presentation/2009/hiv-aids/ihra-conference/Does_drug_rehabilitation_in_closed_settings_work_in_Viet_nam_Duc.pdf.

Mathers, Bradley, Louisa Degenhardt, Benjamin Phillips, Lucas Weissing, Matthew Hickman, Steffanie Strathdee, Alex Wodak, Samiran Panda, Mark Tyndall, Abdalla Toufik, and Richard Mattick. "Global Epidemiology of Injecting Drug Use and HIV among People who Inject Drugs: a Systematic Review." *The Lancet* 372, no. 9651 (2008): 1733–45.

Mattick, Richard, Courtney Breen, Jo Kimber, and Marina Davoli. "Methadone Maintenance Therapy versus no Opioid Replacement Therapy for Opioid Dependence." *Cochrane Database of Systematic Reviews* 3, no. CD002209 (2009): DOI: 10.1002/1465-1858.CD002209.pub2.

Michels, Ingo, Min Zhao, and Lin Lu. "Drug Abuse and its Treatment in China." *Journal of Addiction and Research Practice* 53, no. 4 (2007): 228–37.

Milloy, M-J., Nadia Fairbairn, Kanna Hayashi, Paisan Suwannawong, Karyn Kaplan, Evan Wood, and Thomas Kerr. "Research Overdose Experiences among Injection Drug Users in Bangkok, Thailand." *Harm Reduction Journal* 7, no. 1 (2010): DOI: 10.1186/1477-7517-7-9.

MOFA (Ministry of Foreign Affairs, Kingdom of Thailand). "Questionnaires for the Secretariat of the Working Group on Arbitrary Detention on the issue of Detention of Drug Users." Accessed October 19, 2012. www.mfa.go.th/humanrights/implementation-of-un-resolutions/66-answers-to-questionnaire-for-the-secretariat-of-the-working-group-on-arbitrary-detention-on-the-issue-of-detention-of-drug-users-.

Mutter, Randal, Richard Grimes, and Darwin Labarthe. "Evidence of Intraprison Spread of HIV Infection." *Archives of Internal Medicine* 154, no. 7 (1994): 793–95.

Nai Zindagi. "Rapid Situation Assessments of HIV Prevalence and Risk Factors among People Injecting Drugs in Four Cities of the Punjab." Islamabad, 2009. Accessed January 10, 2013.www.naizindagi.com/reports/rsabsmall.pdf.

Obert, Jeanne, Michael McCann, Patricia Marinelli-Casey, Ahndrea Weiner, Sam Minsky, Paul Brethen, and Richard Rawson. "The Matrix Model of Outpatient Stimulant Abuse Treatment: History and Description." *Journal of Psychoactive Drugs* 32, no. 2 (2000): 157–64.

Parry, Jane. "Vietnam is Urged to Close Drug Detention Centers after Widespread Abuse is Discovered." *BMJ* 8, no. 343 (2011): DOI: 10.1136/bmj.d5739.

Quan, Vu, Apinun Aramrattana, Tasanai Vongchak, Carl Latkin, Deborah Donnell, Ting-Yuang Liu, Kanokporn Wiboonnatakul, and David Celentano. "Mortality among Injection Drug Users in Northern Thailand: A Prospective Cohort Study." *Journal of Addiction Medicine* 4, no. 4 (2010): 217–22. DOI: 10.1097/ADM.0b013e3181c78bf4.

Reid, Gary, Adeeba Kamarulzaman, and Sangeeta Sran. "Malaysia and Harm Reduction: the Challenges and Responses." *International Journal of Drug Policy* 18, no. 2 (2007): 136–40.

Rosmarin, Ari and Niamh Eastwood. "Quiet Revolution: Drug Decriminalisation Policies in Practice across the Globe." Release, London, 2012. Accessed October 19, 2012. www.release.org.uk/downloads/publications/release-quiet-revolution-drug-decriminalisation-policies.pdf.

Rutter, Scott, Kate Dolan, and Alex Wodak. "Sex, Drugs and Viruses in Sin City Sydney. Report on Australian Study of HIV and Injecting Drug Use." National Drug and Alcohol Research Center Technical Report No. 37, Sydney: University of New South Wales (UNSW), 1996.

Rydell, C. Peter and Susan S. Everingham. "Controlling Cocaine: Supply versus Demand Programs." RAND Monograph Report, RAND Corporation, Santa Monica, California, 1994. www.rand.org/pubs/monograph_reports/MR331.

Saucier, Roxanne, Nancy Berlinger, Nicholas Thomson, Michael Gusmano, and Daniel Wolfe. "The Limits of Equivalence: Ethical Dilemmas in Providing Care in Drug Detention Centers." *International Journal of Prisoner Health* 6, no. 2 (2010): 37–43.

Singleton, Nicola, Michael Farrell, and Howard Meltzer. "Substance Misuse among Prisoners in England and Wales." *International Review of Psychiatry* 15 (2003): 150–52.

Singleton, Nicola, Elizabeth Pendry, Tracy Simpson, Eileen Goddard, Michael Farrell, John Marsden, and Colin Taylor. "The Impact of Mandatory Drug Testing in Prisons." London: Home Office Online Report 03/05, Home Office, 2005.

Solomon, Sunil, David Celentano, Aylur Srikrishnan, Conjeevaram Vasudevan, Santhanam Anand, Muniratnam Kumar, Suniti Solomon, Gregory Lucas, and Shruti Mehta. "Mortality among Injection Drug Users in Chennai, India (2005–2008)." *AIDS* 23 (2009): 997–1004.

Stark, Klaus, Ute Herrmann, Stephan Ehrhardt, and Ulrich Bienzle. "A Syringe Exchange Programme in Prison as Prevention Strategy against HIV Infection and Hepatitis B and C in Berlin, Germany." *Epidemiology and Infection* 134, no. 4 (2006): 814–19.

Stoove, Mark, Paul Dietze, Campbell Aitken, and Damien Jolley. "Mortality among Injecting Drug Users in Melbourne: A 16-year Follow-up of the Victorian Injecting Cohort Study (VICS)." *Drug and Alcohol Dependence* 96 (2008): 281–85.

Stöver, Heino, ed. *Overview Study. Assistance to Drug Users in European Prisons.* Lisbon: EMCDDA, 2001.

Swanstrom, Niklas and Yin He. *China's War on Narcotics: Two Perspectives.* Washington, DC: Central Asia–Caucasus Institute and Silk Road Studies Program, 2006.

Taylor, Avril, David Goldberg, John Emslie, Laurence Gruer, Sheila Cameron, James Black, Barbara Davis, James McGregor, Edward Follet, Janina Harvey, John Basson, and James McGavigan. "Outbreak of HIV Infection in a Scottish Prison." *BMJ* 310, no. 289 (6975) (1995): 289.

Thaisri, Hansa,John Lerwitworapong, Suthon Vongsheree, Pathom Sawanpanyalert, Chanchai Chadbanchachai, Archawin Rojanawiwat, Wichuda Kongpromsook, Wiroj Paungtubtim, Pongnuwat Sri-ngam and Rachaneekorn Jaisue "HIV Infection and Risk Factors among Bangkok Prisoners, Thailand: A Prospective Cohort Study." *BMC Infectious Diseases* 3, no. 25 (2003): DOI: 10.1186/1471-2334-3-25.

Tilson, Hugh, Apinun Aramrattana, Samuel Bozzette, David Celentano, Mathea Falco, Theodore Hammett, Andrei Kozlov, Shenghan Lai, Ajay Mahal, Richard Schottenfeld, and S. Solomon. (Committee on the Prevention of HIV Infection among Injecting Drug Users in High-Risk Countries). "Preventing HIV Infection among Injecting Drug Users in High-Risk Countries. An Assessment of the Evidence." Washington, DC: Global Board of Health, Institute of Medicine of the National Academies, 2006.

UNAIDS (Joint United Nations Committee on HIV/AIDS). *Global Report: UNAIDS Report on the Global AIDS Epidemic.* Geneva: UNAIDS, 2010.

UNDP (United Nations Development Programme). *Global Commission on HIV and the Law: Risks, Rights and Health.* New York: UNDP, 2012.

UNODC (United Nations Office of Drugs and Crime). *HIV Prevention, Treatment and Care in Prisons and other Closed Settings: a Comprehensive Package of Interventions.* Vienna: UNODC, 2012.

Vlahov, David, Cunlin Wang, Danielle Ompad, Crystal M. Fuller, Wendy Caceres, Lawrence Ouellet, Peter Kerndt, Don Des Jarlais, and Richard Garfein. "Mortality Risk among Recent-Onset Injection Drug Users in Five U.S. cities." *Substance Use and Misuse* 43 (2008): 413–28.

WHO (World Health Organization). *Model List of Essential Medicines, 2011.* Geneva: WHO, 2011. Accessed August 2012. http://whqlibdoc.who.int/hq/2011/a95053_eng.pdf.

WHO-WPRO (World Health Organization-Western Pacific Regional Office). *Assessment of Compulsory Treatment of People who use Drugs in Cambodia, China, Malaysia and Viet Nam: An Application of Selected Human Rights Principles.* Manila: WHO-WPRO, 2009. Accessed December 8, 2011. www.wpro.who.int/publications /PUB_9789290614173.htm.

World Bank. *Afghanistan HIV/AIDS Prevention Project:* June 2008.

Chapter Five

Law Enforcement and Drug Policy in Southeast Asia

Nick Crofts, Geoff Monaghan, Steve James, Nicole Turner, and Mohd Zaman Khan

In many countries in Southeast Asia (SEA) illicit drug use is commonly seen *publicly* by many state officials and politicians as a "social" or "health" issue rather than a matter for criminal justice agencies, and these sentiments are increasingly reflected in SEA law. Indeed, many countries in the region have passed laws that define drug use as an "illness" or "disease" rather than a crime and emphasize the need for treatment and rehabilitation programs. For instance, Cambodian Prime Minister Hun Sen stated in 2003 that, "In accordance with the drug control law of Cambodia, drug addicted people must have received consultation, treatment and rehabilitation rather than being taken to court. Drug addicted people badly need health support and support from society rather than leaving them as outlawed people of society."[1]

However, belying these stances, state responses to the phenomenon in the SEA region have been historically and still are largely dominated by penal considerations: arrest, fines, and varying periods of detention, criminal or administrative (whether in jail or under the guise of "compulsory rehabilitation"). Compared with health imperatives, the drug control and supply reduction agenda remains much more important politically, for many reasons which cannot be examined here; suffice to say, with Lee, "The 'fear of crime' is a key constituent of governance. . . ."[2] National drug control agencies, often purportedly multisectoral but in reality more often arms of state security and police, and often chaired by a deputy prime minister or equivalent, are far more influential than are the health or social sectors of government.[3] Despite a lack of criminal sanctions, many of the countries in this region use civil or administrative law to involuntarily incarcerate drug users in compulsory drug detention centers.[4] In reality, in keeping with other regions across the globe, measures to counter drug trafficking,[5] possession, and use in SEA have been generally treated as a law enforcement or public security responsibility. Illicit drug use is rarely socially constructed as primarily a social or health issue and until recently has not been a province in which the health or social welfare sectors have had *real* legitimacy or involvement.

Drug control laws are often seen as the major barriers to effective harm reduction interventions,[6] and studies in Vietnam as elsewhere see police behavior toward IDUs as the major factor which impair confidence in accessing harm reduction services.[7]

"Crackdowns" on users and relatively small-scale traffickers are commonplace—perhaps more so than in Western countries because they are more likely to be linked to ministerial whims on the back of quotas, rather than responses to justifiable community concerns over acquisitive crime rates or public order considerations. At the same time as Hun Sen was making the humane pronouncement quoted above, increasing availability and use of drugs in Cambodia was leading to a proliferation and use of compulsory drug treatment centers, documented centers of inhuman practice.[8]

Many countries in SEA have prosecuted their local version of the "War on Drugs," such as the "Strike-Hard" campaigns in China (*Yanda*) and the "war on drugs" in Thailand (*Songkram Yaseptid*).[9] Vietnam's approach has since World War II concentrated on deterrence through punishment and supply-side measures, undergoing a variety of metamorphoses but always with the same goal of eradication of drugs[10] (also see Baldwin's chapter in this book). There are many law enforcement agencies involved, from street-level police to higher levels, special narcotics police, and the army and other public security.[11] At the regional level, policy remains unchanged: in June 2012, for instance, the ASEAN Ambassadors Group in Laos announced that it was aiming to make the ASEAN region a drug-free zone by 2015,[12] despite all the evidence of mounting quantities and diversity of illicit drugs being produced and consumed in the region.

While tackling drug production and trafficking has been the province solely of law enforcement in its police and public security guises in all SEA countries, responses to the use of illicit drugs are rather more difficult to classify and compartmentalize, because "use" is usually classified as an "administrative" or "regulatory" violation rather than a criminal offense and is therefore the province of a range of other authorities (as well as of police). Essentially, however, these are also law enforcement agencies, in different cloaks. For example, in Vietnam the Ministry of Labour, Invalids and Social Affairs (MoLISA) has overall responsibility for enforcing primary and delegated legislation relating to the running of the so-called drug treatment detention centers for drug users (not necessarily drug dependents) (see Baldwin et al. in this book).

THE ROLE OF POLICE

While there has been research into the adverse impact of policing practices and behaviors on risk and risk environments in a number of countries in SEA, the role of police in enforcing drug laws in most SEA countries has been little studied. In any examination of police activities and impact on illicit drug sale and use, it is apparent that they can be viewed from several broad perspectives.

First, and ingenuously, police practices can be viewed as activities designed to enforce laws through coercive powers—identifying those breaking the laws and applying the relevant sanctions. This process is modified by the use of discretion in the application of these powers—on the basis of class (treating the poor offender more harshly than the middle-class), prejudice (sharing social prejudices against certain groups, especially stereotypical "junkies"), income source (treating differently those from whom income can be derived), and so forth. The application of discretion by police in SEA has not been systematically studied, especially in relation to drug-use issues. One rare in-depth study of influences on police behavior at street level in Hanoi found that "Despite the view that drug control was their primary responsibility, ward police reported exercising considerable discretion for a variety of reasons. These included maintaining good relationships with the community through demonstrating a level of latitude."[13] The same study found the exercise of discretion around decisions to send apprehended drug users to compulsory rehabilitation or to the methadone program, on the basis of whether they were "good" or "bad" (see below).

Second, there is the perspective of police activities within a cultural milieu, one formed by the passing on of cultural mores from generation to generation of police, responding to a range of influences including societal values (as expressed in the values they bring with them when they join the police, and the social and political pressures on police, including local community pressures), self-interest (especially including career advancement and financial considerations), and institutionalization of accepted practice.

Third, there is the perspective of the police and the drug users and traffickers being engaged in an intertwined market economy, interdependent. Police factor income from traffickers and users into their planning; to the traffickers, police and the need to bribe them are part of the business planning process; to the user, police are one part of a largely hostile environment with which they must cope.[14]

Fourth, there is ample anecdotal evidence which supports the view that many police officers drug target users simply on the basis that they are seen to commit high numbers of crimes, primarily acquisitive (e.g., theft, burglary, fraud) but also violent crime (street robberies, armed robberies, and assaults committed in order to evade being detained by members of the public when caught stealing, etc.). Given the available research on the numbers of crimes committed by users of opiates, crack cocaine, and methamphetamine, from the police perspective there is an immediate perceived rationale for arresting users in their thousands. [15, 16, 17, 18, 19, 20]

And last there is the use of drug crime as a coverall for other motives, including political corruption, as exemplified by Thailand's notorious War on Drugs of 2003 and the incarceration of non-drug users for drug crimes in Cambodia. [21]

Each particular situation involves different mixes of these perspectives, with varying emphasis; though there are certainly examples where the entire nexus can be satisfactorily understood through the lens of corruption or business.

ADVERSE IMPACT

Since the advent of HIV infection associated with injecting drug use, there has been an increasing number of studies of the impact of policing on heightened HIV risk. The counterproductive impacts of drug law enforcement have been much studied especially the harmful public health outcomes for PWID. [22, 23, 24, 25] Significant barriers to the success of HIV prevention programs reside in the use of drug registries by the police [26, 27] and the fear of negative repercussions from police among PWID accessing HIV prevention programs. Such barriers also exist in relation to access of PWID to drug treatment programs, and "the use of police registries and harassment of patients, detention of PWIDs, and harassment of physicians who prescribe opioids" have been documented in China, Vietnam and Malaysia. [28] A disparity between policy and practice often exists in the area of HIV treatment, as in China's disproportionately low access to ART among PWIDs despite a national policy of free universal access. [29]

The tension and conflict between public health strategies and law enforcement strategies toward PWIDs has been identified as a reality in many countries and at many levels. [30, 31] It has been recognized repeatedly that resolving this conflict is critical to addressing the HIV epidemic and that effective approaches to minimize HIV risk among and from PWID must occur within the context of supportive law enforcement policy and practice. [32]

THE PERCEIVED CONFLICT IN THE DUAL ROLES OF POLICE

While the impact of police behaviors on HIV risk environments is much studied, little is known about how harm reduction programs impact law enforcement policy and practice in SEA. Are the programs and approaches (including advocacy) which are aimed at fostering an environment supportive of harm reduction for all people who used drugs, effective at influencing law enforcement policy and practice?[33] Where this has been studied, the overwhelming finding is of a perceived and often severe conflict between unresolved and competing imperatives of the dual roles police are asked to fulfill—drug crime policing and support for harm reduction.

The Cambodian government has explicitly recognized that drug users are a key target group in prevention of HIV; the responsibility for harm reduction, however, is largely with the National Authority for Combating Drugs (NACD), which is, in Cambodia, as are similar bodies in neighboring countries, primarily responsible for dealing with drug production, trafficking, and use. The NACD has great difficulty simultaneously promoting harm reduction and controlling drugs using law enforcement approaches; to most members of the NACD the two approaches are incompatible, politically, socially, and culturally. This situation has been exacerbated by the institution of a comprehensive crackdown policy directed against all disruptions of social order, including drug users—the Commune and Village Safety Policy—has created or crystallized these competing policy objectives. That this policy has had deleterious effects on HIV prevention efforts among HIV risk groups, including harm reduction programs, is a fact not lost on the government of Cambodia. There has been overt acknowledgment the policy has made it much more difficult to access people who use drugs and has made "service provision for their benefit very difficult due to the misunderstanding of the law enforcement officers, especially at the commune level."[34, 35]

In Vietnam, many police at many levels have what they perceive to be a dual responsibility: preventing and controlling drug use on the one hand and supporting harm reduction on the other. They have multiple roles in relation to drug-related crime but often perceive their tasks as contradictory, are skeptical about the morality and effectiveness of harm reduction, and see it as contradictory to their main task—fighting drug trafficking. In part this is because of the demands of their employment, and in part from pressures from the communities within which they work. This contradiction creates tension for the individual police officer, and between them and their communities: "Working in such a web of overlapping and sometime conflicting policies, police at street level find themselves inextricably entangled and conflicted."[36, 37]

Even where harm reduction is national policy, and where it is supported by the police establishment, its operationalization at the level of the street is usually absent or incomplete. "The practices of street police challenge harm reduction policies, entirely understandably given the competing pressures on them. For harm reduction to be effective in Vietnam, it is essential that the ambiguities and contradictions between laws to control HIV and to control drugs be resolved for the street-level police."[38]

The work cited here illustrates the importance of gaining the perspective of police on their situation—of perceiving and understanding their inability to lead in the fight against HIV, as the front line in dealing with drug users, because of the conflicting policy imperatives—although many *are* aware of the need and of their key role.[39] The published literature offers little explanation of why law enforcement agencies, and particularly individual police, support or impede the lawful implementation of harm reduction policies and practices.

In Laos, where the context is one of little recognized injecting drug use, little overt harm reduction response and early days in advocacy, law enforcement officers have limited understanding of harm reduction approaches, and on the whole do not accept the feasibility and appropriateness such approaches in the Lao context.[40]

CHANGING ROLES FOR POLICE

There has been a slowly growing awareness across the region, however, that zero-tolerance policing and mass imprisonment are crime control policies which are themselves criminogenic—that harsh anti-crime measures actually increase the problems of crime rather than reducing them.[41] In large part, in relation to drug policy, as well as being part of a broader policy reform agenda, this realization has been driven by the imperatives of the HIV epidemic associated with injecting drug use. However, the majority of SEA drug policies acknowledge the fact that prevention, treatment and care are also important and in recent years a number of SEA countries have been ready to adopt harm reduction approaches (e.g., the provision of sterile injecting equipment to persons who inject drugs [PWIDs] and methadone and/ or buprenorphine to opiate-dependent people).

However, the health and social problems associated with illicit drug use tend not to have been well recognized, and police have generally had little training in dealing with these aspects—especially those, such as the use of amphetamine type substances, which are often accompanied by mental health issues—nor in working with health authorities.

THE FUTURE: POLICE COLLABORATIONS

Latterly, a few studies have begun in understanding better how police can operate in collaboration with health authorities in controlling the use of drugs and reducing the harm associated with their use. Some have found positive relationships between IDUs and police;[42, 43] these and other studies conclude that engaging with law enforcement agencies, especially at local level, is essential to the success of harm reduction programs.[44, 45]

Essentially, the imperative for both more effective drug control and for full implementation and success of harm reduction is reconciliation of the drug control and HIV control policies. For police, this means moving from institutionalized antagonism toward drug users—"antagonism" in the sense of a context of conflict resulting from law, regulation, operational impera- tives, and community pressure as well as culture—to an accommodation with harm reduction (in the sense of "first, do no harm"), to positive facilitation and leadership. Reconciling policy imperatives and changing operational goals and police cultures does not happen easily nor is it disconnected from wider changes in society, crime patterns, and policing approaches.

The research cited above of the impact of harm reduction on law enforce- ment gave some insight into what is needed in SEA to bring police through these transitions.[46] In particular, and a key point more often forgotten than acknowledged, is the need for the police role to make sense *to police* and *in policing terms*—"Solutions must be practical and be seen to be of worth by police—police responses and responsibilities in the partnership must be oper- ationalised."[47]

For instance, the implementation of methadone maintenance therapy pro- grams in Hai Phong in Vietnam was driven by the need for HIV prevention and effective drug treatment; that it has been not only accepted but is strong- ly supported by police is gratifying. But when one looks at the reasons *why* police support the programs, their responses are about improved social order and lowered crime rates—*not* about the health outcomes.[48] There is a lesson here: advocates for drug treatment, for harm reduction, for HIV prevention must learn to advocate for their programs in terms that make sense to po- lice—not that demand they move away from their professional and statutory obligations.

Training of police is critical: simply in understanding the law and in understanding the goals and meaning of the law, in relation to effective drug policing and harm reduction, to ensure that positive policy change and law reform is translated into the operational consciousness of police. Increasingly such training is being integrated into police Academies and other training institutions across the region.[49, 50] However, the quality and effectiveness of much of the current training has never been evaluated, and attempts to provide ongoing education and support for police are very rare and often simply one-off sensitization workshops whose value is suspect.

Because of their position in relation to complex social issues, police can be facilitators to attempts to address the; in other public health issues, such as road trauma, police have led responses. If we do not understand the police culture and perspective, if we do not promote common goals and collaborative initiatives, the fields of drug policy reform and harm reduction will not only continue to battle against a much stronger opponent—they will fail to bring on side a potentially powerful ally.

NOTES

1. Kannarath Chheng, Supheap Leang, Nick Thomson, Timothy Moore, and Nick Crofts, "Harm Reduction in Cambodia: a Disconnect between Policy and Practice," *Harm Reduction Journal* 9 (2012): DOI:10.1186/1477-7517-9-30. www.harmreductionjournal.com/series/policing.

2. Murray Lee. *Inventing Fear of Crime: Criminology and the Politics of Anxiety* (Cullumpton Devon: Willan, 2007).

3. Mukta Sharma and Anindya Chatterjee, "Partnering with Law Enforcement to Deliver Good Public Health: The Experience of the HIV/AIDS Asia Regional Program," *Harm Reduction Journal* 9 (2012) : 24. Accessed September 21, 2012. DOI: 10.1186/1477-7517-9-24.

4. HRW (Human Rights Watch). "Drug Treatment Centres Offer Torture not Treatment." New York: HRW, 2012. Accessed September 18, 2012. www.hrw.org/news/2012/07/24/drug-detention-centers-offer-torture-not-treatment.

5. For the purposes of this chapter, the term "drug trafficking" includes the production, manufacture, extraction, offering, offering for sale, distribution, sale, delivery on any terms whatsoever, brokerage, dispatch in transit, transport, importation or exportation of any narcotic drug or psychoactive substance contrary to the provisions of the 1961 United Nations Single Convention on Narcotic Drugs, the 1961 Convention as amended or the 1971 United Nations Convention on Psychotropic Substances (see Article 3, paragraph 1 (a) (i) of the 1988 United Nations Convention Against Illicit Traffic in Narcotic Drugs and Psychotropic Substances).

6. Tim Rhodes, Gerry V. Stimson, Chris Fitch, Andrew Ball, and Adrian Renton, "Rapid Assessment, Injecting Drug Use, and Public Health," *Lancet* 354, no. 9172 (1999): 65–68.

7. Lisa Maher, Heidi Coupland, and Rachel Musson, "Scaling up HIV Treatment, Care and Support for Injecting Drug Users in Vietnam," *International Journal of Drug Policy* 18, no. 4 (2006): 296–305.

8. Nick Thomson, "Detention as Treatment: Detention of Methamphetamine Users in Cambodia, Laos, and Thailand" (Open Society Institute, New York, 2010).

9. OSI (Open Society Institute). *At What Cost? HIV and Human Rights Consequences of the Global "War on Drugs."* International Harm Reduction Development Program, Public Health Program. New York: OSI, 2009.

10. Theodore M. Hammett, Zunyou Wu, Tran Tien Duc, David Stephens, Sheena Sullivan, Wei Liu, Yi Chen, Doan Ngu, and Don C. Des Jarlais, "'Social Evils' and Harm Reduction: The Evolving Policy Environment for Human Immunodeficiency Virus Prevention among Injection Drug Users in China and Vietnam," *Addiction* 103 (2008): 137–45.

11. Melissa Jardine, Nick Crofts, Geoff Monaghan, and Martha Morrow, "Harm Reduction and Law Enforcement in Vietnam: Influences on Street Policing," *Harm Reduction Journal* 9 (2012): 27. DOI: 10.1186/1477-7517-9-27.

12. Khonesavanh Latsaphao, "Asean Targets Drug Free Status by 2015," *Vientiane Times*, June 25, 2012. Accessed 25 September 2012. www.unodc.org/laopdr/en/stories/asean-targets-drug-free-status-by-2015.html.

13. Jardine et al., *Harm Reduction and Law Enforcement in Vietnam.*

14. Thomas Kerr, Will Small, and Evan Wood, "The Public Health and Social Impacts of Drug Market Enforcement: a Review of the Evidence." *International Journal of Drug Policy* 16 (2005): 210–20.

15. Trevor Bennett and Katy Holloway, "Disaggregating the Relationship between Drug Misuse and Crime." *Australian and New Zealand Journal of Criminology* 38, no. 1 (2005): 102–21.

16. Bronwyn Lind, Shuling Chen, Don Weatherburn, and Richard Mattick, "The Effectiveness of Methadone Maintenance Treatment in Controlling Crime: An Australian Aggregate-Level Analysis," *British Journal of Criminology* 45, no. 2 (2005): 201–11. DOI: 10.1093/bjc/azh085.

17. Kora DeBeck, Thomas Kerr, Kathy Li, M-J. Milloy, Julio Montaner, and Evan Wood, "Incarceration and Drug Use Patterns among a Cohort of Injection Drug Users," *Addiction* 104 (2009): 69–76.

18. Kate Dolan, Alex Wodak, Wayne Hall, Matthew Gaughwin, and Fiona Rae, "HIV Risk Behaviour of IDUs before, During and After Imprisonment in New South Wales," *Addiction Research* 4, no. 2 (1996): 151–60.

19. Natalie Gately, Jennifer Fleming, Robyn Morris, and Catherine McGregor, "Amphetamine Users and Crime in Western Australia, 1999–2009," *Trends & Issues in Crime and Criminal Justice* no. 437 Canberra: Australian Institute of Criminology, 2012 www.aic.gov.au/documents/4/4/E/%7B44EF7F96-BB91-41CB-AF45-FEFDEC9E9CCA%7Dtandi437.pdf.

20. Michelle Torok, Shane Darke, Sharlene Kaye, Joanne Ross, and Rebecca McKetin, "Comparative Rates of Violent Crime amongst Methamphetamine and Opioid Users: Victimisation and Offending," *Monograph Series* 32 (Sydney, Australia: National Drug and Alcohol Research Centre, University of New South Wales, Sydney, 2008). www.ndlerf.gov.au/pub/Monograph_32.pdf.

21. Thomson, "Detention as Treatment."

22. David Dixon and Lisa Maher, "Policing, Crime and Public Health: Lessons for Australia from the 'New York miracle.'" *Criminal Justice* 5, no. 2 (2005): 115–43.

23. Lisa Maher and David Dixon, "Policing and Public Health: Law Enforcement and Harm Minimization in a Street-Level Drug Market," *British Journal of Criminology* 39 (1999): 488–512.

24. Kerr et al., "The Public Health and Social Impacts of Drug Market Enforcement," 210–20.

25. Kora DeBeck, Evan Wood, Ruth Zhang, Mark Tyndall, Julio Montaner, and Thomas Kerr, "Police and Public Health Partnerships: Evidence from the Evaluation of Vancouver's Supervised Injection Facility," *Substance Abuse Treatment, Prevention, and Policy* 3 (2008): 11.

26. Acacia Shields, "The Effects of Drug User Registration Laws on People's Rights and Health: Key Findings from Russia, Georgia, and Ukraine" (New York: Open Society Institute, Public Health Program, International Harm Reduction Development Program, 2009).

27. Daniel Wolfe, M. Patrizia Carrieri, and Donald Shepard, "Treatment and Care for Injecting Drug Users with HIV Infection: a Review of Barriers and Ways Forward," 376, no. 9738 (2010): 355–66.

28. Wolfe, Carrieri, and Shepard, *Treatment and Care*, 355–66.

29. Wolfe, Carrieri and Shepard, *Treatment and Care*, 355–66.

30. Andrea Krusi, Evan Wood, Julio Montaner, and Thomas Kerr, "Social and Structural Determinants of HAART Access and Adherence among Injection Drug Users," *International Journal of Drug Policy* 21 (2010): 4–9.

31. Wolfe, Carrieri, and Shepard, *Treatment and Care*, 355–66.

32. Nick Thomson, Timothy Moore, and Nick Crofts, " Assessing the Impact of Harm Reduction Programs on Law Enforcement in Southeast Asia: a Description of a Regional Research Methodology," *Harm Reduction Journal* 9 (2012): 23. DOI:10.1186/1477-7517-9-23.

33. Thomson, Moore, and Crofts, *Assessing the Impact.*

34. NAA (National AIDS Authority). *Cambodia Country Progress Report: Monitoring the Progress towards the Implementation of the Declaration of Commitment on HIV/AIDS.* Phnom Penh: NAA, 2012. www.aidsdatahub.org/dmdocuments/UNGASS_2012_Cambodia_Narra-

tive_Report.pdf .

35. Chheng et al., *Harm Reduction in Cambodia.*

36. Thu Hong Khuat, Van Anh Thi Nguyen, Melissa Jardine, Timothy Moore, Thu Huong Bui, and Nick Crofts, "Harm Reduction and 'Clean' Community: Can Viet Nam Have Both?" *Harm Reduction Journal* 9 (2012): 25. DOI: 10.1186/1477-7517-9-25.

37. Jardine et al., *Harm Reduction and Law Enforcement in Vietnam.*

38. Jardine et al., *Harm Reduction and Law Enforcement in Vietnam.*

39. Jardine et al., *Harm Reduction and Law Enforcement in Vietnam.*

40. Vanphanom Sychareun, Visanou Hansana, Sysavanh Phommachanh, Vathsana Somphet, Phouthong Phommavongsa, Brigitte Tenni, Timothy Moore, and Nick Crofts. "Defining and Redefining Harm Reduction in the Lao Context," *Harm Reduction Journal* 9 (2012): 28. DOI: 10.1186/1477-7517-9-28.

41. James Sheptycki, "Transnationalisation, Orientalism and Crime," *Asian Journal of Criminology* 3, no. 1 (2008): 13–35. Accessed September 21, 2012. DOI: 10.1007/s11417-008-9049-0.

42. Theodore M. Hammett, Don C. Des Jarlais, Wei Liu, Doan Ngu, Nguyen Duy Tung, Tran Vu Hoang, Ly Kieu Van, and Meng Donghua, "Development and Implementation of a Cross-Border HIV Prevention Intervention for Injection Drug Users in Ning Ming County (Guangxi Province), China and Lang Son Province, Vietnam." *International Journal of Drug Policy* 14, nos. 5–6 (2003): 389–98.

43. Don C. Des Jarlais, Ryan Kling, Theodore M. Hammett, Doan Ngu, Wei Liu, Yi Chen, Kieu Thanh Binh, and Patricia Friedmann, "Reducing HIV Infection among New Injecting Drug Users in the China - Vietnam Cross Border Project." *AIDS* 21, no. 8 (2007): S109–S114.

44. Anh D. Ngo, Lucina Schmich, Peter Higgs, and Andrea Fischer, "Qualitative Evaluation of a Peer-based Needle Syringe Programme in Vietnam." *International Journal of Drug Policy* 20 (2009): 179–82.

45. Jardine et al., *Harm Reduction and Law Enforcement in Vietnam.*

46. LEHRN (Law Enforcement and Harm Reduction at the Nossal Institute), "Sleeping with the Enemy: Engaging with Law Enforcement in Prevention of HIV among and from Injecting Drug Users in Asia," *HIV Matters* 2, no. 1 (2010): 14-16

47. LEHRN, "Sleeping with the Enemy."

48. Jardine et al., *Harm Reduction and Law Enforcement in Vietnam.*

49. Mukta Sharma and Anindya Chatterjee, "Partnering with Law Enforcement to Deliver Good Public Health: The Experience of the HIV/AIDS Asia Regional Program," *Harm Reduction Journal* 9 (2012) : 24. Accessed September 21, 2012. DOI: 10.1186/1477-7517-9-24.

50. WHO (World Health Organisation). *Good Practices in Asia: Effective Paradigm Shifts towards an Improved National Response to Drugs and HIV/AIDS. Scale up of Harm Reduction in Malaysia.* Geneva: WHO, 2011. www.wpro.who.int/publications/docs/GoodPracticesinAsia_WEB_270411.pdf.

BIBLIOGRAPHY

Bennett, Trevor and Katy Holloway. "Disaggregating the Relationship between Drug Misuse and Crime." *Australian and New Zealand Journal of Criminology* 38, no. 1 (2005): 102–21.

Chheng, Kannarath, Supheap Leang, Nick Thomson, Timothy Moore, and Nick Crofts. "Harm Reduction in Cambodia: A Disconnect between Policy and Practice." *Harm Reduction Journal* 9 (2012): 30. DOI: 10.1186/1477-7517-9-30. www.harmreductionjournal.com/series/policing.

DeBeck, Kora, Thomas Kerr, Kathy Li., M-J. Milloy, Julio Montaner, and Evan Wood. "Incarceration and Drug Use Patterns among a Cohort of Injection Drug Users." *Addiction* 104 (2009): 69–76.

DeBeck, Kora, Evan Wood, Ruth Zhang, Mark Tyndall, Julio Montaner, and Thomas Kerr. "Police and Public Health Partnerships: Evidence from the Evaluation of Vancouver's Supervised Injection Facility." *Substance Abuse Treatment, Prevention, and Policy* 3 (2008): 11.

Des Jarlais, Don C., Ryan Kling, Theodore M. Hammett, Doan Ngu, Wei Liu, Yi Chen, Kieu Thanh Binh, and Patricia Friedmann. "Reducing HIV Infection among New Injecting Drug Users in the China—Vietnam Cross Border Project." *AIDS* 21, no. 8 (2007): S109–S114.

Dixon, David and Lisa Maher. "Policing, Crime and Public Health: Lessons for Australia from the 'New York Miracle.'" *Criminal Justice* 5, no. 2 (2005): 115–43.

Dolan, Kate, Alex Wodak, Wayne Hall, Matthew Gaughwin, and Fiona Rae. "HIV Risk Behaviour of IDUs before, During and After Imprisonment in New South Wales." *Addiction Research* 4, no. 2 (1996): 151–60.

Gately, Natalie, Jennifer Fleming, Robyn Morris, and Catherine McGregor. "Amphetamine Users and Crime in Western Australia, 1999–2009." *Trends & Issues in Crime and Criminal Justice* no. 437 Canberra: Australian Institute of Criminology, 2012. www.aic.gov.au/documents/4/4/E/%7B44EF7F96-BB91-41CB-AF45-FEFDEC9E9CCA%7Dtandi437.pdf.

Hammett, Theodore M., Don C. Des Jarlais, Wei Liu, Doan Ngu, Nguyen Duy Tung, Tran Vu Hoang, Ly Kieu Van, and Meng Donghua. "Development and Implementation of a Cross-Border HIV Prevention Intervention for Injection Drug Users in Ning Ming County (Guangxi Province), China and Lang Son Province, Vietnam." *International Journal of Drug Policy* 14, nos. 5–6 (2003): 389–98.

Hammett, Theodore M., Zunyou Wu, Tran Tien Duc, David Stephens, Sheena Sullivan, Wei Liu, Yi Chen, Doan Ngu, and Don C. Des Jarlais. "'Social Evils' and Harm Reduction: the Evolving Policy Environment for Human Immunodeficiency Virus Prevention among Injection Drug Users in China and Vietnam." *Addiction* 103 (2008): 137–45.

HRW (Human Rights Watch). "Drug Treatment Centres Offer Torture not Treatment." New York: HRW, 2012. Accessed September 18, 2012. www.hrw.org/news/2012/07/24/drug-detention-centers-offer-torture-not-treatment.

Jardine, Melissa, Nick Crofts, Geoff Monaghan, and Martha Morrow. "Harm Reduction and Law Enforcement in Vietnam: Influences on Street Policing." *Harm Reduction Journal* 9 (2012): 27. DOI: 10.1186/1477-7517-9-27.

Kerr, Thomas, Will Small, and Evan Wood. "The Public Health and Social Impacts of Drug Market Enforcement: A Review of the Evidence." *International Journal of Drug Policy* 16 (2005): 210–20.

Khuat, Thu Hong, Van Anh Thi Nguyen, Melissa Jardine, Timothy Moore, Thu Huong Bui, and Nick Crofts. "Harm Reduction and "Clean" Community: Can Viet Nam Have Both?" *Harm Reduction Journal* 9 (2012): 25. DOI: 10.1186/1477-7517-9-25.

Krusi, Andrea, Evan Wood, Julio Montaner, and Thomas Kerr. "Social and Structural Determinants of HAART Access and Adherence among Injection Drug Users." *International Journal of Drug Policy* 21 (2010): 4–9.

Latsaphao, Khonesavanh. "Asean Targets Drug Free Status by 2015." *Vientiane Times* , June 25, 2012. Accessed 25 September 2012. www.unodc.org/laopdr/en/stories/asean-targets-drug-free-status-by-2015.html.

Lee, Murray. *Inventing Fear of Crime: Criminology and the Politics of Anxiety*. Cullumpton Devon: Willan, 2007.

LEHRN (Law Enforcement and Harm Reduction at the Nossal Institute). "Sleeping with the Enemy: Engaging with Law Enforcement in Prevention of HIV among and from Injecting Drug Users in Asia." *HIV Matters* 2, no. 1 (2010): 14–16.

Lind, Bronwyn, Shuling Chen, Don Weatherburn, and Richard Mattick. "The Effectiveness of Methadone Maintenance Treatment in Controlling Crime: An Australian Aggregate-Level Analysis." British Journal of Criminology 45, no. 2 (2005): 201–11. DOI: 10.1093/bjc/azh085.

Maher, Lisa and David Dixon. "Policing and Public Health: Law Enforcement and Harm Minimization in a Street-Level Drug Market." *British Journal of Criminology* 39 (1999): 488–512.

NAA (National AIDS Authority). *Cambodia Country Progress Report: Monitoring the Progress towards the Implementation of the Declaration of Commitment on HIV/AIDS*. Phnom Penh: NAA, 2012. www.aidsdatahub.org/dmdocuments/UNGASS_2012_Cambodia_Narrative_Report.pdf.

Ngo, Anh D., Lucina Schmich, Peter Higgs, and Andrea Fischer. "Qualitative Evaluation of a Peer-based Needle Syringe Programme in Vietnam." *International Journal of Drug Policy* 20 (2009): 179–82.

OSI (Open Society Institute). *At What Cost? HIV and Human Rights Consequences of the Global "War on Drugs."* International Harm Reduction Development Program, Public Health Program. New York: OSI, 2009.

Sharma, Mukta and Anindya Chatterjee, "Partnering with Law Enforcement to Deliver Good Public Health: the Experience of the HIV/AIDS Asia Regional Program." *Harm Reduction Journal* 9 (2012): 24. Accessed September 21, 2012. DOI: 10.1186/1477-7517-9-24.

Sheptycki, James. "Transnationalisation, Orientalism and Crime." *Asian Journal of Criminology* 3, no. 1 (2008): 13–35. Accessed September 21, 2012. DOI: 10.1007/s11417-008-9049-0.

Shields, Acacia. "The Effects of Drug User Registration Laws on People's Rights and Health: Key Findings from Russia, Georgia, and Ukraine." New York: Open Society Institute, Public Health Program, International Harm Reduction Development Program, 2009.

Sychareun, Vanphanom, Visanou Hansana, Sysavanh Phommachanh, Vathsana Somphet, Phouthong Phommavongsa, Brigitte Tenni, Timothy Moore, and Nick Crofts. "Defining and Redefining Harm Reduction in the Lao Context." *Harm Reduction Journal* 9 (2012): 28. DOI: 10.1186/1477-7517-9-28.

Thomson, Nick. "Detention as Treatment: Detention of Methamphetamine Users in Cambodia, Laos, and Thailand." New York: Open Society Institute, 2010.

Thomson, Nick, Timothy Moore, and Nick Crofts. " Assessing the Impact of Harm Reduction Programs on Law Enforcement in Southeast Asia: A Description of a Regional Research Methodology." *Harm Reduction Journal* 9 (2012): 23. DOI: 10.1186/1477-7517-9-23.

Torok, Michelle, Shane Darke, Sharlene Kaye, Joanne Ross, and Rebecca McKetin. "Comparative Rates of Violent Crime amongst Methamphetamine and Opioid Users: Victimisation and Offending." *Monograph Series* 32. Sydney, Australia: National Drug and Alcohol Research Centre, University of New South Wales, 2008. www.ndlerf.gov.au/pub/Monograph_32.pdf.

WHO (World Health Organisation). *Good Practices in Asia: Effective Paradigm Shifts towards an Improved National Response to Drugs and HIV/AIDS. Scale up of Harm Reduction in Malaysia.* Geneva: WHO, 2011. www.wpro.who.int/publications/docs/GoodPracticesinAsia_WEB_270411.pdf.

Wolfe, Daniel, M. Patrizia Carrieri, and Donald Shepard. "Treatment and Care for Injecting Drug Users with HIV Infection: a Review of Barriers and Ways Forward." 376, no. 9738 (2010): 355–66.

Chapter Six

Effective Development and Effective Drug Control Are Interdependent

The Example of Southeast Asia

Priya Mannava, Sasha Zegenhagen,
Nick Crofts, and Nick Thomson

Socioeconomic development is associated with illicit drugs—production, trade, and consumption—through complex intertwined and often opposing connections. These associations can be unraveled by considering "drugs" and "socioeconomic development" as independent variables, thus enabling us to look at the impact of socioeconomic development on illicit drugs and the converse, in this instance specifically in South East Asia.

Rural underdevelopment, conflict, and economic crises can drive illicit drug production, while poverty, unemployment, marginalization, and changing social norms create vulnerability to drug consumption. At the same time, free trade, open markets, and greater disposable income resulting from enhanced socioeconomic development may encourage consumption of illicit drugs and facilitate trafficking. Illicit drug economies can sustain and boost economic development in the short term; however, this is likely to be offset by longer-term consequences of corruption, crime, erosion of social capital, increased health costs, and reduced productivity.

Yet these interrelationships are not well acknowledged, if not actually often ignored—as illustrated by the fact that illicit drugs figure nowhere within the Millennium Development Goals. Traditionally, approaches to enhancing socioeconomic development have generally focused on boosting economic growth and generating additional income; illicit drug control has not typically been a factor taken into consideration. Rather, illicit drugs have primarily been considered as a domain of law enforcement and public security, though the past few decades have seen increased recognition of drug use as a public health issue. As such, policies which aim to control the harms associated with illicit drugs may cause more damage to societies than the drugs themselves. Human rights violations continue to be a casualty of such policies.

The evidence strongly indicates that, to be effective, illicit drug control strategies need to be mainstreamed within broader development strategies, such as national development or poverty reduction strategies. Similarly, development policies need to take into account the social and economic disparities that create vulnerabilities to illicit drug economies.

INTRODUCTION

In spite of the complex interrelationships between illicit drug production, trade and use, and socioeconomic development, drug control and socioeconomic development policies tend to occur in isolation of each other, as exemplified by the lack of inclusion of illicit drugs in the Millennium Development Goals. The failure to acknowledge the interconnections between these two areas hinders the effectiveness of both drug control and socioeconomic development policies, and also undermines a human-rights-based approach to both illicit drug policy and development policies and programs.

We examine in this chapter the multifaceted relationships between illicit drug production, trade and use, on the one hand, and socioeconomic development on the other, and then demonstrate the ways in which the implementation of illicit drug control policies often hinders development sector gains, and furthermore, the ways in which many development sector policies actually *increase* vulnerability to illicit drug production, trade and use in Southeast Asian countries. By raising awareness of the links between drugs, drug policy, and socioeconomic development, our aim is to initiate and facilitate needed dialogue and collaboration between development and drug control agencies.

Our original hypothesis was that *"Equitable socioeconomic development is necessary for successful control of illicit drugs,* while *effective and human-rights-based illicit drug control is required to foster sustainable socioeconomic development."* To test this hypothesis, we examined the impact of socioeconomic development on illicit drug production, trade, and consumption, and then conversely the effect of the three processes on socioeconomic development.

We define "socioeconomic development" as the processes of social and economic development in a society, whereby the "socio" consists of "social change designed to promote the well-being of a population as a whole"[1] while the "economic" refers to "qualitative change and restructuring in a country's economy in connection with technological and social progress."[2]

"Control" is referred to here as the processes undertaken in order to minimize the harms associated with the availability and use of drugs in a community at a given point of time, including the minimization of availability. In line with the United Nations Office for Drugs and Crime, "illicit drugs" are defined as drugs produced, traded, and consumed for purposes prohibited by law, as outlined by the international drug control conventions.

This chapter is based on a report prepared as part of a larger project examining these relationships.[3] We conducted a review of formal and non-formal English language literature published between 1990 and 2010 on the relationships between illicit drug production, trade, and consumption, illicit drug policies, socioeconomic development, and human rights.

THE IMPACT OF SOCIOECONOMIC DEVELOPMENT ON ILLICIT DRUGS

Conditions of Poor Social and Economic Development Create Vulnerabilities to Illicit Drugs

Conditions which contribute to weak socioeconomic development often create vulnerabilities for illicit drug consumption. Communities suffering from high unemployment, poverty, and social marginalization will have much higher likelihoods of high consumption of illicit drugs. Rhodes et al. (2003)[4] summarized findings from the United States and the United Kingdom which demonstrated that poverty, unemployment, crime, poor housing, and low levels of education are associated with illicit drug use and diffusion of illicit drugs; the same holds in Southeast Asia, though not yet as well documented. For instance in Indonesia, psychotropic drug (especially marijuana) consumption increased in youth and laborers following unemployment.[5]

Rural underdevelopment and poverty are similarly associated with illicit drug production. Illicit drugs are cultivated in the poorest, often isolated, regions of low-income countries,[6] where agriculture is the main economic activity but infrastructure and facilities are inadequate for commercial agricultural production. These regions are characterized by soils unsuitable to many licit crops, poor irrigation systems, weak transport systems, and lack of access to markets and credit facilities—in addition to broader social issues such as poor access to health or education.[7, 8] In such conditions, the characteristics of illicit drug crops make them a more viable farming option in comparison to other crops: they grow in a range of soils, altitudes, and temperatures, do not perish quickly, and often sell at prices higher than licit crops.[9, 10, 11, 12, 13, 14] In addition, farmers do not need to worry about transport or access to markets, as illicit drug traders have established routes and networks and often provide credit.

For example, in Myanmar, poppy farmers have tried to grow alternative crops such as corn, tea, and sugarcane. Lengthy yield times and the prohibitive cost of initial capital investment have meant that the long-term sustainable development of these crops is uncertain. Furthermore, mountainous geography, lack of access to land, irrigation, and sedimentary and poor nutrient soil make it impossible to grow corn successfully.[15] Unlike corn, opium grows well in mountainous area without irrigation, and farmers do not have to worry about access to market as opium traders from other places will come and buy opium right at the farm gates. Farmers have turned to non-timber forest products (NTFP), such as roots and tree bark from forests, to sell to Chinese traders; but this is not a sustainable solution as NTFPs become depleted and difficult to find.[16] Some farmers in the Wa region have sold livestock, such as pigs and cattle, to generate income, but lack of credit and animal husbandry technologies limit their possibilities.[17]

Failure of alternative forms of income generation has adverse implications on food security. In the East Shan State of Myanmar, 79 percent of households in villages where opium was not farmed were food secure for twelve months as opposed to 52 percent in villages growing opium, while in North Shan State the difference was as wide as 65 percent versus 11 percent.[18] Thus with few other economic alternatives available, farmers in these regions turn to farming of illicit drug crops out of the need to earn a livelihood and maintain food security.[19, 20, 21]

ILLICIT DRUG ECONOMIES AND CONFLICT ARE CLOSELY LINKED

In settings with a history of illicit drug production or trade, violent conflict facilitates growth of drug economies.[22] The vast majority of opium production occurs in countries currently experiencing war or with long histories of war, such as Myanmar.[23] The damage to infrastructure and social instability caused by conflict means that production of illicit drugs becomes a viable source of income.[24] In the Wa region of eastern Myanmar, for example, rice-growing farmers began producing opium poppies to counter-balance increased food insecurity caused by armed conflict and resultant weak economic development in the region.[25]

Sales of narcotics form the basis of a black market economy to fund both the military regime and the pro-independence armies. The military has significantly profited from involvement in the illicit drug economy. For example, SHAN Drug Watch has reported recently that the military is forcing many townships in Shan State to pay heavy taxes to the military with farmers noting that it is impossible to meet the tax load without growing opium. It has been equally reported that armed ethnic armies are involved in illicit drug production, with sales used to fund their armed struggle against the military. In effect, conflict and illicit drug economies engage in a mutually reinforcing cycle, whereby conflict helps to facilitate growth of the economies, which in turn, help to sustain the conflict. This vicious cycle poses considerable challenges to socioeconomic development.[26, 27, 28, 29]

MODERNIZATION CREATES VULNERABILITIES TO ILLICIT DRUG USE

Socioeconomic development is accompanied by significant cultural and political change, including modernization.[30] While definitions vary, modernization is generally characterized by the creation of a consumer society centered around individual choice and pleasure.[31, 32] Traditional norms are replaced with new identity formations and values, which in turn may influence vulnerabilities and decisions to consume illicit drugs. In many societies, economic growth has resulted in the emergence of a new middle class who with a sudden increase in disposable income are able to access new forms of leisure—including psychotropic drugs.[33, 34] At the same time, globalization of Western popular culture has resulted in illicit drugs being associated with modernity and wealth, regardless of whether the dangers of illicit drug use have been communicated.[35] In Indonesia, for example, a 7 percent growth of the economy between 1968 and 1981 gave rise to a new affluent class of society which had the financial and social means to access illicit drugs.[36] The types of drugs being used were reported to have been influenced by Western popular culture.[37]

At the other end of the spectrum are the traditional and isolated societies who have to suddenly cope with new values and practices—a social dislocation which may create vulnerabilities to illicit drug use. In Laos, for instance, the Akha who had faced decades of discrimination and isolation suddenly had to abandon subsistence economies to participate in the nation's new market economy.[38] In order to cope with the demands of a new lifestyle, members of the tribe have often resorted to consumption of amphetamine-type stimulants and heroin to enhance physical strength and psychosocial pleasure.[39]

THE IMPACT OF ILLICIT DRUGS ON SOCIOECONOMIC DEVELOPMENT

Illicit Drug Economies Are Closely Linked to Corruption

Noting the difficulties in determining causality, as well as issues with defining corruption and thereby obtaining appropriate data,[40] illicit drug producing and trading countries are plagued by chronic corruption, which is exacerbated by the drug industry regardless of whether it is the root cause.[41] The profitability and accessibility of the illicit drug trade encourages government officials and law enforcement employees to engage in corruption to supplement their wages. For example, law enforcement officials in countries world-over have been known to intentionally hold people on suspicion of possession, even when this is not the case, and then release them in exchange for money.[42] Corruption is a severe impediment to sustained socioeconomic growth since, as the above examples demonstrate, it can penetrate the political system, as well as judicial and economic structures, thereby weakening social integrity. This, in turn, can further fuel the drug trade, thus creating a vicious circle.[43, 44] The rise of both production of illicit drugs—the waves of opium, then heroin, then amphetamine-type substances—and their consumption across Southeast Asia have been paralleled by rises in organized crime and institutionalized corruption.[45] This is possibly the most difficult to study and intransigent aspect of the relationship we are studying, but also, perhaps the most important from the point of view of impairment of socioeconomic development.

Illicit Drug Economies Disrupt Social Structures and Are Associated with Violence

Two examples of well-documented and critically important aspects of the relationship show the degree to which there has been neglect of these issues in Asia.

The illicit drug trade disrupts social structures. Families are torn apart and struggle socially and financially when the primary care giver is incarcerated for drug-related offenses.[46] Children left behind may then engage in criminal activity or drug use as they struggle to cope with living in institutions, foster care, or with relatives.[47] Female involvement in drug trading has also been steadily increasing due to economic circumstances;[48] as a result, women are more likely to be subject to violence or harassment including invasive searches.[49] Power structures within communities may also be disturbed as a result of widening income disparities caused by the illicit drug trade. Moreover, visible income differences encourage more people to enter the illicit drug industry.[50]

Numerous studies have found a correlation between illicit drug markets and violence.[51] Drug gangs often engage in violence to protect and control the production and trade of illicit drugs.[52] Innocent civilians suffer the most from drug-fuelled violence.[53] As violence continues in a particular area, wealthier inhabitants and businesses leave for safer environments, in turn leaving behind a poorer segment of the community to face deteriorating facilities and infrastructure, increased unemployment, and decreased social mobility due to fear of bloodshed.[54] Violence caused by illicit drug econo- mies threatens peace and security, weakens social institutions, and under- mines state legitimacy—which together prevent socioeconomic develop- ment.[55]

There has been very little research or documentation of any of these issues in the Asian regions, despite their importance and much anecdotal evidence of their existence.

Illicit Drug Use Has Important Social and Economic Costs

There are also considerable social and economic costs associated with illicit drug use, both at the individual and societal level. The health effects of illicit drug consumption are numerous, including blood-borne infections such as hepatitis C virus and HIV infection, bacterial infections, cardiovascular com- plications, mental illness, overdose, and suicide.[56, 57, 58] Of the health conse- quences, viral infections are widely recognized. Risk of transmission of HIV is high among injecting drug users, due to sharing of contaminated injection equipment and engagement in unprotected sex, and a lack of policies and programs of proven effectiveness to stop their transmission (see Des Jarlais et al. chapter in this book). Drug overdose is another significant health issue associated with drug use. Drug-related suicide is also a risk, estimated to be fourteen times more likely to occur among drug users compared to the gener- al population.[59]

Drug users are likely to be less productive due to increased occupational injuries and absenteeism.[60, 61] A decrease in productivity also occurs among drug producers, who are affected by hazardous work conditions and exposure to chemicals, with side effects including asthma, diarrhea, and gastro prob- lems.[62, 63] In Hai Phong, productivity losses have been estimated to be US $8,611 per case of HIV/AIDS and include reduced employment for caregiv- ers ($351) during the most severe phase of illness, and a permanent reduction in employment ($8,260) due to the premature death as a result of AIDS.[64] At a national level, illicit drug consumption is particularly prevalent among fifteen- to forty-four-year-olds, which is also the most productive sector of an economy. According to Singer, this means that rather than contributing to the national economy, an important source of a country's productivity is instead becoming a financial and social burden.[65] Considering that the majority of the people in drug detention in Southeast Asia are young people, the implications for the development of these young people is dire. Removing young people from their communities and families and placing them in detention also removes them from formal education systems and workforces, placing further pressures on fragile labor markets. Exacerbating this, many drug traders are also within this productive age group and are often arrested while smuggling, further reducing the size of the population of productive labor. [66]

Illicit Drug Economies Erode the Potential for Long-term Sustainable Development

Financial and human resources invested in the illicit drug sector erode the potential for long-term sustainable development. [67] Finances earned through the illicit drug industry are largely invested in unproductive sectors based primarily on the potential to launder money. [68, 69, 70] As a result of factors such as violence, money laundering, and corruption that are often associated with the illicit drug industry, private investment in licit and productive areas of the economy may decrease. [71] Decreased investment serves to hinder economic industrialization and employment opportunities within the licit sector, thereby increasing individual incentive to partake in the illicit drug economy. [72]

POLICY IMPLICATIONS

The evidence strongly indicates that to be effective illicit drug control strategies need to be mainstreamed within broader development strategies, such as national development or poverty reduction strategies. Similarly, development policies need to take into account the social and economic disparities that create vulnerabilities to illicit drug economies. Development agencies and governments would be well advised, following the evidence, to investigate and account for the impact of development on vulnerabilities to drug production, trade, and use. All aspects of development, ranging from infrastructure projects to education programs, especially if donor funded, should consider the implications for illicit drug production, trade, and use, as is often already done with respect to the environment, HIV/AIDS, or gender dynamics.

Social Impact Assessments

The adverse impacts of failing to incorporate illicit drugs in social impact assessments in development policies is exemplified through numerous infrastructure projects in Southeast Asia. The Asian Development Bank, the World Bank, and bilateral donors have embraced the development of large-scale infrastructure projects in Southeast Asia as means of increasing the socioeconomic development of both individual countries within the region and the region as a whole. Examples of these projects include the Nam Thuen hydropower dams in Laos and the north-south and east-west corridor highway systems built to connect the countries of the Mekong to improve transport, trade and therefore economic development. The social impact of infrastructure projects on illicit drug use trends has not been adequately included in the social impact assessment framework. The ADBI recently released a report that examined twenty-six infrastructure projects in the Mekong spanning across transport, energy, and information technology projects. In addition to citing the positive impacts of the infrastructure projects on enhanced development opportunities, their report also suggests multiple negative social impacts.[73] These impacts have included HIV/AIDS vulnerability, increased numbers of casinos, increases in human trafficking, drug trafficking, and illegal logging. The impact on drug use has not been explicitly measured, but the report notes that the poor and vulnerable people living around transport intersections are vulnerable to turn to drug trafficking. Furthermore, the report notes that migrant workers are susceptible to drug use, particularly methamphetamines, given by their employers in order to improve "strength" associated with the labor-intensive nature of the infrastructure building. In 1997, a highway was constructed between Mandalay and Muse; UNDP noted that a year after the construction had finished, HIV prevalence rates among injecting drug users in three towns along the highway had significantly increased. While it was noted that drug use was rampant in these three provinces prior to the road building, enhanced drug trade expanded along the highway and one year after construction ended, HIV prevalence in three provinces along the highway in Myanmar—Mandalay, Lashio, and Muse—rose from 51 percent to 88 percent, 34 percent to 74 percent, and 86 percent to 92 percent, respectively.[74]

Given that these reports implicating infrastructure projects with increases in vulnerabilities associated with drug use have been documented for over ten years, it seems unfortunate that public health responses to illicit drug use associated with infrastructure have not been forthcoming. The responsibility for documenting the potential impact on illicit drug use should come from the donors and implementers. Through the design and implementation of a social impact assessment that notes potential implications of large-scale infrastructure projects on illicit drug use trends, donors, contractors, the UN, and NGOs would be in a much better position to design systems and programs that mitigate the negative implications of illicit drug use associated with infrastructure projects. Considering the billions of US dollars associated with the implementation of these projects, donors need to also fund not only the social impact assessments on illicit drug use but also the necessary public-health- and human-rights-based responses.

Alternative Development

The development dialogue around illicit drugs has largely centered on HIV/ AIDS or alternative development projects. As opium eradication continues in Southeast Asia, "alternative development" strategies have been increasingly viewed as the optimum method of creating alternative economic opportunities in order to reduce the farming of illicit drug crops. The reality, however, is that in the pursuit of the "alternative development" model, livelihoods have often been significantly worsened, as can be seen in the case of Myanmar.

With significant support from UNODC, phased opium eradication began in northern Shan State 1999–2004, eastern Shan State and Wa region in 2004–2009, and parts of southern Shan State in 2009–2014.[75] The bans have had devastating effects on farmers who cultivate opium as their main cash crop; nearly two million people in Shan State lost their primary source of income, while 90 percent did in Kokang.[76][77] In the Wa region, 82 percent of farmers use money from opium poppy cultivation to buy food, and 73 percent of household income is attributed to sales of opium; eradication has resulted in widespread food shortages.[78] In Shan State it has been reported that many farmers have only enough rice to feed their family from six to eight months and are therefore dependent on opium as a cash crop to fund extra food, medicines, clothing, and access to education. This is similarly the case in the Wa region where 89.5 percent of people report food insecurity.[79]

Furthermore, an assessment conducted in Kokang reported that nearly sixty thousand people have migrated to other areas to seek alternative livelihoods.[80] This is exacerbated by a stark lack of investment in "alternative development," including in the Wa region, where local authorities believed that it was easier to relocate ex-farmers from mountainous northern areas to lowlands where people can find alternative livelihoods, than providing infrastructure such as road, school, clinics to mountainous and scattered villages in the region.[81] The relocation itself resulted in a larger number of people dying from malaria.

In Song Khie villages, 108 people out of an original population of 370 died in first three years during the resettlement.[82] When arriving in the lowlands, many people did not have enough seeds and other resources to make a living, leading to prolonged suffering from food insecurity.[83] While UN agencies and international NGOs attempt to address issues of food insecurity, the levels of assistance are insufficient compared to the magnitude of affected population. Despite providing food to nearly 160,000 people in Wa region in 2004, and 100,000 people in Kokang region in 2003, the World Food Programme (WFP) acknowledged that the assistance reached only 40 percent of the people in need.[84][85] Unless ongoing efforts are increased to bring about a stable political environment, where fundamental human rights are recognized, opium eradication and "alternative development" will continue to fail.

This also highlights the need for integration of illicit drug and development policies and strategies, through increased dialogue and collaboration between drug control and development agencies. To date, traditional development agencies, such as the United Nations Development Program (UNDP), have rarely invested in drug control, while drug control agencies, like the UNODC, lack the capacity to design and implement large-scale development programs. Acknowledgment that illicit drugs and socioeconomic development are inherently linked and the resultant increased cooperation between such agencies will enable the UNODC, for example, to capitalize on the comparative advantage that UNDP has in implementation of development programs. Enhanced linkages between development and drug entities will, however, require widespread acknowledgment of the interrelationships between both fields.

Law Enforcement

Most illicit drug policies focus on reducing demand and supply through law enforcement. These strategies seemed to have largely failed in reducing illicit drug use, trade, or production because they have failed to address the broader environmental, economic, and socio-cultural factors that lead to production, trade, or consumption of illicit drugs. Most countries in the region today still rely on punitive drug control measures and treat all those involved in drug economies as criminals. The default response for amphetamine-type substance users, for instance, has been the funding and building of an increasing number of compulsory drug detention centers where they are held in violation of international law and even sometimes contrary to specific national law, such as in Cambodia, for example.[86] This response is widely recognized as being inhumane, lacking an evidence base, and placing vulnerable people at risk of infectious disease and violence through their interactions in prison and compulsory drug treatment center environments. Exacerbating this issue is the fact that in national and regional forums there appears to be almost no distinction made between recreational ATS users and ATS users who would be considered dependent. Considering only a small number of ATS users experience negative health outcomes, the inherent idea that treatment options need to be applied broadly for all ATS users is fundamentally flawed. This also in part explains the problem agencies have in knowing how to respond with evidenced-based interventions.[87]

Harm Reduction

Implementing effective policies without criminalizing drug use can have important economic benefits to the community, as exemplified in the case of

Hai Phong, the third most populous city in Vietnam (population about two million) and an important commercial and transportation hub for Northern Vietnam due to its seaport. Hai Phong has also been significantly affected by injecting drug use and HIV. According to surveillance data, about 50 percent of people who injected drugs surveyed in 2009 were HIV positive, and there are somewhere between seven thousand to fifteen thousand people who regularly inject drugs.[88, 89] In response, methadone maintenance therapy (MMT) has been implemented, estimated at averting approximately 598 HIV cases each year for every ten thousand people on MMT, leading to a lifetime cost saving of over twelve million dollars. Participants also reported to be dropping their heroin spending from $10.50 per day prior to the treatment to less than 10 cents per day. Thus it can be estimated that MMT reduces heroin expenditure by about $3,832 per person on the program per year. At the time of writing, there were 2,271 people on MMT in Hai Phong, resulting in a reduction of $8.5 million dollars being spent on heroin.

This has implications on the local economy. Over half of the drug users on the program in Hai Phong moved from informal jobs and crime to more formal jobs after being on the program. They also report having more disposable income than they did while using drugs.[90] The shift away from informal economic activity to more formal activity has also been accompanied by a significant reduction in crime. According to police data, crime has reduced by 80 percent in areas with MMT clinics and family conflicts (and conflicts with neighbours and friends) also dropped from 20 percent prior to treatment to 3.56 percent after nine months.[91] The final way in which MMT has impacted on the economic development of Hai Phong is through the investment made by the international donor community including money spent on renovations and long-term employment for staff within the health sector.

However it is important to tailor the policy response to the situation, as the significant rise in ATS usage in Southeast Asia demonstrates. It has become increasingly clear that the sheer number of ATS users in the Southeast Asian region dwarfs the number of injecting opiate users.[92] This has created a situation where the traditional harm reduction responders—including NGOs, human rights activists, some government officials, national and regional UNAIDS/UNODC, and WHO bodies and the host of bilateral and regional harm reduction programs active in the region—are struggling to come to terms with the implications for harm reduction activities and indeed treatment options for the large number of ATS users in the region. While the direct implications for HIV of ATS are somewhat unclear, ATS users are increasingly being exposed to HIV risk and acquisition through their detention in prisons and compulsory drug treatment centers. ATS users also have multiple HIV risk behaviors, including unprotected sex, high rates of STIs, and transition to injection of ATS. In addition to responding to the HIV risk behavior, community-based harm reduction strategies are urgently needed in

Southeast Asia that work across the spectrum of drug use and sexual risk reduction and consider the appropriate role of law enforcement and public health in the context of ATS. Regionally, UNODC has become the UN focal point for ATS, both anti-trafficking and treatment. This approach means that what is essentially a public health and development issue is dominated not by health and development experts but by agencies whose mandate is primarily law enforcement. The result has been that many prisons in the region are overcrowded with ATS users and small-time dealers and judicial systems and police efforts clogged with ATS-related cases.[93] Unless a multi-sectoral approach is championed between health, education, and law enforcement, this situation will only continue to get worse and solutions will be further away, not closer. Focusing on community-based drug use and sexual risk reduction will help foster an environment where young ATS users can manage and cease their use without being placed in detention, lost to the education system, or being rendered invalid by the workforce.

Adopting a development-oriented approach to drug control, underpinned by a fundamental respect for human rights, will require a major shift in mindset but likely result in both enhanced illicit drug control and socioeconomic development.

CONCLUSION

As demonstrated by evidence within the literature, socioeconomic development and illicit drug production, trade, and use are associated in complex and intertwined ways. That poor socioeconomic development, including conflict, drives illicit drug production, trade, and use, and that modernization and greater disposable income resulting from enhanced socioeconomic development create vulnerabilities to illicit drug use, is evident. Similarly, that illicit drug economies negatively impact socioeconomic development due to corruption, crime, erosion of social capital, increased health costs, and aggregate effects at the national level of reduced productivity of individuals using illicit drugs is also evident. That these connections are not adequately made by policymakers, development agencies, or drug control agencies severely undermines the effectiveness of both areas—drug control and development. And the fact that there is a relative dearth of research in these connections and relationships indicates that the research communities have partitioned their activities—and their consciousnesses—in the same manner as the policy makers and agencies.

Equitable socioeconomic development is clearly essential for controlling the harms associated with illicit drugs, while effective control of these harms is necessary for sustainable socioeconomic development. There is a need for increased dialogue and cooperation between drug and development agencies to ensure that development policies consider vulnerabilities to illicit drug production, trade, and use, and that drug policies are aligned with development strategies.

ACKNOWLEDGMENTS

This research was funded by a grant from Global Drug Policy Program of the Open Society Institute. The research was assisted by Deepankar Malik, Ashok Agarwal, Simon Baldwin; the report writing by Arunkumar Moirangthem Cha, Patrick O'Gorman, Michelle Kermode, Martina Melis, Irene Salam Singh, Richard Tanter, Brigitte Tenni; the project by Jennifer Sainsbury at the Nossal Institute and Kasia Malinowska-Sempruch at the Open Society Institute.

NOTES

1. James Midgley, *Social Development: the Developmental Perspective in Social Welfare* (London: Sage, 1995).
2. Tatyana P. Soubbotina, *Beyond Economic Growth: An Introduction to Sustainable Development* (USA: The World Bank, 2004). Accessed October 18, 2012. www.worldbank.org/depweb/english/beyond/global/glossary.html.
3. Priya Mannava, Sasha Zegenhagen, and Nick Crofts, "Dependent on Development: the Interrelationships between Illicit Drugs and Socioeconomic Development" (Melbourne: Nossal Institute for Global Health, 2011).
4. Tim Rhodes, Robert Lilly, Cesareo Fernández, Enzo Giorgino, Uwe E. Kemmesis, Hans C. Ossebaard, Nacer Lalam, Imar Faasen, and Karen Ellen Spannow, "Risk Factors Associated with Drug Use: The Importance of Risk Environment." *Drugs: Education, Prevention, and Policy* 10, no. 4 (2003): 303–29.
5. Irwanto Irwanto, "Indonesia: Facing Illicit Drug Abuse Challenges." *Development Bulletin* 69 (2006): 44–48.
6. Martina Melis and Marie Nougier, "Drug Policy and Development: How Action against Illicit Drugs Impacts on the Millennium Development Goals" (London: International Drug Policy Consortium, 2010). Accessed November 1, 2010.http://idpc.net/sites/default/files/library/Drug%20policy%20and%20development%20briefing.pdf?utm_source=IDPC+Monthly+Alert&utm_campaign=5a7b06b62a-IDPC_October_2010_Alert10_27_2010=email.
7. Pierre Arnaud Chouvy and Laurent R. Laniel, *Production De Drogue Et Stabilité Des Etats* (Secrétariat Général de la Défense Nationale, 2006). Accessed October 18, 2012. http://laniel.free.fr/INDEXES/PapersIndex/SGDN/DrugProductionStateStabilityChouvyLanielSGDN-CERI-2006.pdf.
8. Melis and Nougier, *Drug Policy and Development*.
9. David Whynes, "Illicit Drug Production and Supply-Side Drugs Policy in Asia and South America," *Development and Change* 22, no. 3 (1991): 475–96.
10. Chouvy and Laniel, *Production De Drogue Et Stabilité*.
11. Michelle L. Dion and Catherine Russler, "Eradication Efforts, the State, Displacement and Poverty: Explaining Coca Cultivation in Colombia During Plan Colombia," *Journal of Latin American Studies* 40, no. 3 (2008): 399–421.
12. William A. Byrd, "Responding to Afghanistan's Opium Economy Challenge: Lessons and Policy Implications." Policy Research Working Paper 4545, The World Bank, South Asia Region, 2008.

13. Julia Buxton, *The Political Economy of Narcotics: Production, Consumption and Global Markets* (Canada: Fernwood Publishing, 2006).

14. Merrill Singer, "Drugs and Development: The Global Impact of Drug Use and Trafficking on Social and Economic Development," *International Journal of Drug Policy* 19, no. 6 (2008): 467–78.

15. Tom Kramer, Martin Jelsma, and Tom Blickman, "Withdrawal Symptoms in the Golden Triangle: A Drug Market in Disarray" (Amsterdam: Drugs and Democracy Programme, Transnational Institute (TNI), 2009). Accessed October 19, 2010. www.tni.org/sites/www.tni.org/archives/reports/drugs/pr090109.pdf.

16. Kramer, Jelsma, and Blickman, "Withdrawal Symptoms in the Golden Triangle."

17. UNODC (United Nations Office of Drugs and Crime), *Opium Cultivation in South East Asia* (Vienna: UNODC, 2006). Accessed October 19, 2010.www.unodc.org/pdf/research/Golden_triangle_2006.pdf.

18. UNODC, *Opium Cultivation in South East Asia*.

19. Chouvy and Laniel, *Production De Drogue Et Stabilité*.

20. GTZ (Deutsche Gesellschaft für Technische Zusammenarbeit), and ADE (Drugs and Development Programme), *Drugs and Poverty: The Contribution of Development-Oriented Drug Control to Poverty Reduction* (Drugs and Development Programme. Bonn: GTZ, 2003b). Accessed October 1, 2010. www.gtz.de/de/dokumente/en-drugs-poverty-english.pdf.

21. UNRISD (United Nations Research Institute for Social Development), "Illicit Drugs: Social Impacts and Policy Responses," UNRISD Briefing Paper No. 2, World Summit For Social Development, 1994. Accessed September 29, 2010. www.unrisd.org/80256-B3C005BCCF9/(httpAuxPages)/4C3D0BE90FAD550480256B6400419B57/$file/bp2.pdf.

22. Cornelius Graubner, "Drugs and Conflict: How the Mutual Impact of Illicit Drug Economies and Violent Conflict Influences Sustainable Development, Peace and Stability" (Eschborn, Germany: Report Commissioned by the German Federal Ministry for Economic Cooperation and Development, GTZ, 2007).

23. UNDP (United Nations Development Program), *Taking Narcotics Out of the Conflict-The War on Drugs.* UNDP, 2003. Accessed November 3, 2010.www.pnud.org.co/2003/EnglishVersion/Chapter13.pdf.

24. Graubner, *Drugs and Conflict.*

25. Graubner, *Drugs and Conflict.*

26. Pierre Arnaud Chouvy, *Opium: Uncovering the Politics of the Poppy* (Massachusetts: Harvard University Press, 2009).

27. Chouvy and Laniel, *Production De Drogue Et Stabilité*.

28. Graubner, *Drugs and Conflict.*

29. GTZ (Deutsche Gesellschaft für Technische Zusammenarbeit), *Drugs and Conflict.* Drugs and Development Programme (Bonn: GTZ, 2003a). Accessed September 30, 2010. / www.gtz.de/de/dokumente/en-drugs-conflict.pdf.

30. Inglehart, Ronald, and Welzel, *Modernization, Cultural Change, and Democracy: The Human Development Sequence* (New York: Cambridge University Press, 2005).

31. Inglehart, Ronald, and Welzel, *Modernization, Cultural Change, and Democracy*.

32. Chris Lyttleton, "Relative Pleasures: Drugs, Development and Modern Dependencies in Asia's Golden Triangle," *Development and Change* 35, no. 5 (2004): 909–35.

33. Michael L. Smith, Charunee N. Thongtham, Najma Sadeque, Alfredo Molano Bravo, Roger Rumrrill, and Amanda Dávila, *Why People Grow Drugs* (Panos Publications: London, 1992).

34. Irwanto, *Indonesia: Facing Illicit Drug Abuse Challenges*, 44–48.

35. Stephen Flynn, "World Wide Drug Scourge: The Expanding Trade in Illicit Drugs," *The Brookings Review* 11, no. 1 (1993): 6–11.

36. Irwanto, *Indonesia: Facing Illicit Drug Abuse Challenges*, 44–48.

37. Irwanto, *Indonesia: Facing Illicit Drug Abuse Challenges*, 44–48.

38. Chris Lyttleton, "Opiates to Amphetamines: Development and Change in the Golden Triangle," *Development Bulletin* 69 (2006): 22–26.

39. Lyttleton, *Opiates to Amphetamines*, 22–26.

40. Francisco E. Thoumi, *Illegal Drugs, Economy and Society in the Andes* (Washington, DC: Woodrow Wilson Center Press, 2003).

41. Peter Reuter, Justin L. Adams, Susan S. Everingham, Robert Klitgaard, J. T. Quinlivan, K. Jack Riley, Kamil Akramov, Scott Hiromoto, and Sergej Mahnovski, "Mitigating the Effects of Illicit Drugs on Development: Potential Roles for the World Bank." Rand Corporation Project Memorandum Series, PM-1645-PSJ, Prepared for the World Bank, 2004. Accessed October 1, 2010. www.gtz.de/de/dokumente/en-wb-effects-drug-dev-afg.pdf.

42. Nancy Lubin, Alex Klaits, and Igor Barsegian, "Narcotics Interdiction in Afghanistan and Central Asia: Challenges for International Assistance." Report to the Open Society Institute, Open Society Institute (OSI), New York, 2002. Accessed September 24, 2010. www.jezail.org/03_archive/01_narcotics_afgh.pdf.

43. GTZ (Deutsche Gesellschaft für Technische Zusammenarbeit), and ADE (Drugs and Development Programme), *Drugs and Poverty -the Contribution of Development-Oriented Drug Control to Poverty Reduction*. Drugs and Development Programme. Bonn: GTZ, 2003b. Accessed October 1, 2010. www.gtz.de/de/dokumente/en-drugs-poverty-english.pdf.

44. Chris Allen, "Africa & the Drugs Trade." *Review of African Political Economy* 26, no. 79 (1999): 5–11.

45. Alan Dupont, "Transnational Crime, Drugs, and Security in East Asia," *Asian Survey* 39, no. 3 (1999): 433–55.

46. Alex Stephens, Dave Bewley-Taylor, and Pablo Dreyfus, "Drug Markets and Urban Violence: Can Tackling One Reduce the Other." Policy paper no. 15, International Drug Policy Consortium, 2009. Accessed October 28, 2010. www.idpc.net/php-bin/documents/BFDPP_UrbanViolence_EN.pdf.

47. Dave Bewley-Taylor, Chris Hallam, and Rob Allen, "The Incarceration of Drug Offenders: An Overview." Report Sixteen, London: The Beckley Foundation Drug Policy Programme, 2009.

48. Lubin, Klaits, and Barsegian, *Narcotics Interdiction*.

49. Lubin, Klaits, and Barsegian, *Narcotics Interdiction*.

50. INCB (International Narcotics Control Board), *Illicit Drugs and Economic Development* (Vienna: INCB, 2002). Accessed October 6, 2010.www.incb.org/documents/Publications/AnnualReports/AR2002/AR_02_Chapter_I.pdf.

51. Stevens, Bewley-Taylor, and Pablo Dreyfus, *Drug Markets and Urban Violence*.

52. Alan A. Block, "Part Five: Africa," *Crime, Law and Social Change* 36, no. 1 (2001): 241–84.

53. GTZ (Deutsche Gesellschaft für Technische Zusammenarbeit), and ADE (Drugs and Development Programme), *Drugs and Poverty -the Contribution of Development-Oriented Drug Control to Poverty Reduction*. Drugs and Development Programme (Bonn: GTZ, 2003b). Accessed October 1, 2010. www.gtz.de/de/dokumente/en-drugs-poverty-english.pdf.

54. Buxton, *The Political Economy of Narcotics*.

55. ICOS (International Council on Security and Development), *Poppy for Medicine* (London: ICOS, 2007). Accessed September 18, 2010. www.icosgroup.net/modules/poppy_for_medicine.

56. Chuan Yu Chen and Keh Ming Lin, "Health Consequences of Illegal Drug Use," *Current Opinion in Psychiatry* 22, no. 3 (2009): 287.

57. Richard Elliott, Joanne Csete, Evan Wood, and Thomas Kerr, "Harm Reduction, HIV/AIDS, and the Human Rights Challenge to Global Drug Control Policy," *Health and Human Rights* 8, no. 2 (2005): 104–38.

58. UNODC (United Nations Office of Drugs and Crime), *Opium cultivation in South East Asia* (Vienna: UNODC, 2007). Accessed October 19, 2010. www.unodc.org/pdf/research/icmp/south_east_asia_report_2007_web.pdf.

59. Trudi Petersen and David Best, "Overdose: Prevalence, Predictors and Prevention," *Injecting Illicit Drugs* (2005): 149–59.

60. UNODC (United Nations Office of Drugs and Crime), *Drugs and Development* (Vienna: UNODC, 1994). Accessed September 18, 2010. www.unodc.org/pdf/Alternative%20-Development/Drugs_Development.pdf.

61. Merrill Singer, *Drugs and Development: The Global Impact on Sustainable Growth and Human Rights* (Illinois: Waveland Press, 2008).

62. Merrill Singer, "Drugs and Development: The Global Impact of Drug Use and Trafficking on Social and Economic Development," *International Journal of Drug Policy* 19, no. 6 (2008): 467–78.

63. Melis and Nougier, *Drug Policy and Development.*

64. Stanley Baldwin, "Cost Effectiveness of Harm Reduction Interventions in Vietnam." Paper presented at the International Harm Reduction Conference, Bangkok, Thailand, April 20–23, 2009.

65. Singer, *Drugs and Development.*

66. Singer, *Drugs and Development.*

67. INCB (International Narcotics Control Board), *Illicit Drugs and Economic Development* (Vienna: INCB, 2002). Accessed October 6, 2010. www.incb.org/documents/Publications/ AnnualReports/AR2002/AR_02_Chapter_I.pdf.

68. Alan Dupont, Transnational Crime, Drugs, and Security in East Asia," *Asian Survey* 39, no. 3 (1999): 433–55.

69. Francisco E. Thoumi, "Why the Illegal Psychoactive Drugs Industry Grew in Colombia," *Journal of Interamerican Studies and World Affairs* 34, no. 3 (1992): 37–63.

70. La Mond Tullis, *Unintended Consequences: Illegal Drugs and Drug Policies in Nine Countries* (Colorado: Lynne Rienner Publishers, 1995).

71. Buxton, *The Political Economy of Narcotics.*

72. GTZ (Deutsche Gesellschaft für Technische Zusammenarbeit), *Drugs and Conflict.* Drugs and Development Programme (Bonn: GTZ, 2003a). Accessed September 30, 2010. www.gtz.de/de/dokumente/en-drugs-conflict.pdf.

73. Miki Fujimuraand Raju Adhikari, "Critical Evaluation of Cross-Border Infrastructure Projects in Asia," *Development Economics Working Papers* (2010).

74. Lee Nah Hsu, *Building an Alliance with Transport Sector in HIV Vulnerability Reduction* (UNDP Thailand, 2001). Accessed February 21, 2012. www.hivdevelopment.org/ Publications_english/Building%20an%20Alliance.htm.

75. TNI (Transnational Institute), *HIV/AIDS and Drug Use in Burma/Myanmar* (Burma Centrum Nederland: TNI, 2006). Accessed October 19, 2010. www.tni.org/sites/www.tni.org/ files/download/brief17.pdf.

76. Martin Jelsma, Tom Kramer, David Aronson, and Fiona Dove, "Downward Spiral: Banning Opium in Afghanistan and Burma," Transnational Institute (TNI) (Amsterdam: Drugs and Democracy Programme, 2005). Accessed October 19, 2010. www.tni.org/sites/www.tni. org/files/download/debate12.pdf.

77. UNODC (United Nations Office of Drugs and Crime), "Sustaining Opium Reduction in Southeast Asia: Sharing Experience on Alternative Development and Beyond" (Vienna: UNODC, 2010). Accessed October 19, 2010. www.unodc.org/documents/alternative-development/Sustaining_Opium_Reduction_in_South_East_Asia.pdf.

78. Tom Kramer, "From Golden Triangle to Rubber Belt?: The Future of Opium Bans in the Kokang and Wa Regions." Transnational Institute, 2009. Accessed October 19, 2010. www.tni. org/sites/www.tni.org/files/download/brief29.pdf.

79. UNODC (United Nations Office of Drugs and Crime), *Opium cultivation in South East Asia*, 2006 (Vienna: UNODC, 2006). Accessed October 19, 2010. www.unodc.org/pdf/ research/Golden_triangle_2006.pdf.

80. Kramer, *From Golden Triangle to Rubber Belt?*

81. UNODC (United Nations Office of Drugs and Crime), *Mainstreaming Alternative Development in Thailand, Lao PDR and Myanmar: A Process of Learning* (Vienna: UNODC, 2010). Accessed October 19, 2010. www.unodc.org/documents/alternative-development/Final_ Published_version_Mainstreaming_AD.pdf.

82. Tom Kramer, Martin Jelsma, and Tom Blickman, "Withdrawal Symptoms in the Golden Triangle: A Drug Market in Disarray," Drugs and Democracy Programme (Amsterdam: Transnational Institute (TNI), 2009). Accessed October 19, 2010. www.tni.org/sites/www.tni.org/ archives/reports/drugs/pr090109.pdf.

83. UNODC. (United Nations of Drugs and Crime) , *Mainstreaming Alternative Development in Thailand, Lao PDR and Myanmar: A Process of Learning* (Vienna: UNODC , 2010a) . Accessed October 19 2010.
www.unodc.org/documents/alternative-development/-
Final_Published_version_Mainstreaming_AD.pdf.
  84. Kramer, Jelsma, and Blickman, *Withdrawal Symptoms*.
  85. UNODC (United Nations Office of Drugs and Crime), *Morocco Cannabis Survey 2005 Executive Summary* (Vienna: UNODC, 2007). Accessed November 10, 2010.www.unodc.org/pdf/research/Morocco_survey_2005_ex_sum.pdf.
  86. WHO (World Health Organisation), "Assessment of Compulsory Treatment of People who use Drugs in Cambodia, China, Malaysia and Viet Nam: An Application of Selected Human Rights Principles" (Western Pacific Region: WHO, 2009). Accessed September 29, 2010.   www.wpro.who.int/publications/docs/FINALforWeb_Mar17_Compulsory_Treatment.pdf.
  87. Nick Thomson,"Detention as Treatment: Detention of Methamphetamine Users in Cambodia, Laos, and Thailand" (New York: Open Society Institute, 2010).
  88. Integrated Biological and Behavioral Surveillance (IBBS), Data sharing Workshop Hanoi: Vietnam, 2009.
  89. UNAIDS (Joint United Nations Programme on HIV/AIDS). Size Estimation Workshop. Hanoi: Vietnam, 2010.
  90. Chemonics. "Job Market Analysis in Hai Phong and Ho Chi Minh City," (Vietnam: FHI, 2010).
  91. Nhu Nguyen, "The Impact of Methadone on Mental Health, Quality of Life and Social Integration of Injecting Drug users in Vietnam." Paper presented at the National AIDS Conference, Hanoi, Vietnam, 2010.
  92. Although exact numbers are difficult to verify data from Cambodia, Laos and Thailand all indicate that the number of ATS users is likely to be at least ten times the number of injecting opiate users. For more detailed figures see: Thomson N. Detention as Treatment: Detention of Methamphetamine Users in Cambodia, Laos, and Thailand (New York: Open Society Institute, 2010).
  93. Thomson, *Detention as Treatment*.

BIBLIOGRAPHY

Allen, Chris. "Africa & the Drugs Trade." *Review of African Political Economy* 26, no. 79 (1999): 5–11.
Baldwin, Stanley. "Cost Effectiveness of Harm Reduction Interventions in Vietnam." Paper presented at the International Harm Reduction Conference, Bangkok, Thailand, April 20–23, 2009.
Block, Alan A. "Part Five: Africa." *Crime, Law and Social Change* 36, no. 1 (2001): 241–84.
Buxton, Julia. *The Political Economy of Narcotics: Production, Consumption and Global Markets*. Canada: Fernwood Publishing, 2006.
Byrd, William A. "Responding to Afghanistan's Opium Economy Challenge: Lessons and Policy Implications." Policy Research Working Paper 4545, The World Bank, South Asia Region, 2008.
Chemonics. "Job Market Analysis in Hai Phong and Ho Chi Minh City." Vietnam: FHI, 2010.
Chen, Chuan Yu and Keh Ming Lin. "Health Consequences of Illegal Drug Use." *Current Opinion in Psychiatry* 22, no. 3 (2009): 287.
Chouvy, Pierre Arnaud. *Opium: Uncovering the Politics of the Poppy*. Massachusetts: Harvard University Press, 2009.
Chouvy, Pierre Arnaud and Laurent R. Laniel. *Production De Drogue Et Stabilité Des Etats*. Secrétariat Général de la Défense Nationale, 2006.
Dion, Michelle L. and Catherine Russler. "Eradication Efforts, the State, Displacement and Poverty: Explaining Coca Cultivation in Colombia During Plan Colombia." *Journal of Latin American Studies* 40, no. 3 (2008): 399–421.

Dupont, Alan. "Transnational Crime, Drugs, and Security in East Asia." *Asian Survey* 39, no. 3 (1999): 433–55.

Flynn, Stephen. "World Wide Drug Scourge: The Expanding Trade in Illicit Drugs." *The Brookings Review* 11, no. 1 (1993): 6–11.

Fujimura, Miki and Raju Adhikari. "Critical Evaluation of Cross-Border Infrastructure Projects in Asia." *Development Economics Working Papers* 2010.

GTZ (Deutsche Gesellschaft für Technische Zusammenarbeit). *Drugs and Conflict*. Drugs and Development Programme. Bonn: GTZ, 2003a. Accessed September 30, 2010. www.gtz.de/de/dokumente/en-drugs-conflict.pdf.

GTZ (Deutsche Gesellschaft für Technische Zusammenarbeit), and ADE (Drugs and Development Programme). *Drugs and Poverty -the Contribution of Development-Oriented Drug Control to Poverty Reduction*. Drugs and Development Programme. Bonn: GTZ, 2003b. Accessed October 1, 2010. www.gtz.de/de/dokumente/en-drugs-poverty-english.pdf.

Graubner, Cornelius. "Drugs and Conflict-How the Mutual Impact of Illicit Drug Economies and Violent Conflict Influences Sustainable Development, Peace and Stability." Report Commissioned by the German Federal Ministry for Economic Cooperation and Development, GTZ, Eschborn, Germany, 2007.

Hsu, Lee Nah. *Building an Alliance with Transport Sector in HIV Vulnerability Reduction*. UNDP Thailand, 2001. Accessed February 21, 2012. www.hivdevelopment.org/Publications_english/Building%20an%20Alliance.htm.

ICOS (International Council on Security and Development). *Poppy for Medicine*. London: ICOS, 2007. Accessed September 18, 2010. www.icosgroup.net/modules/poppy_for_medicine.

INCB (International Narcotics Control Board). *Illicit Drugs and Economic Development*. Vienna: INCB, 2002. Accessed October 6, 2010. www.incb.org/documents/Publications/AnnualReports/AR2002/AR_02_Chapter_I.pdf.

Inglehart, Ronald, and Christian Welzel. *Modernization, Cultural Change, and Democracy: The Human Development Sequence*. New York: Cambridge University Press, 2005.

Integrated Biological and Behavioral Surveillance (IBBS) Data sharing Workshop, Hanoi: Vietnam, 2009.

Irwanto, Irwanto. "Indonesia: Facing Illicit Drug Abuse Challenges." *Development Bulletin* 69 (2006): 44–48.

Jelsma, Martin, Tom Kramer, David Aronson, and Fiona Dove. "Downward Spiral: Banning Opium in Afghanistan and Burma." Transnational Institute (TNI), Amsterdam: Drugs and Democracy Programme, 2005. Accessed October 19, 2010. www.tni.org/sites/www.tni.org/files/download/debate12.pdf.

Kramer, Tom. "From Golden Triangle to Rubber Belt?: The Future of Opium Bans in the Kokang and Wa Regions." Transnational Institute, 2009. Accessed October 19, 2010. www.tni.org/sites/www.tni.org/files/download/brief29.pdf.

Kramer, Tom, Martin Jelsma, and Tom Blickman. "Withdrawal Symptoms in the Golden Triangle: A Drug Market in Disarray." Drugs and Democracy Programme, Transnational Institute (TNI): Amsterdam 2009. Accessed October 19, 2010. www.tni.org/sites/www.tni.org/archives/reports/drugs/pr090109.pdf.

Lubin, Nancy, Alex Klaits, and Igor Barsegian. "Narcotics Interdiction in Afghanistan and Central Asia: Challenges for International Assistance." Report to the Open Society Institute, Open Society Institute (OSI), New York, 2002. Accessed September 24, 2010. www.jezail.org/03_archive/01_narcotics_afgh.pdf.

Lyttleton, Chris. "Relative Pleasures: Drugs, Development and Modern Dependencies in Asia's Golden Triangle." *Development and Change* 35, no. 5 (2004): 909–35.

Lyttleton, Chris. "Opiates to Amphetamines: Development and Change in the Golden Triangle." *Development Bulletin* 69 (2006): 22–26.

Mannava, Priya., Sasha Zegenhagen., and Nick Crofts. "Dependent on Development: the Inter-relationships between Illicit Drugs and Socioeconomic Development." Melbourne: Nossal Institute for Global Health, 2011.

Melis, Martina and Marie Nougier. "Drug Policy and Development: How Action against Illicit Drugs Impacts on the Millennium Development Goals" International Drug Policy Consor-

tium, London, 2010. Accessed November 1, 2010. http://idpc.net/sites/default/files/library/
Drug%20policy%20and%20development%20briefing.pdf?utm_source=IDPC+Monthly+Al
ert&utm_campaign=5a7b06b62a-IDPC_October_2010_Alert10_27_2010&
utm_medium=email.

Midgley, James. *Social Development: The Developmental Perspective in Social Welfare.* London: Sage, 1995.

Nguyen, Nhu. "The Impact of Methadone on Mental Health, Quality of Life and Social Integration of Injecting Drug users in Vietnam." Paper presented at the National AIDS Conference, Hanoi, Vietnam, 2010.

Petersen, Trudi and David Best. "Overdose: Prevalence, Predictors and Prevention." *Injecting Illicit Drugs* (2005): 149–59.

Rhodes, Tim, Robert Lilly, Cesareo Fernández, Enzo Giorgino, Uwe E. Kemmesis, Hans C. Ossebaard, Nacer Lalam, Imar Faasen, and Karen Ellen Spannow. "Risk Factors Associated with Drug Use: The Importance of Risk Environment." *Drugs: Education, Prevention, and Policy* 10, no. 4 (2003): 303–29.

Singer, Merrill. *Drugs and Development: The Global Impact on Sustainable Growth and Human Rights.* Illinois: Waveland Press Inc., 2008.

Singer, Merrill. "Drugs and Development: The Global Impact of Drug Use and Trafficking on Social and Economic Development." *International Journal of Drug Policy* 19, no. 6 (2008): 467–78.

Soubbotina, Tatyana P. *Beyond Economic Growth: An Introduction to Sustainable Development.* USA: The World Bank, 2004. Accessed October 18, 2012. www.worldbank.org/depweb/english/beyond/global/glossary.html.

Smith, Michael L., Charunee N. Thongtham, Najma Sadeque, Alfredo Molano Bravo, Roger Rumrrill, and Amanda Dávila. *Why People Grow Drugs.* Panos Publications: London, 1992.

Thomson, Nick. "Detention as Treatment: Detention of Methamphetamine Users in Cambodia, Laos, and Thailand." Open Society Institute, New York, 2010.

Thoumi, Francisco E. "Why the Illegal Psychoactive Drugs Industry Grew in Colombia." *Journal of Interamerican Studies and World Affairs* 34, no. 3 (1992): 37–63.

Thoumi, Francisco E. *Illegal Drugs, Economy and Society in the Andes.* Washington, DC: Woodrow Wilson Center Press, 2003.

TNI (Transnational Institute). *HIV/AIDS and drug use in Burma/Myanmar.* Burma Centrum Nederland: TNI, 2006. Accessed October 19, 2010. www.tni.org/sites/www.tni.org/files/download/brief17.pdf.

Tullis, La Mond. *Unintended Consequences: Illegal Drugs and Drug Policies in Nine Countries.* Colorado: Lynne Rienner, 1995

UNAIDS (Joint United Nations Programme on HIV/AIDS). 2010. Size Estimation Workshop. Hanoi: Vietnam.

UNDP (United Nations Development Program). *Taking Narcotics Out of the Conflict-The War on Drugs.* UNDP, 2003. Accessed November 3, 2010.www.pnud.org.co/2003/EnglishVersion/Chapter13.pdf.

UNODC (United Nations Office of Drugs and Crime). *Opium C ultivation in South East Asia .* Vienna: UNODC, 2006. Accessed October 19, 2010. www.unodc.org/pdf/research/Golden_triangle_2006.pdf.

UNODC (United Nations Office of Drugs and Crime). *Morocco Cannabis Survey 2005 Executive Summary.* Vienna: UNODC, 2007. Accessed November 10, 2010. www.unodc.org/pdf/research/Morocco_survey_2005_ex_sum.pdf.

UNODC. (United Nations of Drugs and Crime). *Mainstreaming Alternative Development in Thailand, Lao PDR and Myanmar: A Process of Learning.* Vienna: UNODC , 2010a . Accessed October 19 2010. www.unodc.org/documents/alternative-development/Final_Published_version_Mainstreaming_AD.pdf.

UNODC (United Nations Office of Drugs and Crime). "Sustaining Opium Reduction in Southeast Asia: Sharing Experience on Alternative Development and Beyond." Vienna: UNODC, 2010b. Accessed October 19, 2010. www.unodc.org/documents/alternative-development/Sustaining_Opium_Reduction_in_South_East_Asia.pdf.

UNRISD (United Nations Research Institute for Social Development). "Illicit Drugs: Social Impacts and Policy Responses." UNRISD Briefing Paper No. 2, World Summit For Social Development, 1994. Accessed September 29, 2010. www.unrisd.org/80256B3C005BCCF9/ (httpAuxPages)/4C3D0BE90FAD550480256B6400419B57/$file/bp2.pdf.

WHO (World Health Organisation). "Assessment of Compulsory Treatment of People who use Drugs in Cambodia, China, Malaysia and Viet Nam: An Application of Selected Human Rights Principles." Western Pacific Region: WHO, 2009. Accessed September 29, 2010. www.wpro.who.int/publications/docs/FINALforWeb_Mar17_Compulsory_Treatment.pdf.

Whynes, David. "Illicit Drug Production and Supply-Side Drugs Policy in Asia and South America." *Development and Change* 22, no. 3 (1991): 475–96.

Chapter Seven

The Asian Network of People Who Use Drugs (ANPUD)

*Illicit Drug Policy in Southeast Asia:
The Users' Perspective*

Jimmy Dorabjee, Mohamad Firdaus Zakaria,
and Dean Lewis

The Asian region is home to more than half the total global population. The two largest illicit opium producing regions of the world, the Golden Triangle and Golden Crescent, are located in Asia, ensuring the abundant and widespread availability of opium and its alkaloids, morphine and heroin. Until the mid-1970s, cannabis and opium were the two most commonly used traditional drugs across Asia, predominantly through oral ingestion. The introduction of strict narcotic laws paved the way for the widespread use of heroin through injection that continues till today. In the past two decades Southeast Asia has witnessed an explosive increase in the manufacture and use of Amphetamine-Type Stimulants (ATS) especially among the younger population, and this trend continues to grow unabated.

With an estimated 5.5 million people who inject drugs (PWID) in the Asian region and poor access to even the most basic of harm reduction tools such as sterile syringes and Opioid Substitution Therapy, the sharing of contaminated injecting equipment has played a driving role in the initiation and spread of HIV epidemics in many Asian countries.[1]

Thailand, Malaysia, Myanmar, Nepal, Cambodia, China, Vietnam, and Indonesia continue to document high prevalence of HIV among PWID.

HISTORICAL PERSPECTIVE

Since time immemorial the use of mind-altering substances was common, and countries in the Asian region including Cambodia, Vietnam, Thailand, Laos, China, India, Nepal, Bangladesh, and Pakistan have been traditional consumers of cannabis and opium, with cultural norms restricting the use of cannabis and opium to the adult male population.[2, 3]

In India and Nepal cannabis use has been linked to Hindu religious festivals like Shiv Ratri and Krishna Ashtami—the birth of Lord Krishna and participation in bhajan (religious chanting) sessions. Indeed, occasions like Holi, "the festival of colors," are not complete without the sharing of a traditional offering of bhang—a drink made with crushed cannabis leaves. Opium is also offered at the harvest festival in a ceremony called "akha teej," intended to strengthen family marital clan bonds and put aside old feuds.[4] In rural Myanmar, opium was an integral part of the culture, used in religious festivals and for medicinal purposes.[5]

While the use of opium and cannabis was culturally accepted, traditional forms of opioids gave way to the aggressive marketing of heroin from the Golden Triangle and Golden Crescent regions. The high purity of heroin manufactured in the Southeast Asian region, coupled with the reduced availability of opium, resulted in a switch from oral use of opium to heroin injecting, a more efficient and cost effective mode of drug use.

DRUG CONTROL LAWS AND POLICIES: MORE HARM THAN GOOD

The legal and political environment determines national responses to drug trafficking and use within their borders. The introduction of punitive drug control laws and policies in Asia resulted in a significant decline in the use of culturally sanctioned traditional drugs and the introduction of harder drugs and the injecting of drugs.

In 1976, over three decades ago, Joseph Westermeyer's prophetic paper titled "Pro Heroin Effects of Anti-Opium Laws" alerted us to the unintended negative consequences of law enforcement initiatives that followed the introduction of strict anti-opium laws in Hong Kong, Laos, and Thailand.[6] Westermeyer commented that all three countries followed a pattern that began with government passing and enforcing laws banning the production, sale, and use of opium under pressure from North American, European, and international interests. He noted that within a decade, most of the former opium users in Hong Kong and Thailand had switched to the use of heroin, and all new recruits began with heroin rather than opium. The pattern was striking as not only did it occur in three different locations but also at three different decades, beginning in Hong Kong during the late 1940s and 1950s, in Thailand during the 1960s, and in Laos during the 1970s, suggesting a causal relationship between the strict new narcotic laws and heroin use.

Since then, other Asian countries including Pakistan, Thailand, India, Nepal, China, and Indonesia have enacted tougher anti-narcotics laws under intense pressure from the West and the UN conventions, resulting in the lower availability of traditional drugs such as opium.[7, 8]

The enforcement of the harsh narcotics and drugs laws and stricter control measures over the traditional drugs that were used orally set the stage for the emergence of widespread heroin injecting, followed years later by the large scale use of Amphetamine-Type Stimulants.

For example, India introduced the Narcotic Drugs & Psychotropic Substances (NDPS) Act in 1985. Within a few years, local opium dens and cannabis outlets disappeared, and reports of the widespread smoking of heroin in major metropolitan cities began to appear, with some heroin injecting. A few years later when law enforcement activities reduced the availability of heroin, the injecting of licit buprenorphine and other pharmaceutical drugs such as diazepam, chlorpheneramine maleate, promethazine, pethidine, and dextropropoxyphene began across the country.[9, 10, 11, 12]

While heroin continued to be freely available in the northeastern states of India bordering Myanmar, drug users in metropolitan cities of Delhi, Chennai, and Kolkata started to inject pharmaceuticals such as buprenorphine, often cocktailing with antihistamines and benzodiazepines which were easily available over the counter in chemists.[13]

The evidence suggests that the new legislation exacerbated the problems arising from such structural changes and far from reaching its goal of eradicating drug use, enforcement appears to have inadvertently facilitated a shift to harder drugs and riskier modes of consumption. In Thailand, enforcement policies against opium in the 1970s led to the substitution of opium with injected heroin.[14, 15]

DRUG POLICY: TRADITIONAL RESPONSES TO DRUG USE

With deterrence and punishment the focus of drug policy and abstinence the predominant philosophy of drug dependence treatment in Southeast Asia, the region has seen a proliferation of compulsory drug treatment centers managed by the police, army, or other uniformed services.

Governments in Southeast Asia have responded to illicit drugs by the criminalization of drug use and have adopted particularly harsh policies in response to drug use and trafficking.[16]

Dependent drug users are considered to be criminals and are subjected to disproportionately severe punishments meted out including detention in compulsory centers for extended periods of time. Even where policy changes have mandated that people who use drugs be viewed as patients in need of medical treatment, regular law enforcement crackdowns have continued, highlighting the disconnect between public health and drug control policies and undermining access to harm reduction services.

International and Regional Drug Control Frameworks (see table 7.1) as well as national drug laws prescribe harsh penalties for possession and use of illicit drugs. Several countries in the region including China, Indonesia, Lao PDR, Malaysia, Singapore, Thailand, and Vietnam still retain the death penalty for drug offenses.[17]

A major barrier to the introduction of evidence informed approaches and harm reduction has been the position taken by influential regional bodies such as the Association of South East Asian Nations (ASEAN) declaring the aspiratory goal "*A drug-free Asia by 2015*," and the UNODC's slogans such as "*A drug free world—we can do it*" that have spurred Asian countries to bear down heavily on the use of drugs and conduct a "war on drugs" approach which has translated into a "war on drug users" across the region.

International Drug Control Frameworks	Regional Drug Control Frameworks
The Single Convention on Narcotic Drugs (1961): All practicable measures for the prevention of abuse of drugs and for the early identification, treatment, education, after-care, rehabilitation and social reintegration of the persons involved.	*ASEAN and China Cooperative Operations in Response to Dangerous Drugs (ACCORD): In Pursuit of a Drug-Free ASEAN and China 2015, a plan of action to address both the demand and the supply of drugs.*
The Convention on Psychotropic Substances (1971): Controls over a number of synthetic drugs according to their abuse potential.	*ASEAN Senior Officials on Drug Matters (ASOD): A plan of action for drug control*
The Convention against Illicit Traffic in Narcotic Drugs and Psychotropic Substances (1988): Appropriate measures which include interventions to counteract the social and health consequences of drug dependence.	*Memorandum of Understanding (MOU) on Drug Control: China, Lao PDR, Myanmar, Thailand, Vietnam and Cambodia - a drug control framework that encompasses the Greater Mekong Region China, Indonesia, Malaysia and Philippines (2004)*

Table 7.1. Drug Control Frameworks

The most infamous example of the "war on drugs" occurred in January 2003, when the Thai government of Prime Minister Thaksin Shinawatra announced an aggressive "War on Drugs" aimed at stopping all illicit drug supply and trafficking in Thailand, treating all known drug users and involving communities in monitoring and preventing drug use. Blacklists containing 329,000 names of people supposedly involved in the drug trade were compiled by the police, village heads, and the Office of the Narcotics Control Board. By the end of April 2003, some 2,637 people had been killed, of whom 68 were shot by the police claiming it was in "self-defense."[18] More than 250,000 drug users were treated in health care settings or military type camps. It is ironic that the International Harm Reduction Association's 14th International Conference on the Reduction of Drug Related Harm was held in early April of 2003 in Chiang Mai, Northern Thailand, while this campaign was at its peak.

Compulsory drug treatment centers for people who use illicit drugs currently exist in eleven countries across Asia. Cambodia, China, Indonesia, the Lao People's Democratic Republic, Malaysia, Thailand, and Vietnam operate compulsory drug treatment centers and re-education through labor centers for drug users that are comparable to prison settings.[19]

As a result of the international treaties, drug prohibition continues to dominate national responses to drug use in most countries of the region. With laws effecting harsh penalties for drug-related offenses such as possession and use of illicit drugs, people who use drugs are liable for punishment. Several countries in the region including China, Indonesia, Lao PDR, Malaysia, Singapore, Thailand, and Vietnam still retain the death penalty for drug offenses.[20]

Drug control policies that rely heavily on incarceration are largely underpinned by the concept of deterrence.[21] If the targeted outcomes of coerced treatment involve stable recovery from dependence and the alleviation of burden to public health and safety, rather than social control or punishment, then the effectiveness of the approach has arguably not been adequately demonstrated to date.[22]

People who use drugs are vastly overrepresented in prisons, often accounting for a significant proportion of all inmates; for example, in Vietnam 37 percent of prisoners were people who inject drugs (PWID). HIV has been identified as a major health concern for prisons. Indonesia, Malaysia, and Vietnam reported HIV prevalence levels greater than 10 percent among the general prison populations. In Cai-Yuan City, China, 42 percent of PWID inmates were HIV positive, whereas in Bali, Indonesia, 56 percent of PWID inmates were HIV positive. Evidence for HIV transmission in prison was found for Indonesia and Thailand.[23]

Country	National drug laws	HIV: Legal and policy provisions
Cambodia	*Law on the Control of Drugs in Cambodia 1997, amended 2005* *The new drugs law is at the final draft stage*	*Law on the Prevention and Control of HIV/AIDS, 2002* *National Strategic Plan for a Comprehensive and Multi-sectoral Response to HIV and AIDS 2006–2010* *National Strategic Plan for Illicit Drug Use Related HIV/AIDS 2008-2010* *Policy provision for needle syringe program*
China	*The Regulations on Prohibition Against Narcotics, 1990* *Anti-Drug Law of the People's Republic of China, June 2008 (Narcotics Control Law 2008)*	*Responsive Measures for HIV/AIDS Prevention in Yunnan Province Law, 2004 (legalized NSP)* *Yunnan Provincial HIV/AIDS Prevention and Treatment Regulations, 2006* *Regulations on AIDS Prevention and Treatment, 2006* *Action Plan for reducing and preventing the spread of HIV/AIDS 2006–2010* *Notification on Opioid Dependence Treatment from MOH, Ministry of Public Security, and National Drug and Food Administration in 2006* *Policy provision for needle syringe program* *Policy provision for opioid substitution therapy (methadone maintenance therapy)*
Indonesia	*Law of the Republic of Indonesia No. 22, 1997, on Narcotics*	*The National Strategy Prevention and Control HIV/AIDS and Drugs Abuse* *Indonesian Correction and Detention Policy provision for needle syringe program* *Policy provision for opioid substitution therapy*
Laos	*Lao PDR Law on Drugs (No. 10/NA), 25 December 2007* *National Program Strategy for the Post-Opium Scenario*	*National Strategic and Action Plan on HIV/AIDS/STIs 2006–2010* *No specific HIV laws* *No policy provisions for harm reduction program*

Table 7.2. Key Laws and Policies Related to Drug Use and HIV in Selected Southeast Asian Countries

Malaysia	Drug Dependants Treatment and Rehabilitation Act, 1983	Policy provision for needle syringe program
		Policy provision for opioid substitution therapy
	Dangerous Drugs Act, 1952	Prescribes the death penalty for drug trafficking.
		Corporal punishment and jail for drug possession.
Myanmar	Narcotic Drugs and Psychotropic Substances Law of 1993 (Ministry of Home Affairs, Notification No. 1/1995, Yangon)	National Strategic Plan on HIV/AIDS 2006–2010
		Policy provision for needle syringe programs
		Policy provision for opioid substitution therapy
Thailand	Narcotic Addict Rehabilitation Act, B.E. 2545 (2002)	Policy provision for opioid substitution therapy
Vietnam	Law on Narcotic Drugs Prevention and Suppression (Narcotics Law), 2001 (2008 revision in force January 2009)	HIV Law: Law on HIV/AIDS Prevention and Control, 2007
	Ordinance on Administrative Violations (No. 44/2002/PL-UBTVQH10 of 2 July 2002)	Decree No. 108/2007/ND-CP
		Policy provision for needle syringe program
	Decree on Post Detoxification 2009	Policy provision for opioid substitution therapy

In Thailand a prospective cohort study of inmates in Bangkok's central prison found that HIV incidence in 2001–2002 was 11.1 per 100 person-years among PWID inmates.[24]

CLASSIFICATION OF DRUGS: LEGAL VERSUS "ILLICIT"

The vast majority of the world's population use alcohol and tobacco which are legal drugs and are easily available everywhere while a small proportion use currently illegal drugs. Current policies mean that different drugs are classified disproportionately to their harms.

For example, WHO reported that the extent of psychoactive substance use worldwide was estimated at 2 billion alcohol users, 1.3 billion tobacco smokers, and 185 million drug users in 2002.[25] WHO reported the impact of drugs on the global burden of disease, and tobacco, alcohol, and illicit drugs contributed together 12.4 percent of all deaths worldwide in the year 2000. Mortality (deaths) related to tobacco was 8.8 percent, 3.2 percent for alcohol, and 0.4 percent for all illicit drugs.[26] It is clear that the vast majority of drug related deaths are related to alcohol and tobacco, and yet these are "legal" drugs. How have we come to this situation?

WE REALLY NEED TO RECLASSIFY DIFFERENT DRUGS ON THE BASIS OF THE HARMS THEY CAUSE

Drug Dependence

The Asian Network of People Who Use Drugs (ANPUD) views drug dependence as a health condition that needs long-term treatment. We believe that treatment for drug dependence should be comprehensive, informed by evidence, offered on a voluntary basis, and respectful of human rights. The responsibility for treatment and rehabilitation of drug dependence should lie with health ministries and not anti-drug agencies or home ministries. Law enforcement agencies, which are administered by criminal law, should focus on supply-reduction activities.

Drug dependence is defined as a chronic relapsing and remitting medical condition. People may need many episodes of treatment in order to overcome their dependence. But we have to acknowledge that some people will never be able to lead a drug-free life and keep going through a circle of using drugs, abstinence, and relapse. These people need to be medically managed, similar to the medical management of other chronic diseases such as diabetes or heart disease. Those who have diabetes need to take their medication every day. We don't tell diabetics that you will get medications for one, two, or six months and then you must stop. So why is it that we tend to impose limits and give low doses of medications such as methadone or buprenorphine when we treat people who use illegal drugs?

If people are forced to undergo treatment and they are not yet ready, the chances of relapse are high. People have to be ready for treatment and must want treatment. Putting them in prison, mental hospitals, or drug detention centers demoralizes the person, and they begin to think there is something very wrong with them as they are unable to stop using drugs. Telling them that they are bad, useless, or unworthy because they use drugs does not allow them to maintain their dignity and self-respect. After spending so much time in drug treatment centers or prison, drug users feel left behind. Their friends and colleagues have all moved on in their lives, while they remain stuck in the cycle of drug dependence.

Because of the stigma associated with illegal drugs, they have to hide the fact that they are using. They begin to lead double lives in which they must lie to their families and friends—no, I don't use drugs! Because it is an illegal drug, they cannot go to the wine or cigarette shop and buy their drug just as alcohol and tobacco users do. Life revolves around a vicious cycle: get money for the drug, find the dealer, buy the drug, and then use it. This cycle is repeated every day and often a few times a day. So drug users are very busy and do not have the time and space for other ordinary, everyday things in life.

Once dependent, the person is only concerned about obtaining the drug, and as a result, they neglect to fulfill social or family obligations.

DRUG DETENTION CENTERS

ANPUD is cognizant and aware of the growing number of compulsory drug detention centers in East and Southeast Asia where people who use drugs are forcibly detained for long periods of time. In the guise of drug treatment, these centers violate basic human rights and personal freedom, and people who use drugs are subjected to torture, poor living conditions, forced HIV testing, and forced labor.

ANPUD denounces the forced detention of people who use drugs in the detention centers. We encourage and support any effort to completely abolish these drug detention centers. Until then, we strongly recommend that existing centers implement the full range of services that make up the comprehensive harm reduction package of services.

ANPUD urges all donors and the UN community to monitor and ensure that their resources are not being used for the establishment, maintenance, and operations of such centers. We recommend that those who are currently resourcing these centers immediately stop funding them and instead redirect the resources to evidence-based community-led responses.

ANPUD also urges international agencies responsible for health and drug dependence to immediately evaluate all detention centers in Asia and issue clear guidelines on the minimum standards of drug dependence treatment based on human rights and evidence.

By forcibly incarcerating people who use drugs in these centers the governments are contributing to the prevailing social stigma and discrimination experienced by people who use illicit drugs.

HUMANE AND EFFECTIVE DRUG TREATMENT IS A RIGHT

When people want to stop using drugs and enter treatment but relapse, they are condemned by society and family. It is not a simple matter of exerting will power or that you are a weak person. Over time, drugs such as heroin alter the brain, and the body stops manufacturing the natural painkillers (endorphins) in our body which results in the body demanding the drug from outside. We must not make them feel guilty or ashamed because of this medical condition. It is better to suggest that the person try some other forms of treatment such as methadone or buprenorphine maintenance.

In places where you can get methadone and the clinicians are understanding and supportive, something remarkable begins to happen. Once drug users are taking OST, they begin to stabilize their lives and make other life changes. They no longer are obsessed or have to worry about finding money to buy drugs or fear that the police will arrest them anymore as they are taking a legal prescribed drug. They now live in a safe environment and have more time for other aspects of their lives that has been neglected for so long. They re-engage with family and society and can tell people that they are undergoing treatment and no longer taking drugs. This makes a huge difference in the mental makeup and impacts positively on their life. Self-esteem rises and they begin to perceive themselves as normal citizens. Methadone or buprenorphine are life-saving medicines and should be made available wherever there is a need.

We should not make people feel ashamed to be on methadone. It is just another medicine, and it is so much better than taking illegal heroin. Once on methadone or buprenorphine, they are on the same level as other members of society. OST helps people in a humane way and gives people who use drugs the opportunity to move on in their lives.

Evidence-based good practice and accumulated scientific knowledge on the nature of drug dependence should guide interventions and investments in drug dependence treatment. The high quality of standards required for approval of pharmacological or psychosocial interventions in all the other medical disciplines should be applied to the field of drug dependence.

WE NEED GOOD POLICY NOW

One hundred years ago many of the drugs that are illegal now were legal. The haphazard classification of drugs has had a severe negative impact on the people that use illegal drugs. Many countries have tried to prohibit or ban certain drugs. For example the United States imposed prohibition of alcohol, but found that criminal syndicates took over and began to supply locally brewed alcohol that caused a great deal of harm.

Prohibition didn't stop the use of alcohol, and the decision was reversed and alcohol was legalized again. Similarly, we need to re-examine our policies in our own contexts. In Asia, opium and cannabis have been the traditional drugs used for hundreds of years, and they were never considered a problem. Society imposed social control, and we didn't read or hear of a "drug menace" or problem until opium and cannabis became illegal. The unintended result was that more potent and harmful drugs such as heroin and ATS replaced opium and cannabis in the Asian region.

We have to change the way we are dealing with illicit drugs because it affects all of us—our brothers and sisters, parents, friends, children—everyone is affected.

NOTES

1. Bradley M. Maters, Louisa Degenhardt, Hammad Ali, Lucas Wiessing, Matthew Hickman, Richard P. Mattick, Bronwyn Myers, Atul Ambekar, and Steffanie A. Strathdee, "HIV Prevention, Treatment and Care for People who Inject Drugs: A Systematic Review of Global, Regional and Country Level Coverage," *Lancet* 375, no. 9719 (2010): 1014–28.

2. Molly Charles, David Bewley-Taylor, and Amanda Neidpath, "Drug Policy in India: Compounding Harm?" Briefing Paper Ten, The Beckley Foundation Drug Policy Programme (Beckley, Oxford, 2005). www.beckleyfoundation.org/pdf/BriefingPaper_10.pdf.

3. WHO-SEARO (World Health Organization South East Asia Region). *Regional Health Forum* 5, no. 1 (India: WHO-SEARO, 2001).

4. WHO-SEARO, *Regional Health Forum.*

5. UNAIDS/UNODC (Joint United Nations Programme on HIV/AIDS/United Nations Office for Drugs and Crime), *Drug Use and HIV Vulnerability: Policy Research Study in Asia, Task Force on Drug Use and HIV Vulnerability* (Bangkok: UNAIDS/UNODC, 2000).

6. Joseph Westermeyer, "The Pro-Heroin Effects of Anti-Opium Laws," *Archives of General Psychiatry* 33 (1976): 1135–39.

7. Alfred W. McCoy, *The Politics of Heroin: CIA Complicity in the Global Drug Trade* (New York: Lawrence Hill Books, 1991).

8. Charles, Bewley-Taylor, and Neidpath, *Drug Policy in India.*

9. Kumar, M. S. and D. Daniels, "HIV Risk Reduction Strategies among IDU's in Madras" (New Delhi, India: CARITAS India, 1994).

10. Jimmy Dorabjee and Luke Samson, "Self and Community-Based Opioid Substitution among Opioid Dependent Populations in the Indian Sub-continent," *International Journal of Drug Policy* 9 (1998): 411–16.

11. A. Bharadwaj, "Self-Injecting of Drugs Gains Popularity in Punjab," *Times of India,* July 1, 1995.

12. S. Biswas, "Hooked to a New High," *India Today,* April 1994.

13. Dorabjee and Samson, *Self and Community-Based Opioid Substitution,* 411–16.

14. McCoy, *The Politics of Heroin.*

15. Westermeyer, *The Pro-Heroin Effects,* 1135–39.

16. WHO-WPRO (World Health Organization Western Pacific Regional Office), *Assessment of Compulsory Treatment of People who use Drugs in Cambodia, China, Malaysia and Viet Nam: an Application of Selected Human Rights Principles* (Manila: WHO WPRO, 2009).

17. HAARP (HIV/AIDS Asia Regional Program), *Law and Policy Review* (HAARP, 2009). www.unodc.org/documents/eastasiaandpacific/topics/hiv-aids/HAARP_Law_and_Policy_Review.pdf.

18. Saksith Saiyasombut and Siam Voices, "Resurrecting Thailand's Brutal 'War on Drugs,'" *Asian Correspondent,* March 10, 2011. http://asiancorrespondent.com/49966/the-war-on-drugs-pheu-thais-democratic-deficit/.

19. WHO-WPRO, *Assessment of Compulsory Treatment.*

20. HAARP, *Law and Policy Review.*

21. Dave Bewley-Taylor, Chris Hallam, and Rob Allen, "The Incarceration of Drug Offenders: an Overview." The Beckley Foundation Drug Policy Program, Report Sixteen, March 2009.

22. Karen A. Urbanoski, "Coerced Addiction Treatment: Client Perspectives and the Implications of their Neglect," *Harm Reduction Journal* 7 (2010): 13–22.

23. Kate Dolan, Ben Kite, Emma Black, Carmen Aceijas, and Gerry V. Stimson, "HIV in Prison in Low-income and Middle-income Countries," *Lancet Infectious Diseases* 7 (2007): 32–41.

24. Hansa Thaisri, John Lerwitworapong, Suthon Vongsheree, Pathom Sawanpanyalert, Chanchai Chadbanchachai, Archawin Rojanawiwat, Wichuda Kongpromsook, Wiroj Paungtubtim, Pongnuwat Sri-Ngam, and Rachaneekom Jaisue, "HIV Infection and Risk Factors among Bangkok Prisoners, Thailand: A Prospective Cohort Study," *BMC Infectious Diseases* 3 (2003): 25.

25. WHO/UNDCP (World Health Organization/UN Drug Control Programme), *Global Initiative on Primary Prevention of Substance Abuse: Overall Evaluation: Baseline Assessment Guidelines and Instruments* (Geneva/Vienna: WHO/UNDCP, 2002).

26. WHO (World Health Organization), "Management of Substance Abuse: The Global Burden." Accessed September 11, 2012. www.who.int/substance_abuse/facts/global_burden/en/index.html.

BIBLIOGRAPHY

Bharadwaj, A. "Self-Injecting of Drugs Gains Popularity in Punjab." *Times of India*, July 1, 1995.

Bewley-Taylor, Dave, Chris Hallam, and Rob Allen. "The Incarceration of Drug Offenders: an Overview." The Beckley Foundation Drug Policy Program, Report Sixteen, March 2009.

Biswas, S. "Hooked to a New High." *India Today*, April 1994.

Charles, Molly, David Bewley-Taylor, and Amanda Neidpath. "Drug Policy in India: Compounding Harm?" Briefing Paper Ten, The Beckley Foundation Drug Policy Programme. Beckley, Oxford, 2005. www.beckleyfoundation.org/pdf/BriefingPaper_10.pdf.

Dolan, Kate, Ben Kite, Emma Black, Carmen Aceijas, and Gerry V. Stimson. HIV in Prison in Low-income and Middle-income Countries." *Lancet Infectious Diseases* 7 (2007): 32–41.

Dorabjee, Jimmy and Luke Samson. "Self and Community-Based Opioid Substitution among Opioid Dependent Populations in the Indian Sub-continent." *International Journal of Drug Policy* 9 (1998): 411–16.

HAARP (HIV/AIDS Asia Regional Program). *Law and Policy Review*. HAARP, 2009. www.unodc.org/documents/eastasiaandpacific/topics/hiv-aids/HAARP_Law_and_Policy_Review.pdf.

Kumar, M. S. and D. Daniels. "HIV Risk Reduction Strategies among IDU's in Madras." CARITAS India, New Delhi, India, 1994.

Mathers, Bradley M., Louisa Degenhardt, Hammad Ali, Lucas Wiessing, Matthew Hickman., Richard P. Mattick, Bronwyn Myers, Atul Ambekar, and Steffanie A. Strathdee. "HIV Prevention, Treatment and Care for People who Inject Drugs: A Systematic Review of Global, Regional and Country Level Coverage." *Lancet* 375, no. 9719 (2010): 1014–28.

McCoy, Alfred W. *The Politics of Heroin: CIA Complicity in the Global Drug Trade*. New York: Lawrence Hill Books, 1991.

Saiyasombut, Saksith and Siam Voices. "Resurrecting Thailand's Brutal 'War on Drugs.'" Asian Correspondent , March 10, 2011. http://asiancorrespondent.com/49966/the-war-on-drugs-pheu-thais-democratic-deficit/.

Thaisri, Hansa, John Lerwitworapong, Suthon Vongsheree, Pathom Sawanpanyalert, Chanchai Chadbanchachai, Archawin Rojanawiwat, Wichuda Kongpromsook, Wiroj Paungtubtim, Pongnuwat Sri-Ngam, and Rachaneekom Jaisue. "HIV infection and risk factors among Bangkok Prisoners, Thailand: a Prospective Cohort Study." *BMC Infectious Diseases* 3 (2003): 25.

UNAIDS/UNODC. (Joint United Nations Programme on HIV/AIDS/United Nations Office for Drugs and Crime). *Drug Use and HIV Vulnerability: Policy Research Study in Asia, Task Force on Drug Use and HIV Vulnerability*. Bangkok: UNAIDS/UNODC, 2000.

Urbanoski, Karen A. "Coerced Addiction Treatment: Client Perspectives and the Implications of their Neglect." *Harm Reduction Journal* 7 (2010): 13–22.

Westermeyer, Joseph. "The Pro-Heroin Effects of Anti-Opium Laws." *Archives of General Psychiatry* 33 (1976): 1135–39.

WHO (World Health Organization). "Management of Substance Abuse: The Global Burden." Accessed September 11, 2012. www.who.int/substance_abuse/facts/global_burden/en/index.html.

WHO-SEARO (World Health Organization South East Asia Region). *Regional Health Forum* 5, no. 1. India: WHO-SEARO, 2001.

WHO/UNDCP (World Health Organization/UN Drug Control Programme). *Global Initiative on Primary Prevention of Substance Abuse: Overall Evaluation: Baseline Assessment Guidelines and Instruments.* Geneva/Vienna: WHO/UNDCP, 2002.

WHO-WPRO (World Health Organization Western Pacific Regional Office). *Assessment of Compulsory Treatment of People who use Drugs in Cambodia, China, Malaysia and Viet Nam: an Application of Selected Human Rights Principles.* Manila: WHO WPRO, 2009.

Chapter Eight

Harm Reduction: The Islamic Perspective

Faisal Ibrahim

A MALAYSIAN EXPERIENCE

Malaysia is one of the many countries whose HIV epidemic has been driven by injecting drug use and continues to suffer the devastating psychosocial and economic consequences associated with the drug-use-related HIV epidemic.

The HIV profile in Malaysia is predominantly male injecting drug users of Muslim Malay ethnicity.[1] However, it has been worryingly noted that women and girls are increasingly getting infected with HIV. They amount to 21 percent of newly infected persons in 2011 compared to being barely 5 percent ten years ago.[2] By age group, 79 percent of the reported cases are young people in their prime productive years (twenty to thirty-nine years). There are rising concerns that the trend of HIV transmission is significantly changing from only one sexual transmission for every nine associated with IDU in 1990, to five sexual transmissions for every five associated with IDU in 2010.[3] It is estimated that Malaysia has about four thousand AIDS orphans whose parents were most likely HIV-infected drug users.[4] The prevalence of HIV among injecting drug users in Malaysia is currently 22.1 percent.[5]

A study conducted by Ministry of Health among 6,326 inmates of twenty-six "Drug Rehabilitation Centers" revealed that 64.6 percent of the drug users were injecting drugs, 77 percent of whom admitted they injected drugs more than three times per day, and ever or always shared needles with more than five others.[6] 28 percent of the injecting drug users were confirmed HIV positive, and almost two-thirds of them were sexually active while 25 percent were married. These injecting drug users practiced dual risk behaviors, but only 19 percent of them used a condom during sexual intercourse. The study also found that the risk of getting HIV infection among IDUs is six times higher than among non-IDUs, while the risk of being infected with HIV among those sharing needles is seven times higher than among those who don't share needles.

THE RESPONSE

In response to the above evidence of an HIV epidemic driven by injecting drug use, the main concern of Muslim policymakers in the country was principally focused on proliferating Muslim ideals, namely abstinence from illicit drug and sexual practices. Sexuality, considered a private matter, was and continues to be a taboo topic for discussion. In Muslim culture, social stigma arising from religious doctrine on premarital sex and drug use prevents those at risk from coming forward for appropriate counseling, testing, and treatment. Harm reduction, as an evidence-based, pragmatic approach for curbing the spread of HIV infection among persons who use drugs, has in the past been misconstrued and misconceptualized away from Islamic principles. It has been perceived as a way of encouraging and condoning further drug use and promoting sexual promiscuity. However, a paradigm shift occurred in 2006 when the National Islamic authority was sensitized and convinced that harm reduction was a necessity in order to reverse and halt the HIV epidemic in the country.

HARM REDUCTION

Harm reduction (or *harm minimization*) is a pragmatic approach that aims to reduce risks to the individual and the community associated with recreational drug use and some often stigmatized, antisocial, or illegal behaviors. The perspective of harm reduction, developed primarily from work on AIDS and drug problems in the Netherlands and United Kingdom,[7, 8] is a pragmatic approach to the social and individual problems associated with the misuse of psychoactive drugs. Harm reduction is put forward as a useful perspective alongside the more conventional approaches of demand and supply reduction.

In public health terms, the term *harm reduction* is used to describe a concept aimed at preventing or reducing negative health consequences associated with certain behaviors, without *necessarily* reducing those behaviors. In relation to HIV and injecting drug use, harm reduction aims at preventing the transmission of HIV and other infections that occur through the most notorious dual risk behaviors of drug users—that is, sharing needles while injecting drugs and practicing unsafe sex. Harm reduction takes a morally neutral stance to drug use, neither condoning nor opposing drug use. It focuses on actual harm and assumes that some people will continue to inject drugs despite government repression and therefore they should be given the possibility to do so in a way that reduces the risks and causes least harm to themselves and others.

Operationally, harm reduction is about making hazardous behavior less hazardous. It is about improving and saving lives. Harm reduction is comprehensive actions that encompasses not just the provision of sterile needles and syringes through needle and syringe exchange programs (NSEP) and drug substitution therapy, but equally important the provision of information, education and communication (IEC) on drug injecting and HIV/AIDS, appropriate and adequate psycho-spiritual counseling, supervised care, life-skill training, and behavioral change services (see Lee et al. in this book).

THE ISLAMIC PERSPECTIVE OF "HARM REDUCTION"

Understanding and internalizing the Islamic perspective of harm reduction is crucial as any supportive response from Islamic authorities and groups will depend solely on the Islamic "Sharia" justification for this program, which essentially should not go against textual evidence (Holy Quran and sunnah). Basically, the Sharia justification of harm reduction program can be based on some of the following fundamentals:

1. The Purpose of Islamic Sharia Makasid Al-Shariah (مقاصد الشريعة) stipulates protection of human body, soul, and mind. The five purposes of shariah are: Protection of Religion (Deen), Life (Nafs), Progeny (Nasl), Mind (Aql), and Wealth (Mal). These five fundamental purposes provide a holistic relationship to preserve the sanctity, dignity, and safety of mankind. Collectively, they have close relationships with the concept of combating an extensive range of psycho-social dilemmas that face humankind, including HIV/AIDS. Thus the concept of improving and saving lives, in the harm reduction approach, is sensibly applicable to the legitimate purposes of Makasid Al-Shariah.

2. Darura (ضرورة) or necessity is also among the principles of Islamic Shariah, stipulating that *necessities permit the prohibitions* (الضرورات تبيح المحظورات). The application of necessity is not only expanded to protect the necessity of an individual person but to protect the necessity of the public at large. Darura concentrates on the removal of hardship which would result in the loss or a great harm to any of these five "Sharia" fundamentals. In line with this notion, the harm reduction approach is justified from the Sharia perspective, based on the

reality that the HIV epidemic in the country is heavily and continuous-
ly driven by large populations of drug users, and hence adopting the
harm reduction approach is deemed crucial to the public at large and
most importantly to protect the life and the health of the concerned
drug users. However, it should be noted that the objectives of Sharia
law are not only to protect human necessities but also human interest,
as long as the interests do not conflict with the textual evidence (Holy
Quran and Hadith).

3. "Rafu'al-Haraj" (رفع الحرج145) or "lifting a burden" that operates to
    prevent a Muslim being harmed, is a basic notion in Islamic law that
    denies heavy burdens on the Muslim. In harm reduction, the main goal
    is to prevent the individual from being further burdened with a fatal
    HIV infection while he is already heavily drained by drug addiction.

4. "Rukhsah" (رخصة) refers to all cases of need or necessity. The defini-
    tion includes all types of legal dispensation regardless of the degree of
    harm, which could imply that drug users who are at high risk of being
    infected or infecting others with HIV might be allowed to acquire their
    own clean needles and syringes. Obviously, this special consideration
    needs to be linked with all the initiatives that the program provides.

5. The principle of harm in Islam (*darar or* ضرر) asserts that no one
    should be hurt or cause hurt to others. This principle has been affirmed
    by Prophet Muhammad (PBUH) in his "Hadith" that states: (لاضرر
    ولاضرار *or No damage and to damage*), in an attempt to reiterate that a
    damage that has occurred should not lead to further damages. A legal
    rule in Islam gives the provision that "a lesser harm may be tolerated
    in order to avoid a greater harm (*the rule of* أخف الضررين)." The basis
    of the harm reduction approach is that it is of greater harm for the
    entire community to allow more injecting drug users to be infected
    with HIV/AIDS.

6. Right to professional counseling: counseling is part and parcel of harm
    reduction programs. From the Islamic perspective, Prophet Muham-
    mad (PBUH) encourages Muslims to sincerely advise each other as is
    evident from his Hadith: Al-Din al-Nasihah (Religion is sincere ad-
    vice).

Sunan Abi Dawud, op. cit. Kitab al-Adab. Hadith no. 59

However, such counseling should not be restricted to making them cope with
the disease, but should also include an element of Islamic ethos. Fundamentally counseling is seen as a matter of inspiring hope and positive thinking.
The Glorious Quran testifies:

Say: O my servants who have transgressed against their souls! Despair not of the Mercy of Allah for Allah forgives all sins for He is Oft Forgiving, Most Merciful.

"Turn you to your Lord in repentance and submit to Him before the chastisement comes on you, after that you shall not be helped."

The Glorious Quran, chapter 39, verses 53–54

1. *Right to be treated*; Therapeutically, there is clear Islamic guidance to seek remedy and cure from all ailments:

Seek cure, for Allah has not established a disease without establishing its cure.
Narrated by Ahmad. Sahih Ibni Hibban no. 1219, Ibni Majah Al-Sunan, no. 2045

Drug users as well as HIV/AIDS patients cannot be refused access to medical care. They should therefore be given both moral and financial support to be in a position to gain access to required medication. This can be inferred from the following Hadith: The believers, in their love and sympathy for one another are like one body; when one part of it is affected with pain, the whole of it responds in terms of wakefulness and fever.
Al-Nawawi, Abu Zakariya Muhyi al-Din Yahya. 1992. Nuzhat al-Mutaqqin Sharh Riyad al-Salihin. vol. 1. Hadith no. 226, p. 199

CONCLUSION

The most prominent feature of the HIV epidemic in Malaysia is its far-reaching spread among injecting drug users, and a substantial proportion of HIV infection in Malaysia is occurring within the Malay community, of which the majority are Muslims. It is therefore crucial that any approach to effectively reverse and halt the epidemic in the country should be based on the most pragmatic approach which has been proven successful, while still adhering to the fundamental principles of Islam.

Like most religions, Islam condemns homosexuality, drug use, and sex outside of marriage. Though the most important means of protection is obviously abstinence from sex and to remain faithful to the marriage partner, however, Muslims must recognize that in many instances there is a gap between religious teaching and practice—that is between reality and morality; risky behaviors that may not be allowed by Islam are indeed practiced. Validating the Islamic justification of the harm reduction approach could be one of the possible pathways to bridge this gap.

NOTES

1. MOH (Ministry of Health Malaysia). Annual Report (Putrajaya: AIDS STD Unit, 2010).

2. MOH (Ministry of Health Malaysia). Country Progress Report (Putrajaya: AIDS STD Unit, 2012).

3. MOH, Annual Report.

4. MOH, Annual Report.

5. MOH, Country Progress Report.

6. Zainuddin Abd Wahab,"Risk Behavior of Drug Users at Drug Rehabilitation Centres." Report, AIDS STD Unit (Kuala Lumpur: Ministry of Health, 1998).

7. Alan G. Marlatt, Mary E. Latimer, and Katie Witkiewitz, *Harm Reduction, Pragmatic Strategies for Managing High Risk Behaviours* (New York: Guildford Press, 2012).

8. James A. Inciardi and Lana D. Harrison, *Harm Reduction: National and International Perspectives* (Thousand Oaks, CA: Sage, 2000).

BIBLIOGRAPHY

Abd Wahab, Zainuddin. "Risk Behavior of Drug Users at Drug Rehabilitation Centres." Report, AIDS STD Unit, Ministry of Health, Kuala Lumpur, 1998.

Inciardi, James A. and Lana D. Harrison. *Harm Reduction: National and International Perspectives*. Thousand Oaks, CA: Sage, 2000.

Marlatt, G. Alan, Mary E. Latimer, and Katie Witkiewitz. *Harm Reduction, Pragmatic Strategies for Managing High Risk Behaviours*. New York: Guildford Press, 2012.

MOH (Ministry of Health Malaysia). Annual Report. Putrajaya: AIDS STD Unit MOH, 2010.

MOH (Ministry of Health Malaysia). Country Progress Report. Putrajaya: AIDS STD Unit, 2012.

Chapter Nine

Epidemiology of HIV and HCV among People Who Inject Drugs in Southeast Asia

Don C. Des Jarlais, Jonathan Freelemyer, Heidi Bramson,[1] and Holly Hagan[2]

The transmission of HIV among people who inject drugs (PWID) in Asia reflects the convergence of a truly international set of factors. Asia has a long, colorful, and often painful history of opiate use, including "Opium Wars" over the control of the highly profitable trade in the drug market.[3, 4] The hypodermic needle and syringe, which provides for a very intense, relatively low-cost opiate drug experience was independently invented by a Scottish (Alexander Wood) and a French physician (Gabriel Pravaz).[5, 6] Heroin was first synthesized from morphine by an English chemist (Charles Romley Alder Wright)[7, 8] and first marketed by a German chemical firm (Bayer).[9] The injection of illicit heroin first became a major social problem in the United States, particularly in New York City.[10] And, of course, HIV, the most lethal virus that is spread through the injection of illicit drugs, evolved in Africa.[11, 12] But it has been the globalization of the international traffic in illicit drugs that has spread HIV to people who inject drugs throughout the world.

1. GLOBALIZATION OF ILLICIT DRUG INJECTION

The recent report of the global epidemiology of injecting drug use identifies the presence of injecting drug use in 148 countries[13] and documents the worrisome extent to which it is spreading throughout the world. Figures 9.1 and 9.2 show the distribution of the estimated sixteen million IDUs through-

113

out the world. The great majority of PWID live in low/middle-income countries (LMICs); the three countries with the largest numbers of PWID—at least 1,000,000 in each country—are China, Russia, and the United States.

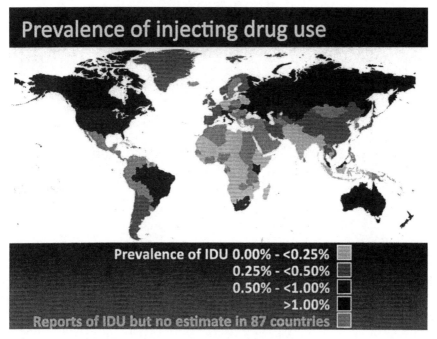

Figure 9.1.   Prevalence of Injecting Drug Use by Country

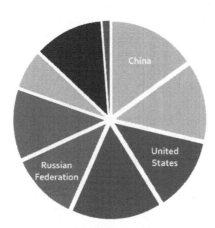

Figure 9.2.   Distribution of People Who Inject Drugs by Geographic Location

High numbers of PWID have now been reported in countries with previously unknown or low rates of injecting drug use. Among the former Soviet Republics, previous estimates were 20,000 PWID in Azerbaijan and 12,000 DWID in Georgia[14] while current estimates, based on more systematic methods, are 300,000 and 127,000 respectively.[15]

The spread of injecting drug use is best understood as an aspect of the globalization of the world economy. The same improvements in transportation and communication, and reductions in barriers to the flow of capital, and economies of scale[16] that have led to the large increases in trade in licit goods have also led to increases in trade of illicit goods. The annual value of the trade in illicit drugs is estimated to be $320 billion.[17] This figure is larger than the gross domestic product of most of the countries in the world.

Law enforcement efforts have not been able to stem the increased distribution of illicit drugs. Indeed, one of the effects of successful law enforcement may paradoxically lead to increased diffusion of illicit drugs. Law enforcement efforts may partially disrupt an established international drug distribution route, but this will not permanently stop the flow of drugs. Rather, a new distribution route will be developed that will often lead to the development of new local drug markets in the areas along the new distribution route. Thus, the local markets along the old distribution route will remain (though possibly at smaller volume) and new local markets will be developed along the new route.

Given the economics of the trade in illicit drugs—low production costs, low transportation costs, large economies of scale, and very high profit margins—it is unlikely that this trade can be eliminated. Public health officials need to plan their activities with the assumption that the international trade in illicit drugs will continue.

2. HIV AMONG PWID: GLOBAL EPIDEMIOLOGY

During the last several decades, HIV infection among PWID has become a worldwide public-health problem. According to the most recent estimate, HIV has been reported in 120 of the 151 countries in which injecting drug use occurs.[18] Figures 9.1 and 9.2 show the distribution of the estimated sixteen million PWID throughout the world. The great majority of PWID live in LMICs. With respect to Asia, China clearly has the largest estimated number of PWID, with over one million.

HIV prevalence among PWID varies greatly among the different countries, from less than 1 percent to more than 72 percent, and an estimated three million of the sixteen million PWID in the world are infected with HIV (see figure 9.3). Approximately 10 percent of all new HIV infections worldwide are among PWID, and approximately 30 percent of all new HIV infections outside of sub-Saharan Africa are among PWID.[19]

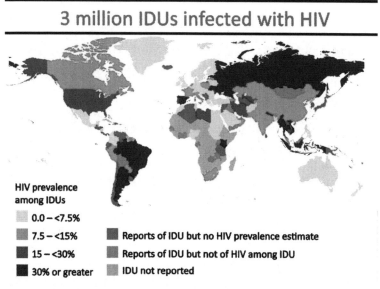

Figure 9.3.   Global HIV prevalence among PWID

The countries of Southeast Asia generally have high rates of HIV prevalence among PWID, from 15 percent to 30 percent or higher than other locations in the world. Indeed Southeast Asian countries, along with Eastern Europe and Central Asia, tend to have among the highest HIV seroprevalence rates among PWID of any regions in the world.

3. GLOBAL ANALYSIS OF HIV AMONG ETHNIC MINORITY GROUPS

In many different countries, substantial proportions of PWID belong to ethnic minority groups. Ethnic minority group members are more likely to be infected with HIV than are ethnic majority group members who inject drugs. A recent systematic review and meta-analysis of the international data on HIV prevalence among minority group PWID compared to ethnic majority group PWID found that on average, minority group members were twice as likely to be HIV seropositive than were ethnic majority group members (Pooled weighted odds ratio = 2.09, 95 percent CI 1.92–2.28).[20] There was great heterogeneity in the comparisons of prevalence among minority to majority group PWID (I^2 = 75.3 percent). The disparity in HIV prevalence, with ethnic minority PWID more likely to be HIV seropositive, was notable in the United States (pooled weighted OR = 2.22, 95 percent CI 2.03–2.44).

There are a number of studies showing high rates of ethnic disparities in HIV prevalence among PWID in China. These disparities were found in various provinces and for various ethnic minorities PWID compared to ethnic majority (Han) PWID. In 2002, Des Jarlais et al., found in Ning Ming County, Guangxi Province, ethnic minorities primarily of Zhuang ethnicity had a HIV prevalence rate of 19 percent compared to 10 percent of the Han majority.[21] Ruan et al.,[22] also found in 2002 in Xichang County, Lianshan Yi Autonomous Prefecture of Sichuan Province, ethnic minorities mostly of Yi descent had an HIV prevalence of 17 percent versus 8 percent prevalence among Han PWID.[23] Additionally, Ruan et al. found incidence rates from data collected during 2002–2005 in Xichang City, Sichuan Province to show ethnic minorities had an HIV incidence rate of 6.5 per 100 person years (95 percent CI 1.1–3.5), RR 7.6 (95 percent CI: 2.4–24.3; p < 0.001), while the Han majority had an incidence rate of 0.9 per 100 person years.

In studies that reported odds ratios, the same pattern of higher HIV prevalence among ethnic minorities was observed, though the odds ratios were not always statistically significant. In 1994, Xia et al., found the Dai minority to have an OR of 1.7 (95 percent CI: 0.04–7.0; p = 0.5) when compared to the Han majority and other ethnic minorities (Jinpo and De'ang) combined.[24] In 2002, Hammett et al. found ethnic minority PWID (defined as non-Han) to be approximately twice as likely as Han PWID of acquiring HIV, OR 2.2 (CI 1.00–5.00; p = 0.050).[25]

Data collected more recently also demonstrates this risk: 2004 data from Xichang City collected by Yin et al., show the Han majority to be at decreased risk of HIV, OR 0.7 (0.4–1.2; p = 0.220) when compared to Yi and other minorities;[26] 2005 data from Urumqui, Xinjiang Province shows the Uighur minority to be at increased risk of HIV, OR 5.9 (CI 3.2–11.1) compared to Han PWID;[27] 2007 data from Kaiyuan, Yunnan Province shows the Han majority to be at decreased risk of HIV, OR 0.7 (0.4–1.2; p = 0.220) compared to ethnic minority PWID.[28]

Although there were fewer studies from other parts of Asia, ethnic disparities have been reported in other countries such as Thailand. Data collected by Perngmark et al., from 1999 to 2000 in numerous provinces throughout southern Thailand found Malaysian PWID to have an HIV prevalence of 64 percent compared to 43 percent of Thai PWID.[29]

As noted above there is great heterogeneity among the ethnic minority/ethnic majority comparisons, including many studies in which there were not significant differences in HIV prevalence between ethnic minority and ethnic majority PWID. For example, in data collected from 2006–2007 in Malaysia by Vicknasingam, et al., there were minimal difference in HIV prevalence between majority Malays and ethnic minorities (comprised of Chinese, Indian, and undefined others). Malays had a RR of 1.06 (CI 0.82–1.37), compared with combined ethnic minorities.[30]

The reasons for these ethnic disparities (and lack of disparities) in HIV prevalence have not been determined, and the causes are likely to be complex rather than single simple causes. One hypothesis that may apply to both the United States and to China, is that drug distribution routes often go through ethnic minority communities, placing those PWID communities at higher risk for HIV infection. Regardless of the causes of the ethnic disparities in HIV infection among PWID, the existence of the disparities can lead to multiple problems, including multiple stigmatization (based on injecting drug use, on risk for HIV and on ethnic minority status) and greater likelihood of sexual transmission from PWID to persons who do not inject drugs in minority communities. A human rights approach to reducing HIV among PWID will need to address these ethnic disparities.

4. HCV EPIDEMIOLOGY FOR SOUTHEAST ASIA

Phylogeographic analysis of HCV in Southeast Asia suggests that endemic genotype 6 strains have been present for perhaps 1,000 years.[31] Unique genotype 6 lineages are historically associated with different locations (for example, 6f in Thailand, 6g in Indonesia, 6d in Vietnam, and 6q in Cambodia). Endemic HCV transmission prior to the introduction of medical injections in the early twentieth century and the spread of injection drug use in the region in the later part of the century is not fully understood. Surveys of PWID indicate more recent introduction of genotypes 1b, 3a and 3b in the region.[32] In the border region near the Golden Triangle there is greater genetic diversity with multiple subtypes of genotype 6,[33] which has been attributed to the a high degree of ethnic diversity, high rates of drug transshipment, and the large and steady influx of migrants to the region.

To characterize the epidemiology of HCV infection in PWID in Southeast Asia, we analyzed data from the HCV Synthesis Project, a global systematic review and meta-analysis of HCV epidemiology and prevention in PWID.[34] The methods have been described in detail elsewhere.[35] To update these data, we searched for more recent publications using the same HCV Synthesis Project search string, and examined the reference list and tables from a systematic review of the global burden of HCV in PWID.[36] As shown in table 9.1, HCV prevalence estimates are available from nine countries (Burma, China, Indonesia, Malaysia, the Philippines, Singapore, Taiwan, Thailand, and Vietnam). No data were found for Cambodia or Laos.

Location	Author, Year	Enrollment Dates	Recruitment Setting	Chars of sample	N IDUs	% HCV+	% HIV+	% HBV+	HCV incidence
BURMA									
China-Burma border region	Zhou YH et al., 2011 [i]	2009	"community"	31.8 yra = median age; 96.5% male	318				
CHINA									
Dehong and Lincang Districts	Baozhing, T et al., 1997	unspecified	Street outreach		88	51.1%	55.7%		
Yunnan Province	Cao, K et al., 1999 [ii]	unspecified	Correctional	26.7 yrs=mean age; 81.7% male	158	86.0%	21.5%	80.0%	
Pingxiang and Binyang	Garten, RJ et al., 2003 [iii]	1999–2000	Street outreach	median IDU duration 2.3 yrs	485	82.9%	19.6%	58.5%	52.6/100PY
Guangxi Province	Lai, S et al., 2001 [iv]	1998	Public Health Clinic		278	68.0%			
Yunnan Province	Li, D et al., 1994 [v]	unspecified	unspecified		507	94.9%	66.7%		
Anhui Province	Liu, H et al., 2006 [vi]	2003	Drug Treatment Center	61.5% male	226	63.3%			

Table 9.1. HCV Infection Rates in Southeast Asia

Location	Author, Year	Enrollment Dates	Recruitment Setting	Chars of sample	N IDUs	% HCV+	% HIV+	% HBV+	HCV incidence
Sichuan Province	Ruan, Y et al., 2004 [vii]	2002	Street outreach	82.6% male	379	71.0%	11.3%		
Nanning, China	Wu, RR et al., 1997 [viii]	unspecified	IDU clinics		85	100.0%	0.0%		
Shanghai, China	Zhao, M et al., 2005 [ix]	2003–2004	Drug Treatment Center	27.3 yrs=mean age; 69.3% male	101	46.5%	0.0%	56.4%	
Shanghai, China	Zhao, M et al., 2006 [x]	2004–2005	Drug treatment center	30.1 yrs=mean age; 72% male;	141	51.8%	0	32%	
INDONESIA									
	Nelwan EJ et al., 2010 [xi]	2007–2009	Incoming prisoners	31.3=mean age; 97% male	686	77.3%			
MALAYSIA									
Kuala Lumpur	Ng, KP et al., 1995 [xii]	1991–1992	Medical Setting		90	30.0%			
Penninsular Malaysia	Vicknasingam B et al., 2009 [xiii]	2006–2007	Street outreach	37.0 yrs=mean age; 95% male; 80% Malay	552	65.40%	42.90%		
Kuala Lumpur	Sinmiah N et al., 1993 [xiv]	1985–2001	Unspecified		190	85.3%		78.8%	
Peninsular Malaysia	Vicknasingam B et al., 2009 [xv]	2006–2007	Unspecified		552	67.10%			

Location	Author, Year	Enrollment Dates	Recruitment Setting	Chars of sample	N IDUs	% HCV+	% HIV+	% HBV+	HCV incidence
PHILLIPINES									
Metro Cebu	Agdamag D et al., 2005 [xvi]	2002	Drug treatment center and Street outreach	30 yrs=mean age; 91.95% male	87	70.0%	0.0%	10.3% HBsAg	
SINGAPORE									
	Winslow M et al., 2007 [xvii]	2005–2006	Drug treatment	39.5 = mean age; 28% Malay; 49% Chinese; 90% male	106	42.50%	0%	8.5% (HBsAG)	
TAIWAN									
Kaohsiung, Taiwan	Chang C-J et al., 1999 [xviii]	1994–1996	Drug treatment center and Correctional	100% male	247	67.2%		96.8%	
Taipei, Taiwan	Huo, TF et al., 2004 [xix]	1985	Drug Treatment Center and Medical Setting	30 years=mean age	115	53.0%			
Taipei, Taiwan	Lee, S et al., 1991 [xx]	1985	Drug Treatment Center	90.4% male; 32.8 yrs=mean age	115	53.0%		16.5%	
Taichung, Taiwan	Liao K et al., 2006 [xxi]	2004–2005	Correctional	100% male	423	89.8%			
Taipei, Taiwan	Wu J et al., 1993 [xxii]	1988–1990	STD Clinic		4	100.0%			

Location	Author, Year	Enrollment Dates	Recruitment Setting	Chars of sample	N IDUs	% HCV+	% HIV+	% HBV+	HCV incidence
THAILAND									
Chaing Rai	Apichartipyakun, C et al., 1999 [xxiii]	1996–1996	Medical Setting	35.5 yrs=mean age; 85% male	79	90.0%			
Chiang Mai	Beyrer C et al., 2005 [xxiv]	1995–2000	Drug Treatment Center	39.5= mean age; 91% male; 49% Chinese, 28% Malay	787	87.7%			
Chiang Mai	Jittwutikarn, J et al., 2006 [xxv]	1999–2000	Drug treatment center	89% male	508	86.0%	30.0%		44.3/100PY
Bangkok, Thailand	Luksamijarulkul, P et al., 1996 [xxvi]	1992	Medical Setting	30.9 yrs=mean age; 100% male	150	95.3%	44.0%		
Chon Buri Province	Paris, R et al., 2003 [xxvii]	1998–2001	Public Health Clinic	100% male	28	96.4%	89.3%		
Chiang Mai	Suganuma N et al., 1998 [xxviii]	1996	Drug treatment center	29 yrs=median age; 98% male	98	84.7%	45.0%	76.5%	
Chaing Mai	Taketa K et al., 2003 [xxix]	1996	Drug treatement center	98% male	98	85.0%	46.0%	77.0%	
VIETNAM									
Ho Chi Minh City	Chau T et al., 2002 [xxx]	1991–1996	Medical Setting	30 yrs=median age; 97% male;	47	96.0%	45.0%	28.0%	
Ho Chi Minh City	Follezou J et al., 1999 [xxxi]	1996	Drug treatment center	39.3 yrs=mean age; 100% male	280	100.0%	83.9%	87.9%	

Location	Author, Year	Enrollment Dates	Recruitment Setting	Chars of sample	N IDUs	% HCV+	% HIV+	% HBV+	HCV incidence
Hanoi, Vietnam	Nakata S et al., 1994 [xxxii]	1993	Drug Treatment Center	29 yrs=mean age; 94% male	200	27.5%		54.0%	
Ho Chi Minh, Vietnam	Nakata S et al., 1994 [xxxiii]	1993	Drug Treatment Center	37 yrs=mean age	67	85.0%		39.0%	
	Quan, VM et al. 2009 [xxxiv]	2003				74.10%			

i. Yan Heng Zhou, Liu Feng-Liang, Yao Zhi-Hong, Hong Li Lin Duo, Yi Sun, and Yong-Tang Zheng, "Comparison of HIV-, HBV-, HCV- and Co-Infection Prevalence between Chinese and Burmese Intravenous Drug Users of the China-Myanmar Border Region," *PLoS One* 6, no. 1 (2011): e16349.

ii. Kun Cao, Masashi Mizokami, Etsuro Orito, Xin Ding, Xian-Min Ge, Guo-Yong Huang, and Ryuzo Ueda, "TT Virus Infection among IVDUs in South Western China," *Journal of Infectious Diseases* 31, no. 1 (1999): 21–25.

iii. Rebecca J. Garten, Shenghan Lai, Jinbing Zhang, Wei Liu, Jie Chen, David Vlahov, and Xiao-Fang Yu, "Rapid Transmission of Hepatitis C virus among Young Injecting Heroin Users in Southern China," *International Journal of Epidemiology* 33, no. 1 (2004): 182–88.

iv. Shenghan Lai, Wei Liu, Jie Chen, Jiye Yang, Zhi-Jun Li, Rong-Jian Li, Fu-Xung Liang, Shao-Ling Liang, Qu-Yang Zhu, and Xiao-Fang Yu, "Changes in HIV-1 Incidence in Heroin Users in Guangxi Province, China," *Journal of Acquired Immune Deficiency Syndromes* 26, no. 4 (2001): 365–70.

v. D. Li, X. Zheng, and G Zhang, "Prevalence of HIV and HCV among injecting drug users (IDUs) in Yunnan, China." *Zhonghua Liu Xing Bing Xue Za Zhi* 15, no. 2 (1994): 74–75.

vi. Hongjie Liu, Oscar Grusky, Xiaojing Li, and Erjian Ma, "Drug Users: A Potentially Important Bridge Population in the Transmission of Sexually Transmitted Diseases, Including AIDS, in China," *Sexually Transmitted Diseases* 33, no. 2 (2006): 111–17.

vii. Yu-Hua Ruan, Kun-Xue Hong, Shi-Zhu Liu, Yi-Xin He, Feng Zhou, Guan-Ming Qin, Kang-Lin Chen, Hui Xing, Jian-Ping Chen, and Yi-Ming Shao, "Community-Based Survey of HCV and HIV Coinfection in Injection Drug Abusers in Sichuan Province of China," *World Journal of Gastroenterology* 10, no. 11 (2004): 1589–93.

viii. Rong-Rong Wu, Masashi Mizokami, Kun Cao, Tatsunori Nakano, Xian-Min Ge, Su-Seng Wang, Etsuro Orito, Ken-ichi Ohba, Motokazu Mukaide, Kazumasa Hikiji, Johnson Y. N. Lau, and Shiro Iino, "GB virus C/hepatitis G Virus Infection in Southern China," *Journal of Infectious Diseases* 175, no. 1 (1997): 168–71.

ix. Min Zhao, Qiu Y. Wang, Guang H. Lu, Ping Xu, Han Xu, and Clyde B McCoy, "Risk Behaviors and HIV/AIDS Prevention Education among IDUs in Drug Treatment in Shanghai," *Journal of Urban Health* 82, nos. 3–4 (2005): 84–91.

x. Min Zhao, Jiang Du, Guang H. Lu, Qiu Y. Wang, Han Xu, Min Zhu, and Clyde B McCoy, "HIV Sexual Risk Behaviors among Injection Drug Users in Shanghai," *Drug and Alcohol Dependence* 82, no. 1 (2006): S43–47.

xi. Erni J. Nelwan, Reinout Van Crevel, Bachti Alisjahbana, Agnes K. Indrati, Reiva F. Dwiyana, Nisaa Nuralam, Herdiman T. Pohan, Ilham Jaya, Andre Meheus, and Andre Van Der Ven, "Human Immunodeficiency Virus, Hepatitis B and Hepatitis C in an Indonesian Prison: Prevalence, Risk Factors and Implications of HIV Screening," *Tropical Medicine & International Health* 15, no. 12 (2010): 1491–98.

xii. K. P. Ng, T. L. Saw, N. W. Wong, K. L. Goh, S. Y. Chuah, and M. Nagaratnam, "The Prevalence of anti-HCV Antibody in Risk Groups and Blood Donors," *Medical Journal of Malaysia* 50, no. 4 (1995): 302–5.

xiii. Balasingam Vicknasingam, Suresh Narayanan, and Visweswaran Navaratnam, "Prevalence Rates and Risk Factors for Hepatitis C among Drug Users Not in Treatment in Malaysia," *Drug and Alcohol Review* 28, no. 4 (2009): 447–54.

xiv. M. Sinniah and B. G. Ooi, "Hepatitis C—The Malaysian Story," *Singapore Medical Journal* 34, no. 2 (1993): 132–34.

xv. Balasingam Vicknasingam, Suresh Narayanan, and Visweswaran Navaratnam, "Prevalence Rates and Risk Factors for Hepatitis C among Drug Users Not in Treatment in Malaysia," *Drug and Alcohol Review* 28, no. 4 (2009): 447–54.

xvi. Dorothy M. Agdamag, Seiji Kageyama, Evelyn T. Alesna, Rontgene M. Solante, Prisca S. Leaño, Anna Marie L. Heredia, Ilya P. Abellanosa-Tac-An, Eutiquio T. Vibal, Lourdes D. Jereza, and Hiroshi Ichimura, "Rapid Spread of Hepatitis C Virus among Injecting-Drug Users in the Philippines: Implications for HIV Epidemics," *Journal of Medical Virology* 77, no. 2 (2005): 221–26.

xvii. M. Winslow, Mythily Subramaniam, W. L. Ng, A. Lee, G. Song, and Y. H. Chan, "Seroprevalence of Hepatitis C in Intravenous Opioid Users Presenting in the Early Phase of Injecting Drug Use in Singapore," *Singapore Medical Journal* 48, no. 6 (2007): 504–8.

xviii. Chai-Jan Chang, Chun-Hui Lin, Chien-Te Lee, Shun-Jen Chang, Ying-Chin Ko, and Hong-Wen Liu, "Hepatitis C Virus Infection among Short-Term Intravenous Drug Users in Southern Taiwan," *European Journal of Epidemiology* 15, no. 7 (1999): 597–601.

xix. Teh-Ia Huo, Jaw-Ching Wu, Shiow-Ing Wu, An-Lung Chang, Shih-Ku Lin, Chun-Hung Pang, Yi-Hsiang Huang, Full-Young Chang, and Shou-Dong Lee, "Changing Seroepidemiology of Hepatitis B, C, and D Virus Infections in High-Risk Populations," *Journal of Medical Virology* 72, no. 1 (2004): 41–45.

xx. Mei-Hsuan Lee, Hwai-I Yang, and C. L. Jen et al., "Community and Personal Risk Factors for Hepatitis C Virus Infection: A Survey of 23,820 Residents in Taiwan in 1991–1992," *Gut* 60, no. 5 (2011): 688–94.

xxi. Kuan-Fu Liao, Shih-Wei Lai, Wu-Long Chang, and Nan-Yung Hsu, "Screening for Viral Hepatitis among Male Non-Drug-Abuse Prisoners," *Scandinavian Journal of Gastroenterology* 41, no. 8 (2006): 969–73.

xxii. Jaw-Ching Wu, Hwa-Chen Lin, Fong-Shya Jeng, Gong-Yih Ma, Shou-Dong Lee, and Wen-Yung Sheng, "Prevalence, Infectivity, and Risk Factor Analysis of Hepatitis C Virus Infection in Prostitutes," *Journal of Medical Virology* 39, no. 4 (1993): 312–17.

xxiii. C. Apichartpiyakul, N. Apichartpiyakul, Y Urwijitaroon et al. "Seroprevalence and subtype distribution of hepatitis C virus among blood donors and intravenous drug users in northern/northeastern Thailand." *Japanese Journal of Infectious*

Diseases 52, no. 3 (1999): 121–23.

xxiv. Chris Beyrer, Teerada Sripaipan, and S. Tovanabutra et al., "High HIV, Hepatitis C and Sexual Risks among Drug-Using Men Who Have Sex with Men in Northern Thailand," *AIDS* 19, no. 14 (2005): 1535–40.

xxv. Jaroon Jittiwutikarn, Satawat Thongsawat, and Vinai Suriyanon et al., "Hepatitis C Infection among Drug Users in Northern Thailand," *American Journal of Tropical Medicine and Hygiene* 74, no. 6 (2006): 1111–16.

xxvi. P. Luksamijarulkul and S. Plucktaweesak, "High Hepatitis C Seroprevalence in Thai Intravenous Drug Abusers and Qualitative Risk Analysis," *Southeast Asian Journal of Tropical Medicine and Public Health* 27, no. 4 (1996): 654–58.

xxvii. Robert Paris, Narongrid Sirisopana, and Michael Benenson et al., "The Association between Hepatitis C Virus and HIV-1 in Preparatory Cohorts for HIV Vaccine Trials in Thailand," *AIDS* 17, no. 9 (2003): 1363–67.

xxviii. Narufumi Suganuma, S. Ikeda, and K. Taketa et al., "Risk Analysis of the Exposure to GB Virus C/Hepatitis G Virus among Populations of Intravenous Drug Users, Commercial Sex Workers and Male Outpatients at STD Clinic in Chiang Mai, Thailand: A Cross-Sectional Case-Control Study," *Acta Med Okayama* 52, no. 3 (1998): 161–67.

xxix. Kazuhisa Taketa, Satoru Ikeda, and Narufumi Suganuma et al., "Differential Seroprevalences of Hepatitis C Virus, Hepatitis B Virus and Human Immunodeficiency Virus among Intravenous Drug Users, Commercial Sex Workers and Patients with Sexually Transmitted Diseases in Chiang Mai, Thailand," *Hepatology Research* 27, no. 1 (2003): 6–12.

xxx. Tran Thi Hong Chau, N. T. Mai, and N. H. Phu et al., "Malaria in Injection Drug Abusers in Vietnam," *Clinical Infectious Diseases* 34, no. 10 (2002): 1317–22.

xxxi. Jane-Yves Follezou, Nguyen Y. Lan, X. Truong, and Lien et al., "Clinical and Biological Characteristics of Human Immunodeficiency Virus-Infected and Uninfected Intravascular Drug Users in Ho Chi Minh City, Vietnam," *American Journal Tropical Medicine and Hygiene* 61, no. 3 (1999): 420–24.

xxxii. Susumu Nakata, Pham Song, and Dao Dinh Duc et al., "Hepatitis C and B Virus Infections in Populations at Low or High Risk in Ho Chi Minh and Hanoi, Vietnam," *Journal of Gastroenterology and Hepatology* 9, no. 4 (1994): 416–19.

xxxiii. Susumu Nakata, Pham Song, and Dao Dinh Duc et al., "Hepatitis C and B Virus Infections in Populations at Low or High Risk in Ho Chi Minh and Hanoi, Vietnam," *Journal of Gastroenterology and Hepatology* 9, no. 4 (1994): 416–19.

xxxiv. Vu Minh Quan, Vivian F. Go, and Le Van Nam et al., "Risks for HIV, HBV, and HCV Infections among Male Injection Drug Users in Northern Vietnam: A Case-Control Study," *AIDS Care* 21, no. 1 (2009): 7–16.

High HCV prevalence has been reported in the Yunnan region of China (up to 95 percent), a rate that corresponds to the excess HIV burden in that province.[37] High prevalence has also been reported in Guangxi Province, which lies just to the east of Yunnan and borders Vietnam. In 2009, 318 Burmese PWID were recruited in a China-Myanmar border region in Yunnan Province;[38] HCV prevalence was 69 percent. Relatively lower prevalence (~50 percent) has been observed in Shanghai.[39] What is remarkable about the epidemic in China is that high prevalence has been observed in very recent-onset injectors, for example, 94 percent prevalence in Yunnan PWID injecting five years on average.[40] The GBD report gave a mid-point estimate of 67 percent for China (Nelson et al. 2011);[41] the great heterogeneity in infection rates across this very large nation suggests that region-specific estimates are more informative. A systematic review and meta-analysis of fifty-three studies of PWID in China calculated a pooled prevalence rate of 61 percent, and also noted wide geographic variability, with HCV prevalence highest along drug transshipment routes (in Yunnan, Xinjiang, Sichuan, Guizhou, Guangxi, and Guangdong).[42] Using data from three studies that reported rates in relation to ethnicity, they calculated that non-Han Chinese were 1.5 times more likely to be HCV seropositive.[43] In a sample of Guangxi PWID, HCV incidence was extremely high, at 53/100PY.[44]

Several studies have been carried out among PWID in Taiwan; prevalence ranges from 53 to 90 percent. In Vietnam, highest prevalence rates have been observed in Ho Chi Minh City (85 to 100 percent). A survey of Hanoi PWID found 28 percent were seropositive. In Bac Ninh Province (just east of Hanoi), prevalence was 74 percent. Uniformly high prevalence has been reported in Thailand PWID (85 to 96 percent). In Chiang Mai, an incidence rate of 44/100PY was reported.[45]

A survey of PWID entering a prison in West Java, Indonesia, found 77 percent were HCV seropositive.[46] In a Singapore study, overall prevalence was in PWID 43 percent; it was six times higher in ethnic Malays, and thirteen times higher in Indian PWID vs. Chinese.[47] In Malaysia, low prevalence was observed in a sample of PWID in a medical setting in Kuala Lumpur (30 percent).[48] A small study of PWID in the Philippines found 70 percent were HCV-positive.[49]

5. COMPREHENSIVE PROGRAMS FOR THE PREVENTION, TREATMENT, AND CARE OF HIV INFECTION AMONG PEOPLE WHO INJECT DRUGS

There are a number of evidence-based programs to address HIV infection among PWID. UNAIDS/WHO have produced a "technical guide for countries to set target for universal access to HIV prevention, treatment, and care for injecting drug users" that lists nine different interventions: Needle and syringe programs (NSP), opiate substitution therapy (OST), HIV testing and counseling, antiretroviral therapy (ART), prevention and treatment of sexually transmitted infections, condom programs for PWID and their sexual partners, targeted information, education and communication for PWID and their sexual partners, vaccination, diagnosis, and treatment of viral hepatitis, and prevention, diagnosis, and treatment of tuberculosis. Of these, needle and syringe programs, opiate substitution therapy, and anti-retroviral therapy for HIV infection are generally considered to be the most important. Recent studies have shown that ART for HIV seropositive persons greatly reduces the likelihood that they will transmit HIV to others. [50, 51] Thus, ART is now also considered a form of HIV prevention.

Small "pilot" programs do not stop epidemics. The levels of "coverage" needed for a combination of different prevention programs to either avert an HIV epidemic among PWID or to "reverse" an ongoing, high seroprevalence HIV epidemic (reduce the rate of new infections to where prevalence declines rapidly) is not yet known. Determining the appropriate levels of coverage for multiple interventions is clearly a complex task but one of great importance in resource-limited settings.

Several brief comments may be helpful here. The levels of coverage needed are likely to vary within the specific epidemiologic settings. HIV prevention programs are generally more effective in low HIV prevalence settings, in which there are relatively few persons capable of transmitting the virus. In such settings, most sharing of needles and syringes is likely to be between HIV seronegatives, so that if the numbers of sharing partners can be limited, HIV transmission may occur, but an outbreak with large numbers of new infections occurring within a short time period is unlikely. In contrast, in a high HIV seroprevalence setting, with large numbers of PWID who are capable of transmitting the virus and large numbers of PWID susceptible to becoming infected, sharing among discordant injecting partners is more likely, and even modest rates of sharing may perpetuate the epidemic.

The desired levels of coverage may also depend upon the level of analysis. To fully protect an individual PWID from becoming infected with HIV, it may be necessary for that person to always be participating in an effective prevention activity. [52] At a population level, however, it may be possible to dramatically reduce HIV transmission while a substantial minority of PWID are not participating in any prevention intervention due to herd protection (herd immunity) effects. [53]

Prevention of HCV in PWID has proven to be quite challenging, owing to the high prevalence of infectious carriers, the fact that HCV is very efficiently transmitted via injection, and the range of injection behaviors that may transmit the virus. [54] A systematic review and meta-analysis of HCV infection rates in relation to time since onset of drug injection showed that in

LMICs, prevalence reaches 50 percent after one year of injecting, versus after five years in high income countries.[55] Recent studies, including a meta-analysis, showed that multicomponent interventions that support a range of risk-reduction strategies (substance use treatment to reduce or eliminate drug injection, adoption of safe injection practices through the provision of sterile syringes and drug-preparation materials, or behavior-change counseling) were highly effective in preventing HCV seroconversion in PWID, reducing HCV transmission by 75–80 percent.[56, 57] With the development of new direct-acting antiviral agents for treatment of HCV infection, there is the prospect of curing infection in the majority of patients; if delivered on a massive scale, this could reduce HCV prevalence and improve effectiveness of harm reduction strategies.[58, 59, 60] At present, however, fewer than 5 percent of HCV-infected PWID receive the current treatment regimen.[61] Additionally, treatment as prevention may be too costly a measure in LMICs.

6. CLOSING

There is considerable variation in the HIV situation among PWID in the different countries in Southeast Asia, and also within countries (China in particular), so that broad generalizations should be avoided. There is much less variation in HCV across the region, with uniformly high rates of HCV prevalence among PWID. We would like to close this chapter with a cautionary tale and a success story from the region.

CAUTIONARY TALE: HIV AND INCARCERATION AMONG PWID IN BANGKOK, THAILAND

Bangkok, Thailand, experienced an extremely rapid period of HIV transmission among PWID in 1989, with seroprevalence rising from 2 percent to over 40 percent in less than a year.[62] Wright and colleagues have argued that this was a "point source" outbreak, originating from a particular location.[63] Specifically, they argue that prisons in Bangkok were the initial location for transmission. HIV was presumably introduced into the prisons where HIV seropositive foreigners were incarcerated. At the time, Bangkok had a plentiful supply of inexpensive, high quality heroin, so that it was a prime location for "drug tourists." Drug injecting with sharing of syringes was common so that HIV would have spread within the prison. In December 1988 there was an amnesty with large numbers of prisoners released back into the community. The release of HIV infected prisoners then set off the local HIV epidemic among PWID in the city. The epidemic continued, with HIV seroprevalence stabilized at approximately 50 percent and incidence of four to six per one hundred person years.[64] Injecting drug use continued in the jails[65] and there were multiple associations between being incarcerated and becoming infected with HIV.[66, 67] Some persons were becoming infected while incarcerated and others formed high-risk social networks with fellow prisoners and became infected after release from incarceration.[68, 69, 70, 71]

The HIV epidemic among PWID in Bangkok has since declined, but it is clear that the incarceration of drug users played multiple important roles in the first large HIV epidemic among PWID in Asia.[72, 73] And incarceration, injecting while incarcerated, and sharing syringes when injecting while incarcerated have continued at high rates among PWID in Bangkok, particularly as a result of the "War on Drugs" in Thailand, described in more detail in Kaplan's chapter in this book.[74]

SUCCESS STORY: THE CROSS-BORDER
HIV PREVENTION PROGRAM

The "Cross-Border" intervention took place in the region of Lang Son Province, Vietnam, and Ning Ming County in the Guangxi province in China. The intervention involved packaged harm reduction services, including a pharmacy-based voucher program for acquiring clean needles/syringes along with clean injecting equipment and condoms. On average, 7,000 to 10,000 needles/syringes were distributed per month at each location, serving a population of approximately 3,000 PWID in each location. Three studies reported on changes in HIV prevalence in these locations, Hammett 2006, Des Jarlais 2007 and Hammett 2012; the Hammett et al. 2012 paper provides the most complete data.[75, 76, 77]

Hammett et al. documented changes in HIV prevalence and HIV incidence among new PWID over an eight-year period in conjunction with NSP expansion in both locations beginning in 2002 of which six years of data was available for Ning Ming while seven years of data was available for Lang Son. 2125 PWID were included in the Ning Ming sample, and 2677 PWID were included in the Lang Son sample.

In Ning Ming, HIV prevalence decreased from 17 percent to 14 percent after twelve months, and then stabilized at 11 percent after seventy-two months ($p = 0.003$). In Lang Son, HIV prevalence decreased to 43 percent after twelve months and decreased further to 23 percent after eighty-four months ($p < 0.001$). When examining only new PWID, defined as injectors that had injected for three years or less, HIV incidence in Ning Ming decreased from 12 percent to 9 percent after twelve months and stabilized at 11 percent after seventy-two months. Among new PWID in Lang Son, the HIV incidence decreased from 22 percent to 16 percent after twelve months and decreased further to 3 percent after eighty-four months ($p < 0.001$).

SUMMARY AND CONCLUSION

There is considerable variation in HIV prevalence among PWID among the different countries in Southeast Asia, though all countries appear to either have high HIV seroprevalence rates or be at risk for HIV epidemics. There is less variation in HCV seroprevalence rates, with uniformly high rates among PWID throughout the region. There are current efforts to scale up evidence-based HIV prevention programs—particularly syringe exchange and methadone maintenance treatment—in the region, but these need to be accelerated.[78] [79] There are good reasons to expect that such programs with be very effective in Southeast Asia, the effective implementation will require cooperation from law enforcement and a basic recognition of the human right of PWID to avoid infection with HIV.

NOTES

1. The Baron Edmond de Rothschild Chemical Dependency Institute, Beth Israel Medical Center New York, NY.

2. NYU College of Nursing New York, NY.

3. James M. Polachek, *The Inner Opium War* (Harvard University Asia Center, 1992).

4. June M. Grasso, Jay P. Corrin, and Michael Kort, *Modernization and Revolution in China: From the Opium Wars to the Olympics* (ME Sharpe Inc, 2009).

5. Diana H. Fishbein and Susan E. Pease, *The Dynamics of Drug Abuse* (Massachusetts: Allyn & Bacon, 1995).

6. MC Corporation MC, *Encyclopedia of Health* (Marshall Cavendish Corporation, 2009).

7. Kenaz Filan, *The Power of the Poppy: Harnessing Nature's Most Dangerous Plant Ally* (Vermont: Park Street Press, 2011).

8. Gulbahar H. Beckett and Charles Romley Alder Wright, "Iv.—Action of the Organic Acids and Their Anhydrides on the Natural Alkaloids. Part Ii. Butyryl and Benzoyl Derivatives of Morphine and Codeine," *Journal of the Chemical Society* 28 (1875): 15–26.

9. Walter Sneader, "The Discovery of Heroin," *Lancet* 352, no. 9141 (1998): 1697–99.

10. David F. Musto, Pamela Korsmeyer, and Thomas W. Maulucci, *One Hundred Years of Heroin* (Connecticut: Auburn House Westport, 2002).

11. John Illife, *The African Aids Epidemic. A History* (Athens: Ohio University Press, 2006).

12. Thomas C. Quinn, Jonathan Mann, James W. Curran, and Peter Piot, "AIDS in Africa: An Epidemiologic Paradigm," *Science* 234, no. 4779 (1986): 955–63.

13. Bradley M. Mathers, Louisa Degenhardt, Benjamin Phillips, Lucas Wiessing, Matthew Hickman, Steffanie A Strathdee, Alex Wodak, Samiran Panda, Mark Tyndall, Abdalla Toufik, Richard P. Mattick, for the 2007 Reference Group to the UN on HIV and Injecting Drug Use, "Global Epidemiology of Injecting Drug Use and HIV among People who Inject Drugs: A Systematic Review," *Lancet* 372, no. 9651 (2008): 1733–45.

14. Carmen Aceijas, Gerry V. Stimson, Matthew Hickman, and Tim Rhodes, "Global Overview of Injecting Drug Use and HIV Infection among Injecting Drug Users," *AIDS* 18, no. 17 (2004): 2295–2303.

15. Mathers et al., *Global Epidemiology*, 1733–45.

16. Thomas L. Friedman, *The Lexus and the Olive Tree* (New York: Anchor Books, 2000).

17. UNODC (United Nations Office of Drugs and Crime), *2005 World Drug Report* (Vienna: UNODC, 2005).

18. Mathers et al., *Global Epidemiology*, 1733–45.

19. UNAIDS/WHO (Joint United Nations Programme on HIV/AIDS), *AIDS Epidemic Update: December 2006* (Geneva: UNAIDS/WHO, 2007).

20. Don C. Des Jarlais, Patrick Johnston, Patricia Friedmann, Ryan Kling, Wei Liu, Doan Ngu, Yi Chen, Tran V. Hoang, Meng Donghua, Ly K. Van, Nguyen D. Tung, Kieu T. Binh, and Theodore M. Hammett, "Patterns of HIV Prevalence among Injecting Drug Users in the Cross-Border Area of Lang Son Province, Vietnam, and Ning Ming County, Guangxi Province, China," *BMC Public Health* 5 (2005): 89.

21. Des Jarlais et al., *Patterns of HIV Prevalence*, 89.

22. Yuhua Ruan, Kanglin Chen, Kunxue Hong, Yixin He, Shizhu Liu, Feng Zhou, Guangming Qin, Jianping Chen, Hui Xing, and Yiming Shao, "Community-Based Survey of HIV Transmission Modes among Intravenous Drug Users in Sichuan, China," *Sexually Transmitted Diseases* 31, no. 10 (2004): 623–27.

23. Ruan, *Community-Based Survey of HIV*, 623–27.

24. Minsheng Xia, Joan K. Kreiss, and King K. Holmes, "Risk Factors for HIV infection among drug users in Yunnan province, China: Association with Intravenous Drug Use and Protective Effect of Boiling Reusable Needles and Syringes," *AIDS* 8, no. 12 (1994): 1701–6.

25. Theodore M. Hammett, Patrick Johnston, Ryan Kling, Wei Liu, Doan Ngu, Nguyen Duy Tung, Binh Thanh Kieu, Ha Viet Dong, Tran Vu Hoang, Ly Kieu Van, Meng Donghua, Yi Chen, and Don C. Des Jarlais, "Correlates of HIV Status among Injection Drug Users in a Border Region of Southern China and Northern Vietnam," *Journal of Acquired Immune Deficiency Syndromes* 38, no. 2 (2005): 228–35.

26. Lu Yin, Guangming Qin, Han Zhu Qian, Yu Zhu, Wei Hu, Li Zhang, Kanglin Chen, Yunxia Wang, Shizhu Liu, Feng Zhou, Hui Xing, Yuhua Ruan, Ning Wang, and Yiming Shao, "Continued Spread of HIV among Injecting Drug Users in Southern Sichuan Province, China," *Harm Reduction Journal* 4, no. 6 (2007). DOI: 10.1186/1477-7517-4-6.

27. Li Zhang, Junling Zhu, Baoling Rui, Yuanzhi Zhang, Lijiang Zhang, Lu Yin, Yuhua Ruan, Han-Zhu Qian, and Yiming Shao, "High HIV Risk among Uigur Minority Ethnic Drug Users in Northwestern China," *Tropical Medicine & International Health* 13, no. 6 (2008): 814–17.

28. Yan Yao, Ning Wang, Jennifer Chu, Guowei Ding, Xia Jin, Yongli Sun, Guixiang Wang, Junjie Xu, and Kumi Smith, "Sexual Behavior and Risks for HIV Infection and Transmission among Male Injecting Drug Users in Yunnan, China," *International Journal of Infectious Diseases* 13, no. 2 (2009): 154–61.

29. Pajongsil Perngmark, David D. Celentano, and Surinda Kawichai, "Risk Factors for HIV Infection among Drug Injectors in Southern Thailand," *Drug and Alcohol Dependence* 71, no. 3 (2003): 229–38.

30. Balasingam Vicknasingam, Suresh Narayanan, and Visweswaran Navaratnam, "The Relative Risk of HIV among IDUs Not in Treatment in Malaysia," *AIDS Care* 21, no. 8 (2009): 984–91.

31. Oliver G. Pybus, Eleanor Barnes, Rachel Taggart, Philippe Lemey, Peter V. Markov, Bouachan Rasachak, Bounkong Syhavong, Rattaphone Phetsouvanah, Isabelle Sheridan, Isla S. Humphreys, Ling Lu, Paul N. Newton, and Paul Klenerman, "Genetic History of Hepatitis C Virus in East Asia," *Journal of Virology* 83, no. 2 (2009): 1071–82.

32. Xueshan Xia, Ling Lu, Kok Keng Tee, Wenhua Zhao, Jianguo Wu, Jing Yu, Xiaojie Li, Yixiong Lin, Muhammad Mahmood Mukhtar, Curt H. Hagedorn, and Yutaka Takebe, "The Unique HCV Genotype Distribution and the Discovery of a Novel Subtype 6u among IDUS Co-Infected with HIV-1 in Yunnan, China," *Journal of Medical Virology* 80, no. 7 (2008): 1142–52.

33. Xia et al., *The Unique HCV Genotype Distribution*, 1142–52.

34. Holly Hagan, Don C. Des Jarlais, Rebecca Stern, Corina Lelutiu-Weinberger, Roberta Scheinmann, Sheila Strauss, and Peter L. Flom, "HCV Synthesis Project: Preliminary Analyses of HCV Prevalence in Relation to Age and Duration of Injection," *International Journal of Drug Policy* 18, no. 5 (2007): 341–51.

35. Rebecca Stern, Holly Hagan, Corina Lelutiu-Weinberger, Don Des Jarlais, Roberta Scheinmann, Shiela Strauss, Enrique Pouget, and Peter Flom, "The HCV Synthesis Project:

Scope, Methodology, and Preliminary Results," *BMC Medical Research Methodology* 8, no. 1 (2008): 62.

36. Paul K. Nelson, Bradley M. Mathers, Benjamin Cowie, Holly Hagan, Don Des Jarlais, Danielle Horyniak, and Louisa Degenhardt, "Global Epidemiology of Hepatitis B and Hepatitis C in People Who Inject Drugs: Results of Systematic Reviews," *Lancet* 378, no. 9791: 571–83.

37. Manhong Jia, Hongbing Luo, Yanling Ma, Ning Wang, Kumi Smith, Jiangyuan Mei, Ran Lu, Jiyun Lu, Liru Fu, Qiang Zhang, Zunyou Wu, and Lin Lu , "The HIV Epidemic in Yunnan Province, China, 1989–2007," *Journal of Acquired Immune Deficiency Syndromes* 53 (2010): S34–S40. DOI: 10.1097/QAI.0b013e3181c7d6ff.

38. Lu Yin, Guangming Qin, Han Zhu Qian, Yu Zhu, Wei Hu, Li Zhang, Kanglin Chen, Yunxia Wang , Shizhu Liu , Feng Zhou , Hui Xing , Yuhua Ruan , Ning Wang , and Yiming Shao , "Continued Spread of HIV among Injecting Drug Users in Southern Sichuan Province, China,." *Harm Reduction Journal* 4, no. 6 (2007). DOI: 10.1186/1477-7517-4-6 .

39. Min Zhao, Qiu Wang, Guang Lu, Ping Xu, Han Xu, and Clyde McCoy, "Risk Behaviors and HIV/AIDS Prevention Education among IDUs in Drug Treatment in Shanghai," *Journal of Urban Health* 82 (2005): iv84–iv91.

40. Xian Xia, Jun Luo, Jianling Bai, and Rongbin Yu, "Epidemiology of Hepatitis C Virus Infection among Injection Drug Users in China: Systematic Review and Meta-Analysis," *Public Health* 122, no. 10 (2008): 990–1003.

41. Paul K. Nelson, Bradley M. Mathers, Benjamin Cowie, Holly Hagan, Don Des Jarlais, Danielle Horyniak, and Louisa Degenhardt, "Global Epidemiology of Hepatitis B and Hepatitis C in People Who Inject Drugs: Results of Systematic Reviews," *Lancet* 378, no. 9791 (2011): 571–83.

42. Xia et al., *Epidemiology of Hepatitis C*, 990–1003.

43. Xia et al., *Epidemiology of Hepatitis C*, 990–1003.

44. Rebecca J. Garten, Sheng-Han Lai, Jin-Bing Zhang, Wei Liu, Jie Chen, and Xiao-Fang Yu, "Factors Influencing a Low Rate of Hepatitis C Viral RNA Clearance in Heroin Users from Southern China," *World Journal of Gastroenterology* 14, no. 12 (2008): 1878.

45. Jaroon Jittiwutikarn, Satawat Thongsawat, Vinai Suriyanon, Niwat Maneekarn, David Celentano, Myat Htoo Razak, Namtip Srirak, Tassanai Vongchak, Surinda Kawichai, David Thomas, Teerada Sripaipan, Dale Netski, Ashwin Ananthakrishnan, and Kenrad E. Nelson, "Hepatitis C Infection among Drug Users in Northern Thailand," *The American Journal of Tropical Medicine and Hygiene* 74, no. 6 (2006): 1111–16.

46. Erni J. Nelwan, Reinout Van Crevel, Bachti Alisjahbana, Agnes K. Indrati, Reiva F. Dwiyana, Nisaa Nuralam, Herdiman T. Pohan, Ilham Jaya, Andre Meheus, and Andre Van Der Ven, "Human Immunodeficiency Virus, Hepatitis B and Hepatitis C in an Indonesian Prison: Prevalence, Risk Factors and Implications of HIV Screening," *Tropical Medicine & International Health* 15, no. 12 (2010): 1491–98.

47. Monte M. Winslow, Malayanna Subramaniam, Wan-Leung Ng, Alice Lee, Gang Song, and Yuk-Hee Chan, "Seroprevalence of Hepatitis C in Intravenous Opioid Users Presenting in the Early Phase of Injecting Drug Use in Singapore," *Singapore Medical Journal* 48, no. 6 (2007): 504.

48. Kee Peng Ng, Teik Leong Saw, Nora W. Wong, Keow Lin Goh, Stew Yeam Chuah, and Mayavaty Nagaratnam, "The Prevalence of Anti-HCV Antibody in Risk Groups and Blood Donors," *The Medical Journal of Malaysia* 50, no. 4 (1995): 302.

49. Dorothy M. Agdamag, Seiji Kageyama, Evelyn T. Alesna, Rontgene M. Solante, Prisca S. Leaño, Anna Marie L. Heredia, Ilya P. Abellanosa-Tac-An, Eutiquio T. Vibal, Lourdes D. Jereza, and Hiroshi Ichimura, "Rapid Spread of Hepatitis C Virus among Injecting-Drug Users in the Philippines: Implications for HIV Epidemics," *Journal of Medical Virology* 77, no. 2 (2005): 221–26.

50. Myron S. Cohen, Ying Q. Chen, Marybeth McCauley, Theresa Gamble, Mina C. Hosseinipour, Nagalingeswaran Kumarasamy, James G. Hakim et al., "Prevention of HIV-1 Infection with Early Antiretroviral Therapy," *New England Journal of Medicine* 365, no. 6 (2011): 493–505.

51. Alison Rodger, Andrew Phillips, Jens Lundgren, Xiaohua Tao, Dan Shao, Wei Xue, Myron S. Cohen, Ying Q. Chen, and Thomas R. Fleming, "Prevention of HIV-1 Infection with Antiretroviral Therapy," *New England Journal of Medicine* 365, no. 20 (2011): 1934–35.

52. Charlotte Van Den Berg, Colette Smit, Giel Van Brussel, Roel Coutinho, and Maria Prins, "Full Participation in Harm Reduction Programmes Is Associated with Decreased Risk for Human Immunodeficiency Virus and Hepatitis C Virus: Evidence from the Amsterdam Cohort Studies among Drug Users," *Addiction* 102, no. 9 (2007): 1454–62.

53. Don C. Des Jarlais, Kamyar Arasteh, Courtney McKnight, Holly Hagan, David C. Perlman, Lucia V. Torian, Sara Beatice, Salaam Semaan, and Samuel R. Friedman, "HIV Infection During Limited Versus Combined HIV Prevention Programs for IDUs in New York City: The Importance of Transmission Behaviors," *Drug and Alcohol Dependence* 109, nos. 1–3 (2010): 154–60.

54. Holly Hagan, "Agent, Host, and Environment: Hepatitis C Virus in People Who Inject Drugs," *Journal of Infectious Diseases* 204, no. 12 (2011): 1819–21.

55. Holly Hagan, Enrique R. Pouget, Don C. Des Jarlais, and Corina Lelutiu-Weinberger, "Meta-Regression of Hepatitis C Virus Infection in Relation to Time since Onset of Illicit Drug Injection: The Influence of Time and Place," *American Journal of Epidemiology* 168, no. 10 (2008): 1099–109.

56. Hagan, *Agent, Host, and Environment*, 1819–21.

57. Katy M. E. Turner, Sharon Hutchinson, Peter Vickerman, Vivian Hope, Noel Craine, Norah Palmateer, Margaret May et al., "The Impact of Needle and Syringe Provision and Opiate Substitution Therapy on the Incidence of Hepatitis C Virus in Injecting Drug Users: Pooling of UK Evidence," *Addiction* 106, no. 11 (2011): 1978–88.

58. Hagan, *Agent, Host, and Environment*, 1819–21.

59. Paul Y. Kwo, Eric J. Lawitz, Jonathan McCone, Eugene R. Schiff, John M. Vierling, David Pound, Mitchell N. Davis et al., "Efficacy of Boceprevir, an Ns3 Protease Inhibitor, in Combination with Peginterferon Alfa-2b and Ribavirin in Treatment-Naive Patients with Genotype 1 Hepatitis C Infection (Sprint-1): An Open-Label, Randomised, Multicentre Phase 2 Trial," *Lancet* 376, no. 9742 (2010): 705–16.

60. John G. McHutchison, Gregory T. Everson, Stuart C. Gordon, Ira M. Jacobson, Mark Sulkowski, Robert Kauffman, Lindsay McNair, John Alam, and Andrew J. McNair, for the PROVE1 Study Team, "Telaprevir with Peginterferon and Ribavirin for Chronic HCV Genotype 1 Infection," *New England Journal of Medicine* 360, no. 18 (2009): 1827–38.

61. Mark A. Stoove, Sandy M. Gifford, and Greg J. Dore, "The Impact of Injecting Drug Use Status on Hepatitis C-related Referral and Treatment," *Drug and Alcohol Depend ence* 77, no. 1 (2005): 81–86.

62. Ministry of Public Health of Thailand, "HIV Epidemiological Situation and Health Sector Response 2010" (Bangkok, 2011).

63. Nicholas H. Wright, Suphak Vanichseni, Pasakorn Akarasewi, Chantapong Wasi, and Kachit Choopanya, "Was the 1988 HIV Epidemic among Bangkok's Injecting Drug Users a Common Source Outbreak?" *AIDS* 8, no. 4 (1994): 529 – 32.

64. Ministry of Public Health of Thailand, *HIV Epidemiological Situation.*

65. Aumphornpun Buavirat, Kimberly Page-Shafer, Godfried J. P. van Griensven, Jack S. Mandel, James Evans, Jaithip Chuaratanaphong, S Chiamwongpat, Rafael Sacks, and Andrew Moss, "Risk of Prevalent HIV Infection Associated with Incarceration among Injecting Drug Users in Bangkok, Thailand: Case-Control Study," *BMJ* 326, no. 7384 (2003): 308.

66. Kachit Choopanya, Don C. Des Jarlais, and Suphak Vanichseni et al., "Incarceration as a continuing HIV risk behavior among injecting Drug Users in Bangkok," Paper presented at: XI International Conference on AIDS, Vancouver, BC, Canada, July 7–12, 1996.

67. Kachit Choopanya, Don C. Des Jarlais, Suphak Vanichseni, Dwip Kitayaporn, Philip A. Mock, Suwanee Raktham, Krit Hireanras, William L. Heyward, Sathit Sujarita, and Timothy D. Mastro, "Incarceration and Risk for HIV Infection among Injection Drug Users in Bangkok," *Journal of Acquired Immune Deficiency Syndromes* 29, no. 1 (2002): 86–94.

68. Buavirat et al., *Risk of Prevalent HIV Infection*, 308.

69. Hansa Thaisri, John Lerwitworapong, Suthon Vongsheree, Pathom Sawanpanyalert, Chanchai Chadbanchachai, Archawin Rojanawiwat, Wichuda Kongpromsook, Wiroj Paung-

tubtim, Pongnuwat Sri-Ngam, and Rachaneekorn Jaisue, "HIV Infection and Risk Factors among Bangkok Prisoners, Thailand: A Prospective Cohort Study," *BMC Infectious Diseases* 3, no. 1 (2003): 25.

70. Kanna Hayashi, M-J. Milloy, Nadia Fairbairn, Karyn Kaplan, Paisan Suwannawong, Calvin Lai, Evan Wood, and Thomas Kerr, "Incarceration Experiences among a Community-recruited Sample of Injection Drug Users in Bangkok, Thailand," *BioMed Central* 9 (2009): 492.

71. Crystal M. Fuller, Carl A. Latkin, Danielle C. Ompad, Sandro Galea, Yingfeng Wu, and David Vlahov, "Social Support and Network Characteristics Soon after Onset of Injection Drug Use: Associations with HIV/HCV Infection," Paper presented at XV International AIDS Conference, Bangkok, Thailand, July 11–16, 2004.

72. Don C. Des Jarlais, Kachit Choopanya, John Wenston, Suphak Vanichseni, Jo L. Sotheran, and K. Phangsringarm, "Risk Reduction and Stabilization of HIV Seroprevalence among Drug Injectors in New York City and Bangkok, Thailand," *Science Challenging AIDS* (1992): 207–13.

73. Dwip Kitayaporn, Chintra Uneklabh, Bruce G. Weniger, and Pongvipa Lohsomboon, "HIV-1 Incidence Determined Retrospectively among Drug Users in Bangkok, Thailand," *AIDS* (1994).

74. Hayashi et al., *Incarceration Experiences*, 492.

75. Theodore M. Hammett, Ryan Kling, Patrick Johnston, Wei Liu, Doan Ngu, Patricia Friedmann, Kieu Thanh Binh, Ha Viet Dong, Ly Kieu Van, Meng Donghua, Yi Chen, and Don C. Des Jarlais, "Patterns of HIV Prevalence and HIV Risk Behaviors among Injection Drug Users Prior to and 24 Months Following Implementation of Cross-border HIV Prevention Interventions in Northern Vietnam and Southern China," *AIDS Education and Prevention* 18, no. 2 (2006): 97–115.

76. Don C. Des Jarlais, "Preventing HIV Transmission among Injecting Drug Users (IDUs) and from IDUs to Non-Injecting Sexual Partners in Sichuan, China," *Sexually Transmitted Diseases* 34, no. 8 (2007): 583–85. DOI:10.1097/OLQ.0b013e3180646412.

77. Theodore M. Hammett, Don C. Des Jarlais, Ryan Kling, Binh Thanh Kieu, Janet McNicholl, Punneeporn Wasinrapee, and J. Steven McDougal et al., "Controlling HIV Epidemics among Injection Drug Users: Eight Years of Cross-Border HIV Prevention Interventions in Vietnam and China," *PLoS One* (2012).

78. Bradley M. Mathers, Louisa Degenhardt, Hammad Ali, Lucas Wiessing, Matthew Hickman, Richard P. Mattick, Bronwyn Myers, Atul Ambekar, and Steffanie A. Strathdee, "HIV Prevention, Treatment, and Care Services for People Who Inject Drugs: A Systematic Review of Global, Regional, and National Coverage," *Lancet* 375, no. 9719 (2010): 1014–28.

79. WHO (World Health Organization), *Report on People who Inject Drugs in the South-East Asia Region* (New Delhi: WHO, 2010).

BIBLIOGRAPHY

Aceijas, Carmen, Gerry V. Stimson, Matthew Hickman, and Tim Rhodes. "Global Overview of Injecting Drug Use and HIV Infection among Injecting Drug Users." *AIDS* 18, no. 17 (2004): 2295–2303.

Agdamag, Dorothy M., Seiji Kageyama, Evelyn T. Alesna, Rontgene M. Solante, Prisca S. Leaño, Anna Marie L. Heredia, Ilya P. Abellanosa-Tac-An, Eutiquio T. Vibal, Lourdes D. Jereza, and Hiroshi Ichimura. "Rapid Spread of Hepatitis C Virus among Injecting-Drug Users in the Philippines: Implications for HIV Epidemics." *Journal of Medical Virology* 77, no. 2 (2005): 221–26.

Beckett, Gulbahar H. and Charles Romley Alder Wright. "Iv.—Action of the Organic Acids and Their Anhydrides on the Natural Alkaloids. Part Ii. Butyryl and Benzoyl Derivatives of Morphine and Codeine." *Journal of the Chemical Society* 28 (1875): 15–26.

Buavirat, Aumphornpun, Kimberly Page-Shafer, Godfried J. P. van Griensven, Jack S. Mandel, James Evans, Jaithip Chuaratanaphong, S. Chiamwongpat, Rafael Sacks, and Andrew Moss.

"Risk of Prevalent HIV Infection Associated with Incarceration among Injecting Drug Users in Bangkok, Thailand: Case-Control Study." *BMJ* 326, no. 7384 (2003): 308.

Choopanya, Kachit, Don C. Des Jarlais, and Suphak Vanichseni et al. "Incarceration as a continuing HIV risk behavior among injecting Drug Users in Bangkok." Paper presented at: XI International Conference on AIDS, Vancouver, BC, Canada, July 7–12, 1996.

Choopanya, Kachit, Don C. Des Jarlais, Suphak Vanichseni, Dwip Kitayaporn, Philip A. Mock, Suwanee Raktham, Krit Hireanras, William L. Heyward, Sathit Sujarita, and Timothy D. Mastro. "Incarceration and Risk for HIV Infection among Injection Drug Users in Bangkok." *Journal of Acquired Immune Deficiency Syndromes* 29, no. 1 (2002): 86–94.

Cohen, Myron S., Ying Q. Chen, Marybeth McCauley, Theresa Gamble, Mina C. Hosseinipour, Nagalingeswaran Kumarasamy, and James G. Hakim et al., "Prevention of HIV-1 Infection with Early Antiretroviral Therapy." *New England Journal of Medicine* 365, no. 6 (2011): 493–505.

Corporation MC. *Encyclopedia of Health*: Marshall Cavendish Corporation, 2009.

Des Jarlais, Don C. "Preventing HIV Transmission among Injecting Drug Users (IDUs) and from IDUs to Non-Injecting Sexual Partners in Sichuan, China." *Sexually Transmitted Diseases* 34, no. 8 (2007): 583–85. DOI: 10.1097/OLQ.0b013e3180646412.

Des Jarlais, Don C., Kachit Choopanya, John Wenston, Suphak Vanichseni, Jo L. Sotheran, and K. Phangsringarm. "Risk Reduction and Stabilization of HIV Seroprevalence among Drug Injectors in New York City and Bangkok, Thailand." *Science Challenging AIDS* (1992): 207–13.

Des Jarlais, Don C., Patrick Johnston, Patricia Friedmann, Ryan Kling, Wei Liu, Doan Ngu, Yi Chen, Tran V. Hoang, Meng Donghua, Ly K. Van, Nguyen D. Tung, Kieu T. Binh, and Theodore M. Hammett. "Patterns of HIV Prevalence among Injecting Drug Users in the Cross-Border Area of Lang Son Province, Vietnam, and Ning Ming County, Guangxi Province, China." *BMC Public Health* 5 (2005): 89.

Des Jarlais, Don C., Kamyar Arasteh, Courtney McKnight, Holly Hagan, David C. Perlman, Lucia V. Torian, Sara Beatice, Salaam Semaan, and Samuel R. Friedman. "HIV Infection During Limited Versus Combined HIV Prevention Programs for IDUs in New York City: The Importance of Transmission Behaviors." *Drug and Alcohol Dependence* 109, nos. 1–3 (2010): 154–60.

Filan, Kenaz. *The Power of the Poppy: Harnessing Nature's Most Dangerous Plant Ally*. Vermont: Park Street Press, 2011.

Fishbein, Diana H. and Susan E. Pease. *The Dynamics of Drug Abuse*. Massachusetts: Allyn & Bacon, 1995.

Friedman, Thomas L. *The Lexus and the Olive Tree*. New York: Anchor Books, 2000.

Fuller, Crystal M., Carl A. Latkin, Danielle C. Ompad, Sandro Galea, Yingfeng Wu, and David Vlahov. "Social Support and Network Characteristics Soon after Onset of Injection Drug Use: Associations with HIV/HCV Infection." Paper presented at XV International AIDS Conference, Bangkok, Thailand, July 11–16, 2004.

Garten, Rebecca J., Sheng-Han Lai, Jin-Bing Zhang, Wei Liu, Jie Chen, and Xiao-Fang Yu. "Factors Influencing a Low Rate of Hepatitis C Viral RNA Clearance in Heroin Users from Southern China." *World Journal of Gastroenterology* 14, no. 12 (2008): 1878.

Grasso, June M., Jay P. Corrin, and Michael Kort. *Modernization and Revolution in China: From the Opium Wars to the Olympics*: ME Sharpe Inc, 2009.

Hagan, Holly. "Agent, Host, and Environment: Hepatitis C Virus in People Who Inject Drugs." *Journal of Infectious Diseases* 204, no. 12 (2011): 1819–21.

Hagan, Holly, Don C. Des Jarlais, Rebecca Stern, Corina Lelutiu-Weinberger, Roberta Scheinmann, Sheila Strauss, and Peter L. Flom. "HCV Synthesis Project: Preliminary Analyses of HCV Prevalence in Relation to Age and Duration of Injection." *International Journal of Drug Policy* 18, no. 5 (2007): 341–51.

Hagan, Holly, Enrique R. Pouget, Don C. Des Jarlais, and Corina Lelutiu-Weinberger. "Meta-Regression of Hepatitis C Virus Infection in Relation to Time since Onset of Illicit Drug Injection: The Influence of Time and Place." *American Journal of Epidemiology* 168, no. 10 (2008): 1099–1109.

Hammett, Theodore M., Ryan Kling, Patrick Johnston, Wei Liu, Doan Ngu, Patricia Fried-mann, Kieu Thanh Binh, Ha Viet Dong, Ly Kieu Van, Meng Donghua, Yi Chen, and Don C. Des Jarlais. "Patterns of HIV Prevalence and HIV risk behaviors among Injection Drug Users prior to and 24 months Following Implementation of Cross-border HIV Prevention Interventions in Northern Vietnam and Southern China." *AIDS Education and Prevention* 18, no. 2 (2006): 97–115.

Hammett, Theodore M., Don C. Des Jarlais, Ryan Kling, Binh Thanh Kieu, Janet McNicholl, Punneeporn Wasinrapee, and J. Steven McDougal et al. "Controlling HIV Epidemics among Injection Drug Users: Eight Years of Cross-Border HIV Prevention Interventions in Vietnam and China." *PLoS One* (2012).

Illife, John. *The African Aids Epidemic. A History.* Athens, Ohio: Ohio University Press, 2006.

Jia, Manhong, Hongbing Luo, Yanling Ma, Ning Wang, Kumi Smith, Jiangyuan Mei, Ran Lu, Jiyun Lu, Liru Fu, Qiang Zhang, Zunyou Wu, and Lin Lu , "The HIV Epidemic in Yunnan Province, China, 1989–2007." *Journal of Acquired Immune Deficiency Syndromes* 53 (2010): S34–S40. DOI: 10.1097/QAI.0b013e3181c7d6ff.

Jittiwutikarn, Jaroon, Satawat Thongsawat, Vinai Suriyanon, Niwat Maneekarn, David Celentano, Myat Htoo Razak, Namtip Srirak, Tassanai Vongchak, Surinda Kawichai, David Thomas, Teerada Sripaipan, Dale Netski, Ashwin Ananthakrishnan, and Kenrad E. Nelson. "Hepatitis C Infection among Drug Users in Northern Thailand." *The American Journal of Tropical Medicine and Hygiene* 74, no. 6 (2006): 1111–16.

Kitayaporn, Dwip, Chintra Uneklabh, Bruce G. Weniger, and Pongvipa Lohsomboon. "Hiv-1 Incidence Determined Retrospectively among Drug Users in Bangkok, Thailand." *AIDS* (1994).

Kwo, Paul Y., Eric J. Lawitz, Jonathan McCone, Eugene R. Schiff, John M. Vierling, David Pound, and Mitchell N. Davis et al. "Efficacy of Boceprevir, an Ns3 Protease Inhibitor, in Combination with Peginterferon Alfa-2b and Ribavirin in Treatment-Naive Patients with Genotype 1 Hepatitis C Infection (Sprint-1): An Open-Label, Randomised, Multicentre Phase 2 Trial." *Lancet* 376, no. 9742 (2010): 705–16.

Mathers, Bradley M., Louisa Degenhardt, Hammad Ali, Lucas Wiessing, Matthew Hickman, Richard P. Mattick, Bronwyn Myers, Atul Ambekar, and Steffanie A. Strathdee. "HIV Prevention, Treatment, and Care Services for People Who Inject Drugs: A Systematic Review of Global, Regional, and National Coverage." *Lancet* 375, no. 9719 (2010): 1014–28.

Mathers, Bradley M., Louisa Degenhardt, Benjamin Phillips, Lucas Wiessing, Matthew Hickman, Steffanie A Strathdee, Alex Wodak, Samiran Panda, Mark Tyndall, Abdalla Toufik, Richard P. Mattick, for the 2007 Reference Group to the UN on HIV and Injecting Drug Use. "Global Epidemiology of Injecting Drug Use and HIV among People who Inject Drugs: a Systematic Review." *Lancet* 372, no. 9651 (2008): 1733–45.

McHutchison, John G., Gregory T. Everson, Stuart C. Gordon, Ira M. Jacobson, Mark Sulkowski, Robert Kauffman, Lindsay McNair, John Alam, and Andrew J. McNair, for the PROVE1 Study Team. "Telaprevir with Peginterferon and Ribavirin for Chronic HCV Genotype 1 Infection." *New England Journal of Medicine* 360, no. 18 (2009): 1827–38.

Ministry of Public Health of Thailand. "HIV Epidemiological Situation and Health Sector Response 2010." Bangkok, 2011.

Musto, David F., Pamela Korsmeyer, and Thomas W. Maulucci. *One Hundred Years of Heroin.* Connecticut: Auburn House Westport, 2002.

Nelson, Paul K., Bradley M. Mathers, Benjamin Cowie, Holly Hagan, Don Des Jarlais, Danielle Horyniak, and Louisa Degenhardt. "Global Epidemiology of Hepatitis B and Hepatitis C in People Who Inject Drugs: Results of Systematic Reviews." *Lancet* 378, no. 9791 (2011): 571–83.

Nelwan, Erni J., Reinout Van Crevel, Bachti Alisjahbana, Agnes K. Indrati, Reiva F. Dwiyana, Nisaa Nuralam, Herdiman T. Pohan, Ilham Jaya, Andre Meheus, and Andre Van Der Ven. "Human Immunodeficiency Virus, Hepatitis B and Hepatitis C in an Indonesian Prison: Prevalence, Risk Factors and Implications of HIV Screening." *Tropical Medicine & International Health* 15, no. 12 (2010): 1491– 98.

Ng, Kee Peng, Teik Leong Saw, Nora W. Wong, Keow Lin Goh, Stew Yeam Chuah, and Mayavaty Nagaratnam. "The Prevalence of Anti-HCV Antibody in Risk Groups and Blood Donors." *The Medical Journal of Malaysia* 50, no. 4 (1995): 302.

Perngmark, Pajongsil, David D. Celentano, and Surinda Kawichai. "Risk Factors for HIV Infection among Drug Injectors in Southern Thailand." *Drug and Alcohol Dependence* 71, no. 3 (2003): 229–38.

Polachek, James M. *The Inner Opium War:* Harvard University Asia Center, 1992.

Pybus, Oliver G., Eleanor Barnes, Rachel Taggart, Philippe Lemey, Peter V. Markov, Bouachan Rasachak, Bounkong Syhavong, Rattanaphone Phetsouvanah, Isabelle Sheridan, Isla S. Humphreys, Ling Lu, Paul N. Newton, and Paul Klenerman. "Genetic History of Hepatitis C Virus in East Asia." *Journal of Virology* 83, no. 2 (2009): 1071–82.

Quinn, Thomas C., Jonathan Mann, James W. Curran, and Peter Piot. "AIDS in Africa: An Epidemiologic Paradigm." *Science* 234, no. 4779 (1986): 955–63.

Rodger, Alison, Andrew Phillips, Jens Lundgren, Xiaohua Tao, Dan Shao, Wei Xue, Myron S. Cohen, Ying Q. Chen, and Thomas R. Fleming. "Prevention of HIV-1 Infection with Antiretroviral Therapy." *New England Journal of Medicine* 365, no. 20 (2011): 1934–35.

Ruan, Yuhua, Kanglin Chen, Kunxue Hong, Yixin He, Shizhu Liu, Feng Zhou, Guangming Qin, Jianping Chen, Hui Xing, and Yiming Shao. "Community-Based Survey of HIV Transmission Modes among Intravenous Drug Users in Sichuan, China." *Sexually Transmitted Diseases* 31, no. 10 (2004): 623–27.

Sneader, Walter. "The Discovery of Heroin." *Lancet* 352, no. 9141 (1998): 1697–99.

Stern, Rebecca, Holly Hagan, Corina Lelutiu-Weinberger, Don Des Jarlais, Roberta Scheinmann, Shiela Strauss, Enrique Pouget, and Peter Flom. "The HCV Synthesis Project: Scope, Methodology, and Preliminary Results." *BMC Medical Research Methodology* 8, no. 1 (2008): 62.

Stoove, M. A., Gifford, S. M., and Dore, G. J. "The Impact of Injecting Drug Use Status on Hepatitis C-related Referral and Treatment." *Drug and Alcohol Dependence* 77, no. 1 (2005): 81–86.

Thaisri, Hansa, John Lerwitworapong, Suthon Vongsheree, Pathom Sawanpanyalert, Chanchai Chadbanchachai, Archawin Rojanawiwat, Wichuda Kongpromsook, Wiroj Paungtubtim, Pongnuwat Sri-Ngam, and Rachaneekorn Jaisue. "HIV Infection and Risk Factors among Bangkok Prisoners, Thailand: A Prospective Cohort Study." *BMC Infectious Diseases* 3, no. 1 (2003): 25.

Turner, Katy M. E., Sharon Hutchinson, Peter Vickerman, Vivian Hope, Noel Craine, Norah Palmateer, and Margaret May et al. "The Impact of Needle and Syringe Provision and Opiate Substitution Therapy on the Incidence of Hepatitis C Virus in Injecting Drug Users: Pooling of UK Evidence." *Addiction* 106, no. 11 (2011): 1978–88.

UNAIDS/WHO (Joint United Nations Programme on HIV/AIDS). *AIDS Epidemic Update: December 2006* . Geneva: UNAIDS/WHO , 2007.

UNODC (United Nations Office of Drugs and Crime). *2005 World Drug Report.* Vienna: UNODC, 2005.

Van Den Berg, Charlotte, Colette Smit, Giel Van Brussel, Roel Coutinho, and Maria Prins. "Full Participation in Harm Reduction Programmes Is Associated with Decreased Risk for Human Immunodeficiency Virus and Hepatitis C Virus: Evidence from the Amsterdam Cohort Studies among Drug Users." *Addiction* 102, no. 9 (2007): 1454–62.

Vicknasingam, Balasingam, Suresh Narayanan, and Visweswaran Navaratnam. "The Relative Risk of HIV among IDUs Not in Treatment in Malaysia." *AIDS Care* 21, no. 8 (2009): 984–91.

WHO (World Health Organization). *Report on People who Inject Drugs in the South- East Asia Region.* New Delhi: WHO, 2010.

Winslow, Monte M., Malayanna Subramaniam, Wan-Leung Ng, Alice Lee, Gang Song, and Yuk-Hee Chan. "Seroprevalence of Hepatitis C in Intravenous Opioid Users Presenting in the Early Phase of Injecting Drug Use in Singapore." *Singapore Medical Journal* 48, no. 6 (2007): 504.

Wright, Nicholas H., Suphak Vanichseni, Pasakorn Akarasewi, Chantapong Wasi, and Kachit Choopanya. "Was the 1988 HIV Epidemic among Bangkok's Injecting Drug Users a Common Source Outbreak?" *AIDS* 8, no. 4 (1994): 529–32.

Xia, Minsheng, Joan K. Kreiss, and King K. Holmes. "Risk Factors for HIV infection among drug users in Yunnan province, China: Association with Intravenous Drug Use and Protective Effect of Boiling Reusable Needles and Syringes." *AIDS* 8, no. 12 (1994): 1701–6.

Xia, Xian, Jun Luo, Jianling Bai, and Rongbin Yu. "Epidemiology of Hepatitis C Virus Infection among Injection Drug Users in China: Systematic Review and Meta- Analysis." *Public Health* 122, no. 10 (2008): 990–1003.

Xia, Xueshan, Ling Lu, Kok Keng Tee, Wenhua Zhao, Jianguo Wu, Jing Yu, Xiaojie Li, Yixiong Lin, Muhammad Mahmood Mukhtar, Curt H. Hagedorn, and Yutaka Takebe. "The Unique HCV Genotype Distribution and the Discovery of a Novel Subtype 6u among Idus Co-Infected with HIV-1 in Yunnan, China." *Journal of Medical Virology* 80, no. 7 (2008): 1142–52.

Yao, Yan, Ning Wang, Jennifer Chu, Guowei Ding, Xia Jin, Yongli Sun, Guixiang Wang, Junjie Xu, and Kumi Smith. "Sexual Behavior and Risks for HIV Infection and Transmission among Male Injecting Drug Users in Yunnan, China." *International Journal of Infectious Diseases* 13, no. 2 (2009): 154–61.

Yin, Lu, Guangming Qin, Han Zhu Qian, Yu Zhu, Wei Hu, Li Zhang, Kanglin Chen, Yunxia Wang, Shizhu Liu, Feng Zhou, Hui Xing, Yuhua Ruan, Ning Wang, and Yiming Shao. "Continued Spread of HIV among Injecting Drug Users in Southern Sichuan Province, China." *Harm Reduction Journal* 4, no. 6 (2007). DOI: 10.1186/1477-7517-4-6.

Zhang, Li, Junling Zhu, Baoling Rui, Yuanzhi Zhang, Lijiang Zhang, Lu Yin, Yuhua Ruan, Han-Zhu Qian, and Yiming Shao. "High HIV Risk among Uigur Minority Ethnic Drug Users in Northwestern China." *Tropical Medicine & International Health* 13, no. 6 (2008): 814–17.

Zhao, Min, Qiu Wang, Guang Lu, Ping Xu, Han Xu, and Clyde McCoy. "Risk Behaviors and HIV/AIDS Prevention Education among IDUs in Drug Treatment in Shanghai." *Journal of Urban Health* 82 (2005): iv84–iv91.

Chapter Ten

Compulsory "Rehabilitation" in Asia

Problems and Possible Solutions

Simon Baldwin and Nicholas Thomson

INTRODUCTION

In Asia, the practice of detaining people who use drugs[1] in compulsory drug rehabilitation centers[2] has increased exponentially over the last decade.[3] This is due, at least in part, to the widespread belief that all people who use drugs require rehabilitation and that if they are unwilling to seek it voluntarily then the state (often co-opting police or locally formed community groups) has the authority to mandate "treatment" in closed settings.

Invariably referred to as "rehabilitation centers," these institutions have been criticized for offering little in the way of evidence-based drug treatment,[4] contravening international (and often national) human rights norms[5] as well as contradicting basic medical principles and voluntariness.[6]

In response to these criticisms several UN agencies recently called on countries to close all compulsory rehabilitation centers and to end the practice of compulsory treatment for drug dependence.[7] This chapter provides a detailed look at the ideological and policy framework underpinning compulsory rehabilitation and proposes answers to a range of difficult ethical dilemmas associated with the use of the centers. This chapter also suggests a range of practical considerations to assist states to move away from the use of compulsory treatment centers.

COMPULSORY DETENTION OF PEOPLE WHO USE DRUGS

Over the past two decades, many national governments in southeast Asia have increasingly turned to compulsory drug treatment.[8] Compulsory drug treatment is currently supported in eleven countries across Asia, including Cambodia, China, Laos, Malaysia, Thailand, and Vietnam. China detains about 330,000 people in compulsory detention centers, Vietnam detains around 60,000, and about 80,000 are detained in Thailand.[9]

Forcing people who use drugs into treatment is based on the premise that people who use drugs lack the internal motivation and mental clarity necessary to seek and persist in voluntarily treatment.[10] In the past, many countries have adopted policies supporting compulsory treatment. For example, during the 1920s and 1930s, the US government supported six months of compulsory treatment in centers for morphine and opium addicts.[11]

Despite recent shifts in drug policy that suggest a more health-oriented approach to drug use in the region, drug prohibition (either through criminal or administrative law) continues to dominate national responses. While countries such as Malaysia, Cambodia, Laos, and Thailand have recently revised their legal statutes to provide for a wider range of non-custodial rehabilitation orders, these laws have not reduced the extent of the interlocking coercive powers of registration, surveillance, and treatment.[12]

In essence, drug policy in Asia has conflated the ideas of treatment and punishment with many countries now supporting a paradoxical position that mandates, most commonly through an extrajudicial process, compulsory rehabilitation to anyone who is unwilling to volunteer to enter a program.

Criticisms of Compulsory Treatment

The virtue of forced rehabilitation can be questioned from two perspectives. The first approach prioritizes whether or not the practice can be considered ethical. The second evaluates compulsory rehabilitation based on its effectiveness. Inherent in this assessment is the need for a clear understanding of the goals of compulsory treatment.

Any assessment of compulsory treatment must first define the criteria by which it will be judged. Assuming that the goal of compulsory treatment is in fact to provide treatment to drug users (and not for ulterior purposes such as obtaining inexpensive labor or imposing extrajudicial detention), the following criteria can be used:

- A reduction or elimination of illicit drug use
- A reduction in the negative health outcomes associated with drug use (e.g., overdose and the transmission of infectious diseases such as HIV, viral hepatitis, and tuberculosis)

• A reduction in the harms to society, primarily in the form of crimes that drug users may commit while under the influence of drugs, in order to buy drugs, or in resolving conflicts in illicit drug markets

ASSESSING COMPULSORY TREATMENT IN ASIA BASED ON ETHICS AND EFFECTIVENESS

As noted by Stevens (2011), the issue of effectiveness is secondary to the issue of ethics because, if a treatment is unethical, it cannot be justified even if it is effective in meeting its goal.[13] Thus the assessment of compulsory treatment in Asia will consider ethical issues first.

Ethics

Compulsory detention clearly breaches a person's right to freedom from arbitrary detention.[14] Second, the principle of informed consent is also breached, as drug users are not provided with the option of refusing treatment. Even in the rare cases that patients provide consent, they are not able to withdraw their consent and leave the center. Further, many have also highlighted that practices common to compulsory detention centers such as detoxification without medical assistance, military-style exercises and initiation rites (such as shaving the heads of new detainees) all breach article 5 of the Universal Declaration of Human Rights, which prohibits inhuman and degrading treatment or punishment. A number of reports have also documented forced labor, systematic beatings, and rape inside the centers.[15]

Finally compulsory rehabilitation is also in breach of the ethical principle of proportionality in sentencing. Stevens (2011) states that there are two ethical limits to the severity of sanctions: first that the sentence should be no more severe than is justified by the harm caused by the offense and second that the sentence should be no more severe than is necessary to achieve its intended purpose.[16] Considering that the majority of people detained in compulsory treatment centers are not serious criminals and that the harm caused by their drug use is limited to the individual and possibly close family members, these harms do not justify the severity of several years of detention. Similarly, if the intended purpose of sentencing is a reduction in drug use and crime, more effective treatments that are less severe can be provided in the community.

Effectiveness

While most proponents claim that compulsory treatment is implemented to provide treatment for people who use drugs, others suggest that motivations for the approach include a more efficient method for "managing" drug users, reducing the strain on increasingly overcrowded prison systems, or providing a cheap workforce. [17, 18]

However, given that most countries in the region classify drug users as patients and not as criminals and that compulsory treatment is provided for the purpose of rehabilitation, [19] the issue of effectiveness will be considered only from this perspective.

First, no evidence exists in Asia to show that compulsory treatment leads to a reduction or elimination of illicit drugs use. Based on government data from a number of countries, the percentage of people returning to drug use upon release ranges between 80 percent and 95 percent. [20, 21] In addition, a number of studies suggest that rather than reducing the negative health consequences of drug use, the system of compulsory treatment in Asia actually increases health harm. [22] The system contributes to health harm in two ways—through poor treatment conditions and through deterring people who use drugs from seeking services.

First, the care provided in compulsory treatment centers in Southeast Asia is often underfunded, of poor quality, and provided by non-qualified staff. Some centers are overcrowded, with inmates living in unsanitary conditions that may be hazardous to health and with little or no medical care. [23, 24] Others have reported being unable to obtain HIV treatment or prevention supplies such as antiretroviral medicines, condoms and sterile injecting equipment while in detention, which has obvious adverse impact on universal access to prevention, treatment, care, and support for people who use drugs and people living with HIV and AIDS.

The second way in which compulsory treatment limits the health of people who use drugs is because the simple threat of being detained deters drug users from accessing community-based services for fear they will be identified. [25, 26]

No published studies look at the impact of compulsory detention on reducing harm to society. On the one hand, it could be argued that this approach would logically lead to a reduction in crime through detainment of a significant proportion of people who use drugs. This idea, however, is based on the largely unfounded premise that the majority of crime is committed by people who use drugs. [27] On the other hand, it could be argued that sending a large number of civilians to compulsory treatment for long periods is extremely disruptive to their lives and has negative consequences for both their families (lack of income, inability to contribute to parenting) and themselves (reduced prospects to reintegrate into the community, lost opportunities for employment and education).

The effectiveness of compulsory treatment is further brought into question by the lack of evidence-based treatment services offered inside compulsory treatment centers. In most cases, compulsory treatment is based on a short period of detoxification followed by a longer period of moral education, drills that focus on instilling discipline, as well as long periods of arduous manual labor, commonly referred to as "labor therapy."[28, 29]

Consequences of Compulsory Rehabilitation

There are three main consequences associated with compulsory detention and forced rehabilitation in Asia.

First, compulsory rehabilitation centers draw considerable resources into a system that is massively ineffective. As discussed above the significant majority of people return to drug use after release and many people leave the centers in worse heath than they entered. One study from Vietnam estimated that it costs $674 dollars per year to detain a person in a compulsory rehabilitation center. It is estimated that this is over three times the cost of maintaining a person on a methadone program for the same period.[30]

The second major consequence of compulsory rehabilitation is a result of the fear it creates among people who use drugs in the community. Most drug users are extremely fearful of being sent to a center. This fear creates a major structural barrier and prevents many people from accessing community-based HIV prevention and other health promotion services. Data from Vietnam suggests that there is a four- to six-year lag between starting injecting drug use and regularly attending community-based HIV prevention services.[31]

The final major consequence of compulsory rehabilitation is that is focuses police resources on arresting street based drug users and away from the most antisocial and harmful elements of the drug market. Many compulsory rehabilitation centers operate on "quota" systems that require police to regularly send a certain number of people to the centers.[32] This focuses their attention on users who generally have little to do with drug manufacturing or distribution.[33, 34, 35]

MOVING BEYOND COMPULSORY TREATMENT

Despite facing increasing criticism from international human rights groups and a call from the United National to close all compulsory rehabilitation centers and to end the practice of compulsory treatment for drug dependence[36] few countries have made significant progress toward this goal.

While some countries, such as Malaysia and Vietnam, have begun converting some compulsory centers to being open and voluntary, progress remains slow and will remain so without changes to their legal frameworks, which still endorse compulsory rehabilitation.[37]

While wholesale agreement on adopting the UN recommendations is unlikely in the short term, organizations working with people who use drugs in the region face a number of difficult questions. Perhaps the most contested issue is how organizations should balance the humanitarian desire to help detainees with the need to also advocate for closure of the centers.

Saucier et al. neatly summarize the ethical conundrum in the following passage:

> We expect good people to do these things, and we believe that human beings need and deserve these social goods. However, ethics also requires the consideration of burdens as well as benefits. An activity ceases to be ethically sound when it harms more than it helps. When health-related resources—including the application of knowledge, as well as personnel, supplies, and funds—are used in ways that perpetuate known harms or that direct limited resources toward the perpetuation of a system that is fundamentally unjust, these resources are supporting interests other than the interests of those who suffer. At some point, these resources are no longer serving health-related ends. [38]

According to this framework, organizations are faced with two potentially competing positions: on the one hand the desire to provide assistance to the several hundred thousand people currently detained in horrific conditions in compulsory centers throughout the region and on the other, ensuring that engagement does not further legitimize or contributing to the longevity of the centers.

This dichotomy leaves organizations with two choices: provide assistance or not. Perhaps a more nuanced and pragmatic position offers a middle ground that focuses on developing programs that address the most significant harms faced by people in compulsory center, while at the same time maintaining a strong commitment to closing them down.

Such solutions will only come about with careful consideration and strong partnerships between a wide array of actors. Ultimately, all activities should focus on closing the centers and developing evidenced based and voluntary alternatives. We argue that it is significantly more difficult to justify engagement inside the centers if equal efforts are not being made to close them down in short to medium term or, at a minimum, scale down their use and negative impacts in the very short term.

When it comes to deciding whether or not to provide services directly to people detained in forced rehabilitation centers, we suggest the follow ethical principles should be considered. Any interventions should first focus in on providing basic health care and protecting human rights. Further, any engagement must not build the capacity of the center or center staff. For example if an organization is considering supporting the provision of ART drugs to people living inside the centers with HIV then this should be implemented through an inreach model with staff and resources controlled by organizations unconnected to the management of the centers.

We also suggest there are three important preconditions before engagement should be considered. The first is guaranteed and unannounced access to monitor the intervention and conditions in the center. The second is an agreed mechanism for dealing with any human rights violations and/or poor monitoring outcomes. The final precondition is a documented strategy for disengagement.

PROPOSING AN ALTERNATIVE TO COMPULSORY DETENTION

While debate has focused on the need to stop compulsory detention, there are also concurrent efforts underway that propose a range of strategies that governments might consider as they move away from the use of compulsory detention. Sustainably moving away from the use of compulsory treatment requires that countries develop coordinated whole-of-government drug policies that focus on ethically diverting people away from the criminal justice system, while at the same time investing in voluntary and community based services. To do this requires the development of an integrated and collaborative mechanism that allows law enforcement and public health to effectively work together.

The collaborative mechanism needs to fundamentally ensure that the role of law enforcement in relation to illicit drugs is focused on the broader enforcement objectives of targeting the most harmful and antisocial elements of drug markets rather than forcing people into treatment. At the same time, this allows for the public health sector oversight of a scaled up and integrated range of complementary social services including community-based harm reduction and medically supervised community-based treatment.

Utilizing and implementing the concept of "justice reinvestment" would see the development and expansion of a range of community-based treatment and social service options for people who use drugs. Justice reinvestment is predicated on the fact that scaling up a range of community-based treatment and social services for people who use drugs means that they are more likely to seek assistance for issues associated with problematic and dependent drug use and are less likely to re-offend or come into contact with the criminal justice system. Increasing access to community-based treatment, especially methadone and social service options has also been shown to reduce the scale of drug markets, reduce crime,[39] reduce HIV risk behavior,[40, 41] and increase the economic productivity of drug users in the criminal justice system.[42]

CONCLUSION

Despite considerable effort across the region to improve access to health care, continued support for forced rehabilitation is a major structural barrier that prevents people who use drugs from accessing these services. Unfortunately while the response to drug possession remains punitive, little wholesale change to the compulsory treatment system will be possible. While change has been slow to this point, a few positive signs are emerging. For example, in July 2012, the National Assembly of Vietnam revised the Ordinance on Administrative Violations to remove compulsory detention and rehabilitation of commercial sex workers. Unfortunately a similar proposal to remove the forced treatment for drug users was defeated. Moving away from the use of compulsory detention in Asia requires policy makers to acknowledge that current approaches do not work and that ethical, evidence-based and community based options actually benefit law enforcement objectives as well as individual and public health outcomes.

ACKNOWLEDGMENT

This chapter is partly based on larger review of compulsory rehabilitation and the subsequent development of a practical guidance document funded by RTI International.

NOTES

1. The United Nations drug control conventions do not recognize a distinction between licit and illicit drugs; rather they describe drug *use* as being licit or illicit. For the purposes of this chapter, the term "illicit drugs" is used to describe drugs that are under international control (and that may or may not have licit medical purposes) but which are produced, trafficked, and/or consumed illicitly. More information can be found at www.unodc.org/unodc/en/illicit-drugs/definitions/index.html (accessed May 5, 2012).

2. This chapter uses the terms *compulsory drug treatment* or *compulsory treatment* or *compulsory drug detention* to describe a process in which people who use drugs—or, in some cases, are suspected of using drugs—and who do not voluntarily opt for drug treatment are sentenced to closed settings for various periods of time. The setting in which the person is detained will be referred to as a *compulsory detention center* or a *compulsory rehabilitation center*. It is also important to note that the term "compulsory treatment" does not imply that internationally recognized drug addiction treatment occurs inside the compulsory detention centers (Wolfe and Saucier, 2010).

3. Adrian Carter, Wayne Hall, and Judy Illes (eds.), *Addiction Neuroethics: The Ethics of Addiction Neuroscience Research and Treatment*: Elsevier Science (reference). Kindle Edition, 2011.

4. Daniel Wolfe and Roxanne Saucier, "In Rehabilitation's Name? Ending Institutionalised Cruelty and Degrading Treatment of People who Use Drugs," *International Journal of Drug Policy* 21, no. 3 (2010): 145–48. DOI: 10.1016/j.drugpo.2010.01.008.

5. HRW (Human Rights Watch), *The Rehab Archipelago* (NYC: HRW, 2011).

6. Alex Stevens, "Policy Analysis: Drug Policy, Harm and Human Rights: A Rationalist Approach," *International Journal of Drug Policy* 22 (2011): 233–38. DOI: 10.1016/j.drugpo.2011.02.003.

7. ILO (International Labour Organisation), Office of the High Commissioner for Human Rights, United Nations Development Programme, United Nations Educational Scientific and Cultural Organisation, United Nations Population Fund, United Nations High Commissioner for Refugees, Joint United Nations Programme on HIV/AIDS (2012). "Compulsory Drug Detention and Rehabilitation Centres." Accessed March 2, 2012.

8. UNODC/ESCAP/UNAIDS (United Nations Office of Drugs and Crime/United Nations Economic and Social Commission for Asia and the Pacific/Joint United Nations Programme on HIV/AIDS), 2011. *Report of the Regional Consultation on Compulsory Centres for Drug Users in Asia and the Pacific 14 – 16 December 2010, Bangkok*, accessed January 21, 2012. www.unescap.org/sdd/meetings/CCDU-Dec2010/index.asp.

9. Nicolas Thomson, "Detention of Methamphetamine Users in Cambodia, Laos, and Thailand" (Open Society Institute, NY, 2010). Accessed 5 October 2012. www.soros.org/sites/default/files/Detention-as-Treatment-20100301.pdf.

10. James A. Inciardi, Duane C. McBride, and James E. Rivers, *Drug Control and the Courts*. (Thousand Oaks, CA: Sage, 1996).

11. David Farabee, Michael Prendergast, and M. Douglas Anglin, "The Effectiveness of Coerced Treatment for Drug-Abusing Offenders," *Federal Probation* 62, no. 1 (1998): 3–10.

12. UNODC/ESCAP/UNAIDS, *Report of the Regional Consultation* .

13. Stevens, *Policy Analysis*, 233–38.

14. HRW, *The Rehab Archipelago*.

15. HRW, *The Rehab Archipelago*.

16. Stevens, *Policy Analysis*, 233–38.

17. HRW, *The Rehab Archipelago*.

18. Thomson, *Detention of Methamphetamine Users*.

19. Thu Vuong, Robert Ali, Simon Baldwin, and Stephen Mills, "Drug Policy in Vietnam: A Decade of Change?" *International Journal of Drug Policy* 23, no. 4 (2012): 319–26. DOI: 10.1016/j.drugpo.2011.11.005.

20. UNODC/ESCAP/UNAIDS, Report of the Regional Consultation.

21. UNODC/WHO (United Nations Office of Drugs and Crime/World Health Organization), 2008. *Principles of Drug Dependence Treatment*, Discussion Paper, accessed April 1, 2012.www.unodc.org/documents/drug-treatment/UNODC-WHO-Principles-of-Drug-Dependence-Treatment-March08.pdf.

22. Wolfe and Saucier, *In Rehabilitation's Name?* 145–48.

23. HRW (Human Rights Watch), *The Rehab Archipelago* (NYC: HRW, 2011).

24. Thomson, *Detention of Methamphetamine Users*.

25. HRW, *The Rehab Archipelago*.

26. Thomson, *Detention of Methamphetamine Users*.

27. David Weisburd, Cody W. Telep, Joshua C. Hinkle, and John E. Eck, "Is Problem-Oriented Policing Effective in Reducing Crime and Disorder?" *Criminology & Public Policy* 9, no. 1 (2010): 139–72. DOI: 10.1111/j.1745-9133.2010.00617.x.

28. HRW, *The Rehab Archipelago*.

29. Thomson, *Detention of Methamphetamine Users*.

30. Simon Baldwin, "Costing Harm Reduction Interventions for Vietnam." Paper presented at the International Conference on Reducing Drug Related Harm, Bangkok, Thailand, April 20–23, 2009.

31. FHI (Family Health International), HIV/STI Integrated Biological and Behavioral Surveillance. Unpublished FHI, 2009.

32. HRW (Human Rights Watch), *Skin on the Cable* (New York: HRW, 2009).

33. Thomas F. Babor, "Drug Policy and the Public Good: A Summary of the Book," *Addiction* 105, no. 7 (2010): 1137–45.

34. Lorraine Mazerolle, David Soole, and Sacha Rombouts, "Drug Law Enforcement," *Police Quarterly* 10, no. 2 (2007): 115–53. DOI: 10.1177/1098611106287776.

35. Alex Wodak and Leah McLeod, "The Role of Harm Reduction in Controlling HIV among Injecting Drug Users," *AIDS* 22 (2008): S81–S92 10.1097/1001.aids.0000327439.0000320914.0000327433.

36. ILO, Compulsory Drug Detention.

37. Suresh Narayanan, Balasingam Vicknasingam, and Noorzurani Robson, "The Transition to Harm Reduction: Understanding the Role of Non-Governmental Organisations in Malaysia," *International Journal of Drug Policy* 22, no. 4 (2011): 311–17.

38. Roxanne Saucier, Nancy Berlinger, Nicholas Thomson, Michael Gusmano, and Daniel Wolfe, "The Limits of Equivalence: Ethical Dilemmas in Providing Care in Drug Detention Centers," *International Journal of Prisoner Health* 6, no. 2 (2010): 37–43.

39. Matthew Epperson, Nabila El-Bassel, Louisa Gilbert, E. Roberto Orellana, and Mingway Chang, "Increased HIV Risk Associated with Criminal Justice Involvement among Men on Methadone," *AIDS and Behavior* 12 (2008): 51–57.

40. Bach Xuan Tran, Arto Ohinmaa, Anh Thuy Duong, Nhan Thi Do, Long Thanh Nguyen, Steve Mills, and Philip Jacobs, "Cost-Effectiveness of Methadone Maintenance Treatment for HIV-Positive Drug Users in Vietnam," *AIDS Care* 24, no. 3 (2011): 283–90. DOI: 10.1080/09540121.2011.608420.

41. Wodak and McLeod, *The Role of Harm Reduction*, S81–S92.

42. Richard P. Mattick, Courtney Breen, Jo Kimber, and Marina Davoli, "Methadone maintenance therapy versus no opioid replacement therapy for opioid dependence" (Review): Cochrane Review, 2009.

BIBLIOGRAPHY

Babor, Thomas F. "Drug Policy and the Public Good: A Summary of the Book." *Addiction* 105, no. 7 (2010): 1137–45.

Baldwin, Simon. "Costing Harm Reduction Interventions for Vietnam." Paper presented at the International Conference on Reducing Drug Related Harm, Bangkok, Thailand, April 20–23, 2009.

Carter, Adrian, Wayne Hall, and Judy Illes (eds.). *Addiction Neuroethics: The Ethics of Addiction Neuroscience Research and Treatment*: Elsevier Science (reference). Kindle Edition, 2011.

Epperson, Matthew, Nabila El-Bassel, Louisa Gilbert, E. Roberto Orellana, and Mingway Chang. "Increased HIV Risk Associated with Criminal Justice Involvement among Men on Methadone." *AIDS and Behavior* 12 (2008): 51–57.

Farabee, David, Michael Prendergast, and M. Douglas Anglin. "The Effectiveness of Coerced Treatment for Drug-Abusing Offenders." *Federal Probation* 62, no. 1 (1998): 3–10.

FHI (Family Health International). HIV/STI Integrated Biological and Behavioral Surveillance Unpublished FHI, 2009.

HRW (Human Rights Watch). *Skin on the Cable*. New York: HRW, 2009.

HRW (Human Rights Watch). *The Rehab Archipelago*. New York: HRW, 2011.

ILO (International Labour Organisation). Office of the High Commissioner for Human Rights, United Nations Development Programme, United Nations Educational Scientific and Cultural Organisation, United Nations Population Fund, United Nations High Commissioner for Refugees, Joint United Nations Programme on HIV/AIDS. (2012). "Compulsory Drug Detention and Rehabilitation Centres." Accessed March 2, 2012.

Inciardi, James A., Duane C. McBride, and James E. Rivers. *Drug Control and the Courts*. Thousand Oaks, CA: Sage, 1996.

Mattick, Richard P., Courtney Breen, Jo Kimber, and Marina Davoli. "Methadone Maintenance Therapy versus No Opioid Replacement Therapy for Opioid Dependence" (Review): Cochrane Review, 2009.

Mazerolle, Lorraine, David Soole, and Sacha Rombouts. "Drug Law Enforcement." *Police Quarterly* 10, no. 2 (2007): 115–53. DOI: 10.1177/1098611106287776.

Narayanan, Suresh, Balasingam Vicknasingam, and Noorzurani Robson. "The Transition to Harm Reduction: Understanding the Role of Non-Governmental Organisations in Malaysia." *International Journal of Drug Policy* 22, no. 4 (2011): 311–17.

Saucier, Roxanne, Nancy Berlinger, Nicholas Thomson, Michael Gusmano, and Daniel Wolfe. "The Limits of Equivalence: Ethical Dilemmas in Providing Care in Drug Detention Centers." *International Journal of Prisoner Health* 6, no. 2 (2010): 37–43.

Stevens, Alex. "Policy Analysis: Drug Policy, Harm and Human Rights: A Rationalist Approach." *International Journal of Drug Policy* 22 (2011): 233–38. DOI: 10.1016/j.drugpo.2011.02.003.

Thomson, Nicholas. "Detention of Methamphetamine Users in Cambodia, Laos, and Thailand." Open Society Institute, NY, 2010. Accessed 5 October 2012.www.soros.org/sites/default/files/Detention-as-Treatment-20100301.pdf.

Tran, Bach Xuan, Arto Ohinmaa, Anh Thuy Duong, Nhan Thi Do, Long Thanh Nguyen, Steve Mills, and Philip Jacobs. "Cost-Effectiveness of Methadone Maintenance Treatment for HIV-Positive Drug Users in Vietnam." *AIDS Care* 24, no. 3 (2011): 283–90. DOI: 10.1080/09540121.2011.608420.

UNODC/ESCAP/UNAIDS (United Nations Office of Drugs and Crime/United Nations Economic and Social Commission for Asia and the Pacific/Joint United Nations Programme on HIV/AIDS). 2011. *Report of the Regional Consultation on Compulsory Centres for Drug Users in Asia and the Pacific 14-16 December 2010, Bangkok.* www.unescap.org/sdd/meetings/CCDU-Dec2010/index.asp. Accessed on 21 January 2012.

UNODC/WHO (United Nations Office of Drugs and Crime/World Health Organization). 2008. *Principles of Drug Dependence Treatment.* Discussion Paper. Accessed April 1, 2012.www.unodc.org/documents/drug-treatment/UNODC-WHO-Principles-of-Drug-Dependence-Treatment-March08.pdf.

Vuong, Thu, Robert Ali, Simon Baldwin, and Stephen Mills. "Drug Policy in Vietnam: A Decade of Change?" *International Journal of Drug Policy* 23, no. 4 (2012): 319–26. DOI: 10.1016/j.drugpo.2011.11.005.

Weisburd, David, Cody W. Telep, Joshua C. Hinkle, and John E. Eck. "Is Problem-Oriented Policing Effective in Reducing Crime and Disorder?" *Criminology & Public Policy* 9, no. 1 (2010): 139–72. DOI: 10.1111/j.1745-9133.2010.00617.x.

Wodak, Alex and Leah McLeod. "The Role of Harm Reduction in Controlling HIV among Injecting Drug Users." *AIDS* 22 (2008): S81–S92 10.1097/1001.aids.0000327439.0000320914.0000327433.

Wolfe, Daniel and Roxanne Saucier. "In Rehabilitation's Name? Ending Institutionalised Cruelty and Degrading Treatment of People who Use Drugs." *International Journal of Drug Policy* 21, no. 3 (2010): 145–48. DOI: 10.1016/j.drugpo.2010.01.008.

Chapter Eleven

Responding to ATS Use in East and Southeast Asia

Rebecca McKetin[1] and Jih-Heng Li[2]

The use of amphetamine-type stimulants (ATS) has become an increasingly important issue in East and Southeast Asia over the past two decades. ATS include methamphetamine, amphetamine, 3- and 4-methelyne-dioxymetham-phetamine (MDMA, or "ecstasy"), and other related synthetic stimulants. These types of drugs have a long history in the region, but their use has burgeoned in recent years, including in regions where opioid drugs (i.e., opium and heroin) have previously dominated the drug situation. Today, ATS form an important component of the drug scene in East and Southeast Asia, and in many countries they are considered to be the leading drug problem. However, most of the responses to the drug situation in the region have been developed in response to opioid use. In fact, East and Southeast Asia are two of the regions most affected by ATS use globally, but the region includes many countries who are also among the least equipped to respond to the ATS situation. ATS present new challenges, both in terms of understanding the nature of use compared to opioid drugs, and also how best to respond to this problem. This chapter presents an overview of ATS use and potential responses to the ATS situation in East and Southeast Asia, drawing off international best practice, and considering some of the issues that are likely to be faced when implementing various responses within the region.

AN OVERVIEW OF ATS USE AND HARMS

ATS are used by an estimated fourteen to fifty-three million people world-wide.[3] Use patterns vary from recreational use through to heavy problematic use. There are no estimates of the how many people experience problematic ATS use.

However, a recent study estimated that half of people who use these drugs five or more times had developed a stimulant use disorder,[4] highlighting the need to be mindful that while these drugs are often seen as "recreational" (e.g., in the case of ecstasy use), they can be associated with significant public health burden. Indeed, in the United States, estimates of the cost of methamphetamine dependence suggest it is at least 75 percent of the cost of heroin dependence per person.[5]

The consequences of ATS use vary greatly depending on the type of ATS. Ecstasy use is mostly used recreationally, and the case for the drug being addictive remains dubious.[6] The nature and severity of harms from using ecstasy is also contentious. There have been concerns around the neurotoxic potential of the drug, corollary changes in memory, and possibly increased risk of depression or other psychiatric conditions.[7] However, it is not clear whether the dosages consumed by recreational users would be sufficient to instate longterm brain changes that would have a significant impact on functioning.[8] While it is appreciated that ingestion of the drug comes with a risk of overdose from toxicity, and that the drug may increase the risk of mortality via its adverse effects on the cardiovascular system,[9] the risk of death is low compared to opioid drugs.

In contrast, methamphetamine can produce a serious dependence syndrome which is associated with chronic relapsing patterns of use and elevated rates of morbidity and mortality. Amphetamine has similar pharmacological properties to methamphetamine but is a less potent euphoriant and is therefore often viewed as a "lesser evil" in terms of its potential to lead to addiction. The major harms associated with both amphetamine and methamphetamine are similar and include a risk of paranoia and aggression and increased risk of stroke and cardiovascular problems. These drugs can also increase the risk of HIV transmission via injecting drug use, increased libido, and associated increases in sexual risk behavior, and compromised immune functioning.[10] Dependence on amphetamine and methamphetamine, as with dependence on any drug, is typically accompanied by poor social and vocational outcomes (e.g., unemployment, relationship breakdowns, and criminal involvement).

A critical factor in determining the health risks associated with these stimulants is how they are taken, for example, whether they are injected, smoked, snorted or swallowed. Injecting tends to be associated with the greatest level of harm, including dependence on the drug, followed by smoking, and then intranasal and oral use.[11, 12, 13] Non-injecting use, which is more often seen among younger recreational drug users, tends to be associated with less frequent use and comparatively fewer harms.[14] In this context, priority needs to be given to minimizing the adverse effects of acute intoxication (e.g., overdose, accidents) and limiting the potential for the development of dependence, because this can lead to more chronic use and significant health problems.

Similar to dependence on other drugs, dependence on ATS typically develops in the late teens through to the early twenties, several years after the onset of use. Around this point in the life-course of ATS use, the frequency of use increases (e.g., at least weekly, if not several days a week) and a transition from swallowing or snorting the drug to more efficient routes of administration, such as smoking or injecting, is often seen.[15] The higher bioavailability afforded by these more efficient routes of administration means that less of the drug is needed to get the same effect (this being cost-efficient for the user). These routes of administration also provide a more rapid and intense high, which can accelerate the development of craving and tolerance, and increases the risk of dependence on ATS.[16]

People who use ATS also use a range of other drugs, most commonly tobacco, alcohol, and cannabis. The use of these drugs typically precedes ATS use and will continue with ATS use, becoming part of a larger milieu of poly-drug consumption.[17] People may take ATS and other drugs concurrently for their joint effects (e.g., stimulant intoxication can facilitate heavy alcohol consumption) or to alleviate the after-effects of ATS (e.g., smoking cannabis). Similarly, people who develop dependence on ATS will be likely to have already developed dependence on cannabis or other drugs, and they may go on to develop dependence on opioid drugs later in their drug-using career.[18] Dependent users may have high levels of prescription sedative use, which they may take to help manage stimulant withdrawal and induce sleep. People who inject opioids may also inject ATS (usually methamphetamine or amphetamine), contingent on what is available.[19, 20]

Finally, people who use ATS, particularly people who are dependent on these drugs, are likely to present to health services with comorbid mental and physical health problems.[21] Mental health problems feature most prominently among stimulant users. High levels of depression are common, which often first occur prior to the onset of drug use but can be exacerbated by the use of ATS. More potent ATS (methamphetamine and amphetamine) can also induce certain types of mental health problems. Most notably, heavy use can precipitate transient psychotic symptoms (paranoia and hallucinations).[22] Intoxication, particularly in the context of paranoia, can be associated with agitation and seemingly unpredictably or irrational acts of violence. These types of irrational violent acts are usually a result of delusional thinking leading to a misinterpretation of events (e.g., the person feeling that they are under threat or in danger) coupled with poor judgement and lack of inhibitions because of intoxication and the stimulating effects of the ATS.[23]

ATS USE IN SOUTHEAST AND EAST ASIA

ATS use has a long history in the Asian region, initially with methamphetamine use in East Asia, more recently with the emergence of ATS pills in Southeast Asia (most of which also contain methamphetamine), and finally with the contemporary popularity of ecstasy and various other synthetic drugs across the entire region. Today the region accounts for almost half of global methamphetamine supply and arguably has the highest rate of ATS use of any region in the world.[24] ATS now challenges the dominance of opium and heroin, which are historically more indigenous to the region. However, ATS use patterns are far more diverse than traditionally seen for opioid drugs, as are the types of people who use these drugs. The market for these drugs is dynamic, with the types of ATS used, and how they are used, varying substantially within the region and changing rapidly over time. This section outlines the long history of ATS use in the region and its lead up to contemporary ATS trends.

The History of ATS Use in East Asia

During World War II, methamphetamine was consumed by both Axis and Allied forces to increase the "war effort."[25, 26] However, because of easy availability from military sources and pharmaceutical companies for general public on a non-prescription basis, Japan suffered the world's first epidemic of methamphetamine use, which occurred from 1945 to 1956.[27, 28] This first epidemic in Japan subsided after various administrative actions, including restriction of its distribution and the enactment of the Stimulants Control Law in 1951 and its amendments in 1954 and 1955, which strengthened the penalties and instigated control of the precursor chemicals used in the drug's manufacture.[29, 30] The methamphetamine epidemic recurred in Japan in 1970 and the Stimulants Control Law was again amended, in 1973, to increase penalties for stimulant drug violations to the same level as those for heroin offences. [31, 32] A temporary 30 percent reduction in stimulant violations was observed in 1974, but the violations bounced back in 1975. [33]

Meanwhile, in the early 1970s, clandestine manufacturing of methamphetamine began to increase in Korea. The phenomenon was attributed, at least in part, to the strict enforcement by the Japanese government that resulted in the shift of methamphetamine production to the neighbor country of Korea.[34] At the initial stage, the methamphetamine problem was believed to be restricted to illegal manufacturing and smuggling destined for export to neighboring Japan. However, by the late 1970s, Korean production also fed a local market for the drug, and soon the nation was affected by a deluge of methamphetamine.[35] In response, the Korean government enacted the Habit-

Forming Medicine Control Act in 1970 which was later replaced by the Psychotropic Medicine Control Act in 1979.

Taiwan was basically drug-free from the 1950s through 1970s, but it witnessed profound methamphetamine use from the early 1990s. Facing the alarming situation, the now obsolete "Act for Eradication of Illicit Narcotics" was revised to become the "Act for Prevention and Control of Drugs Hazard" in 1998. The new Act differed from its previous version in that the control applied not only for traditional narcotics (i.e., opioids and cannabis) but also for psychotropic agents such as methamphetamine, benzodiazepines, and their precursors.[36]

Since 1970s, Japan has subsequently experienced several epidemics, including a recent peak in 1999–2000 that has since stabilized.[37] Although lifetime prevalence in the general population is relatively low (0.4 percent), methamphetamine remains the most widely used illicit drug in Japan.[38] In Korea, the local market began to absorb a greater quantity of drugs in the late 1980s, and use has expanded to affect all levels of society since the 1990s.[39] Recently, the range of drugs used by adolescents has expanded to include methamphetamine pills (*ya ba*), lysergic acid diethylamide (LSD), ecstasy (MDMA) and other new designer drugs, and potent analgesics like nalbuphine HCl.[40] In Taiwan, although it remains a major concern, there has been a steady decrease in the proportion of methamphetamine psychiatric admissions and of urine drug screens testing positive for methamphetamine.[41] By contrast, use of club drugs such as MDMA, ketamine, flunitrazepam (Rohypnol, also known as FM2), and amphetamines have been common in local rave parties and dance clubs.[42, 43]

THE RISE OF ATS USE IN SOUTHEAST ASIA

Southeast Asia remained relatively unaffected by ATS until the 1990s, when there was a dramatic shift in drug use patterns with the emergence of ATS pills in the Mekong subregion. This trend first emerged in Thailand from around 1995 and was underpinned by the trafficking of large quantities of methamphetamine pills from neighboring Myanmar. Associated with international pressure to quell the opium trade, the drug trade in the northeast of the country (Shan state) became marked by large-scale production of methamphetamine.[44] Methamphetamine produced in this region was pressed into pills which were characteristically uniform in their appearance: each contained approximately 5 mg of methamphetamine, usually together with ketamine, was an orange/pink color, and carried the Wa State Army logo, "WY."[45] At this time, it was estimated that several hundred millions of pills were produced in the Shan State region of Myanmar each year. These methamphetamine pills were trafficked overland and then along the Mekong river into Thailand and other neighboring countries.[46, 47]

Methamphetamine quickly rose to epidemic proportions in Thailand, culminating with the so-called "Thai war on drugs" (described in the chapter by Kaplan et al. in this book).[48, 49] Pills were usually smoked, up to several times a day among habitual users. Methamphetamine succeeded heroin as the main drug for which young people were entering drug treatment facilities. Arrests for methamphetamine also quickly overtook other drugs. Use of methamphetamine pills, or "*ya ba*" (meaning crazy medicine), remains a pressing issue today, although the situation has been complicated by a broader range of ATS which have become available in the country, including crystalline methamphetamine and ecstasy.

The shift to methamphetamine use in Thailand portended a cascade of ATS production and use across the Mekong sub-region.[50] Cambodia, Laos, and Vietnam all saw increases in supply and use of ATS, and in both Cambodia and the Lao PDR, methamphetamine became the primary drug of concern. ATS pills in this region included methamphetamine, but pills were more varied in their content and appearance, suggesting that they were not originating from the northeast of Myanmar, as were the original *ya ba* pills that became prolific in Thailand.[51]

CONTEMPORARY TRENDS AND ISSUES

Contemporary ATS trends have become more homogenous across the region with the proliferation of ATS pills and an increasing market for ecstasy. Indicators of ATS use continue to increase, despite stabilizing global trends, with 136 million ATS tablets being seized in 2010. Methamphetamine remains by far the most common drug detected in police seizures of ATS,[52] with an estimated twenty tons of methamphetamine seized in East and Southeast Asia in 2010, accounting for almost half of the global total.[53] While ecstasy remains less common than methamphetamine, the increase in its popularity has affected most countries to some extent. Because ATS pills can contain various types of ATS (ecstasy, methamphetamine), often in combination with other synthetic drugs (e.g., ketamine), there is a less clear division between the use of ecstasy and ATS than seen in other parts of the world. The availability of crystalline methamphetamine is no longer isolated to East Asia, with its trafficking having spread into the Southeast Asian region.[54] Southeast Asia has also become a destination market for ATS produced in other parts of the world (e.g., ATS produced in the Middle East has been trafficked into East and Southeast Asia and was believed to be destined for local markets).[55] While opioids still dominate the drug situation in some countries, ATS have clearly made their mark in East and Southeast Asia and are now a major drug of concern for many countries.[56]

As with other parts of the world, ATS use patterns range from recreational consumption of ecstasy in bars and nightclubs, to problems from methamphetamine dependence and related incidents of psychosis and violent behavior. A pattern of use that probably affects this region more than most Western countries is the use of ATS pills in an occupational context. The availability of methamphetamine in pill form (e.g., *ya ba*) makes the drug accessible as a stay-awake energy promoting agent in the labor market, particularly among long-distance drivers.[57] While there is limited evidence of injecting ATS in the region,[58, 59] smoking the drug (both crystalline methamphetamine and ATS pills) has increased the harms associated with ATS (e.g., methamphetamine psychosis) beyond what might have been seen with oral consumption of ATS pills.

The region has also been affected by the spread of ATS production. Methamphetamine available in the 1990s largely originating from the Shan State and surrounding areas,[60] whereas today production has spread to affect much more of the region and now includes industrial-size production facilities being detected in Malaysia, Indonesia, China, and Cambodia.[61] Production of ecstasy in the region has also become apparent, as has the harvesting of safrole-rich oils, which are used in the production of ecstasy, from forests in Cambodia (from the roots of the *Dysoxylum loureiri* tree).[62] In many countries there is limited capacity to police clandestine drug manufacture and criminal syndicates are capitalizing on this vulnerability. This exposes vulnerable local communities to drug manufacturing and trafficking and potentially to high rates of drug use, where members of the local community become involved in supply chains.

There are flow-on effects from the establishment of ATS manufacture in the region. High levels of ATS use have been documented in ATS trafficking routes—for example, among villages along the border regions of the Cambodia.[63] The lack of infrastructure in these regions makes responding to ATS use and related problems a particular challenge. People living in these areas are also afflicted by a range of vulnerabilities that increase the risk of drug dependence, such as poverty, lack of educational and vocational opportunities, and psychological vulnerabilities (e.g., trauma) among displaced people living along border regions (Mannava et al. in their chapter in this book discuss contextual factors influencing drug use further). High rates of ATS use have also been documented among vulnerable populations (e.g., street children, sex workers) in major cities in Cambodia and the Lao PDR as well.[64, 65, 66] Essentially these more vulnerable groups, particularly in regions affected by drug trafficking, are at high risk for ATS use, and therefore they should be the target of interventions to reduce ATS use and related harms.

The transmission of HIV has also been shown to follow drug trafficking routes through Asia.[67] While this problem has been documented in the context of heroin injection, there is emerging evidence of ATS injection in the region,[68, 69] and ATS use carries an additional risk of increasing HIV transmission through increased libido, sexual risk behavior, and pathological immune processes.[70] With limited knowledge about ATS use and HIV transmission in some of the most vulnerable areas, and with existing HIV prevention strategies focusing largely on the injection of heroin or other opioid drugs, there is limited capacity to respond to the additional risk posed by ATS use.

RESPONSES TO ATS USE

This section examines some of the potential response to ATS use, drawing from international experience, to understand what evidence exists about best practice, and to consider some of the implementation issues that are likely to be encountered within East and Southeast Asia, particularly in regions were infrastructure is less developed and resources are constrained. The section is divided broadly into supply reduction strategies, treatment approaches, and prevention of ATS use (issues concerning responses to the HIV situation are considered in Des Jarlais's chapter in this book). In addition, we discuss the use of "enforcement" strategies to police the use of drugs (particularly drug testing). While these strategies are not exclusive to this region, they are less commonly used in other parts of the world.

Supply Reduction Strategies

The machinery in place to reduce drug supply in East and Southeast Asia has largely been derived from a culture of opium cultivation and efforts to combat the opium trade through crop eradication. The shift to synthetic drugs has occurred only relatively recently even on an international level. Consequently, international drug control conventions around these drugs, their implementation within East and Southeast Asia, and the development of related policing capacity, is a more recent phenomenon and still comparatively limited. The issues involved in controlling synthetic drugs are different from the strategies traditionally used to control opium supply, as they rely heavily on the regulation of chemicals used in the illicit production of ATS (also known as "precursor chemicals"), as discussed below.

International Conventions on ATS

ATS came under international control a decade after heroin, cannabis, and cocaine, with the introduction of the 1971 convention on psychotropic substances.[71] One of the challenges that emerged in attempting to control synthetic drugs was that traditional approaches used to control other narcotics were not appropriate. Specifically, efforts to control heroin, cocaine and cannabis had all focused on crop eradication. In contrast, the production of synthetics drugs utilizes chemical precursors, making it more portable and less visible than the cultivation of opium, cocaine, and cannabis crops.

In recognition that synthetic drugs could not be controlled with the same approach as that used for crop-based drugs, the Convention Against Illicit Traffic in Narcotic Drugs and Psychotropic Substances was adapted in 1988,[72] which sought to tighten regulations around chemicals used in the manufacture of illicit synthetic drugs. Substances that were used as the chemical starting point to make ATS, or so-called "precursor chemicals," were listed under this convention (along with other chemical reagents used in the manufacturing process, often referred to as "essential chemicals"). For example, safrole can be used for MDMA manufacture and pseudoephedrine and ephedrine for methamphetamine manufacture.

Some of these precursors have legitimate uses (e.g., pseudoephedrine and ephedrine are used as decongestants in cold-and-flu remedies), creating a need to maintain their availability through regulated channels. The purpose of precursor regulations is to prevent the diversion of these chemicals from their legitimate use into clandestine drug manufacture. Reducing the availability of precursor chemicals is postulated to "tax" the supply of illicit ATS, increasing their price and reducing their availability. However, the control of these over-the-counter drugs may also add the processing time and costs to both the pharmacies and consumers.

Precursor Regulations as a Means of Reducing Methamphetamine Supply and Use

There is good evidence that these regulations can work to reduce methamphetamine use: evaluations of precursor regulations in North America have found up to 77 percent reductions in methamphetamine-related indicators,[73] including reductions in methamphetamine-related hospital admissions[74] and arrests for methamphetamine-related offences.[75] These reductions appeared to be mediated by reductions in purity and increases in price per pure gram of methamphetamine.[76] Encouragingly, precursor regulations appear not to increase the number of people injecting methamphetamine,[77] alleviating concern that people may take up injecting drug use to compensate for the lower purity of drugs.

While precursor regulations provide promise in reducing harms from methamphetamine use, their implementation is lagging in some of the countries heavily affected by ATS production and trafficking. For example, Lao PDR, Cambodia, and Thailand, which have all been subject to substantial increases in ATS supply since the mid-1990s, have signed up to the 1988 convention on precursor controls only in the past decade (table 11.1)

Within the less developed parts of the region, there are likely to be considerable challenges for the implementing successful precursor regulation, including a lack of governmental and judicial instrumentation to support the policing of precursor chemicals. Corruption and weak governance have also

Year of accession	Convention on Psychotropic Substances, 1971	Convention against illicit traffic in narcotic drugs and psychotropic substances, 1988
1971	(convention instated)	
1972		
1973		
1974	Philippines	
1975	Thailand	
1976		
1977		
1978	Republic of Korea	
1979		
1980		
1981		
1982		
1983		
1984		
1985	China	
1986	Malaysia	
1987	Brunei Darussalam	
1988		(convention instated)
1989		China[a]
1990	Japan[a], Singapore	
1991		Myanmar
1992		Japan[a]
1993		Malaysia[a], Brunei Darussalam[a]
1994		
1995	Myanmar	
1996	Indonesia	Philippines[a]
1997	Lao People's Democratic Republic, Viet Nam	Singapore, Viet Nam
1998		Republic of Korea
1999		Indonesia[a]
2000		
2001		
2002		Thailand
2003		
2004		Lao People's Democratic Republic
2005	Cambodia	Cambodia
2006		
2007	Democratic People's Republic of Korea	Democratic People's Republic of Korea

Table 11.1. Year of Accession for International Conventions to Control ATS Supply. [a] **Year of ratification subsequent to signing convention.**

been argued to undermine the effectiveness of precursor regulations.[78] Patterns of ATS use also differ from those seen in North America, with a greater variety of ATS and other synthetic drugs being available and with plant products used to derive precursor chemicals being indigenous to the region (e.g., *Ma Haung,* or *Ephedra sinica,* from which ephedrine can be derived, and safrole from the *Dysoxylum loureiri* tree). Importantly, the impact of precursor regulations has been tested mainly in the context of methamphetamine use, and it is not clear whether these regulations are effective for other synthetic drugs or indeed what impact they have on the broader synthetic drug market (e.g., whether they produce displacement to production of alternative synthetic drugs).

The effectiveness of precursor regulations, in any context, requires that they are comprehensive. Specifically, for precursor regulations to be effective, they need to cover all major avenues of diversion (e.g., illegal import through to retail level diversion), as regulations that are not comprehensive are readily subverted by obtaining precursors through alterative channels. Regulations often need to extend beyond those that relate directly to the illicit handling of precursor chemicals. For example, rogue pharmaceutical companies have been one of the more significant conduits for precursor diversion in the past,[79, 80] and therefore successful regulations need to govern the operating principles of legitimate companies handling precursors (e.g., import, export, and distribution). Regulations around the use of industrial space, including pharmaceutical industrial facilities, can also play a role in facilitating (or restricting) the use of this space for clandestine drug manufacture.

Finally, regulations also need to be implemented comprehensively in all countries across the region, as their impact can easily be undermined by the availability of precursors from neighbouring countries where regulations are more lax. This has been seen in the case of importation of both precursor chemicals and methamphetamine into North America, undermining the impact of domestic precursor regulations.[81, 82] Indeed, the trafficking of precursor chemicals has become a lucrative criminal enterprise in its own right.[83] Regulations also need to be coupled with a capacity for their enforcement, including broader border control enforcement to reduce trafficking of ATS within the region, and also to guard against importation from outside the region. This is a particularly critical issue in East and Southeast Asia because of the potential for cross-border movement of precursor chemicals and drugs within the region, and the geographic proximity to other countries that are major precursor producers (e.g., India).

TREATMENT

When Is Treatment Appropriate for ATS Use?

As with all drug types, treatment can be used to alleviate dependence on ATS and in turn, reduce harms associated with using the drug. Like other drugs, regular use of ATS can lead to dependence or addiction. This involves escalating use, in which people develop tolerance and need to take more of the drug to get the same effect: they start using higher doses more often, and the use of the drug starts to supersede other aspects of the person's life and reduce their level of functioning. For example, someone who is developing dependence will tend to spend more time with other people who use, spend less time on other non-drug-related activities, and they may fail to fulfill their normal obligations (e.g., fail to attend work). Importantly, people who are dependent on drugs will continue to use despite the fact that they are experiencing problems from their use, be they mental health, occupational, or social problems. In this sense, it is dependence on drugs that drives many of the problems from drug use, and the poor quality of life that goes with dependence is a primary contributor to the "burden of disease" attributable to drug use. This is as true for ATS as it is for other drugs. [84]

An important issue with ATS use is that not all users are dependent on the drug, and therefore treatment may not always be appropriate. Dependence is most often seen with methamphetamine or amphetamine use (cf. ecstasy use), particularly when these drugs are smoked or injected. Dependence typically involves using ATS daily or almost daily, often several times a day. Less intense use patterns, such as occasional recreational use, are unlikely to require or benefit from treatment. Lighter patterns of use are better dealt with by prevention and harm reduction, with time-consuming and costly treatments that are needed for ATS dependence being reserved for those who are most in need of help and likely to reap more substantive benefits from reducing their drug use.

A broader issue is exactly what constitutes "treatment." In most contexts, the goal of treatment is to reduce a person's dependence on drugs. This in turn should improve their capacity to function and engage with society in a healthy and productive way. Some types of treatment are abstinence focussed, aiming to get their clients to cease use altogether. Indeed, this is often the goal of the person seeking treatment, and in keeping with the illegality of many drugs. However, in other contexts, treatment can aim to reduce the level of use below a threshold where the drug presents a problem. That is, the person may still be using the drug but is no longer dependent. This can be helpful in situations where use of a drug is socially acceptable (e.g., alcohol), or an inevitable part of the person's lifestyle (e.g., if the person is using stimulants to assist with shift work).

Treatment of ATS Dependence: What the Evidence Says

There has been less research on what treatment approaches work for ATS dependence than for alcohol, opioids, or tobacco dependence. Not only is the research limited, but there is even less evidence supporting the utility of specific treatment approaches, which means there is scant information to guide the types of treatment that should be implemented at a community level.[85] [86] In short, there are no readily scalable interventions that could be rolled out in resource poor settings that have been proven effective.[87] In particular, there are no pharmacotherapy options, akin to opioid maintenance therapy, that could be promoted to alleviate harms from ATS use. However, there are some specific approaches to treating ATS use that have shown promise (e.g., structured psychological/behavioral therapies), and which could be integrated into routine drug treatment practices. There are also significant developments in the delivery of these interventions (e.g., using novel media, such as the internet, to deliver interventions) which may improve their scalability. The evidence base for treating dependence on ATS, and these newer technological developments, is discussed below.

Pharmacotherapy

The aim of substitution pharmacotherapy is to reduce illicit drug use and thereby alleviate the harms associated with using an illegal substance and stabilize the person's lifestyle to improve their health and well-being. This approach has worked well to alleviate harms associated with heroin dependence, by increasing employment, reducing the risk of fatal overdose, and reducing drug-related crime. While efforts have been made to develop a pharmacotherapy for ATS use, akin to opioid substitution therapy, most of the work in this area remains in the pre-clinical stages.[88]

Specifically, a number of pharmaceutical agents have been trialed as substitution therapies among ATS users, mostly to treat methamphetamine or amphetamine dependence,[89] most of which have been pilot studies or feasibility trials.[90] The small numbers of patients used in these trials limits inferences that can be drawn about the effectiveness of medications.[91] Bearing this in mind, most trials have failed to find a significant improvement of the trialled pharmacotherapy over placebo[92] and some have resulted in increases in health problems due to adverse side effects from the medication.[93] However, two trials have reported significant reductions in amphetamine use with the opioid antagonist naltrexone.[94, 95] There has also been a trial supporting the use of methylphenidate to treat methamphetamine dependence[96] but these findings have not been replicated to date.

Even with some promising pharmacotherapy trials, there are significant impediments to the development and implementation of effective pharmacotherapy for ATS, and it is likely to be some time before this becomes a feasible approach to reducing harms from ATS dependence. Impediments to development of effective pharmacotherapy for methamphetamine dependence include the complex pharmacology of the drug.[97] There are also broader safety concerns, such as the risk of side effects from combination of medications with illicit stimulant use (e.g., exacerbation of stimulant psychosis, increased risk of stroke), the effects of chronic dosing with stimulants, and managing the risk of diversion.[98] These factors are likely to impede the widespread implementation of pharmacotherapy, particularly agonist therapies, in the immediate future.

MANAGING WITHDRAWAL FROM ATS

A more pressing need from a clinical perspective, and perhaps more achievable, is the development of pharmacotherapy that can be used to manage methamphetamine withdrawal symptoms. Ceasing ATS use, particularly heavy methamphetamine or amphetamine use, can elicit a strong withdrawal syndrome that is characterized by extreme mood swings, lethargy and depression, intense cravings for the drug, appetite changes, and sleep disturbances.[99] These symptoms can be severe and can act as a barrier to successfully engaging clients in ongoing drug treatment.

As with substitution therapy, none of the medications trialed for withdrawal has proven particularly promising.[100] Current best practice is to treat withdrawal symptomatically using medications (e.g., benzodiazepines). Withdrawal is usually done within an inpatient medical facility, although where dependence is less severe and withdrawal symptoms are expected to be milder, withdrawal can be managed through outpatient services, with toxicology used to confirm detoxification.

While management of withdrawal symptoms is often necessary, this detoxification process alone does little to alleviate drug dependence in the longer term. Evaluation of detoxification for ATS use shows that within several months after detoxification, the person will show similar ATS use patterns to what would be expected if they had not undergone detoxification.[101] This is because detoxification addresses only the physical changes that occur with heavy drug use, and not the complex array of psychological and social/contextual factors that are at play in the development and maintenance of a drug using habit. Therefore, while detoxification may be a necessary process to help people cope with the withdrawal syndrome that occurs when they stop using ATS, further treatment is needed to help the person reduce their drug use in the longer term. Further treatment could include structured psychological/behavioral therapies, the benefits of which have been shown to be more durable and which are discussed below.[102]

PSYCHOLOGICAL AND BEHAVIORAL TREATMENTS

The intensive application of structured psychological interventions (e.g., cognitive behavioral therapy, contingency management) can reduce ATS use.[103] The most commonly trialled psychological interventions are cognitive behavioral therapy, for which treatment manuals are available[104] and which can be tailored to meet the needs of specific groups of ATS users. For example, in the United States, cognitive behavioral therapy has been tailored to the needs of men in the gay community, particularly to address the relationship between methamphetamine use and sexual risk behavior in this population.[105] Contingency management, which involves providing incentives (e.g., monetary rewards) for ceasing drug use or engaging in other pro-social behaviors, has also been used successfully to reduce methamphetamine use among people who are dependent on methamphetamine.[106] Contingency management can be used in conjunction with cognitive behavioral therapy, particularly to enhance treatment compliance.[107]

A systematic review of these types of psychological interventions found that, across a number of studies, they had a moderate impact on ATS use when implemented intensively (e.g., 10+ sessions over 2-3 months).[108] While less intense application (e.g., brief interventions of one to two sessions of CBT) has produced promising results in specific studies, the overall finding from the meta-analysis conducted by Colfax and colleagues was that minimal application of psychosocial interventions did not produce significant reductions in ATS use.[109]

What Happens in Practice: Community-Based "Treatment as Usual" for Drug Use

What happens in routine practice when treating ATS users is often very different from the types of approaches that have been evaluated in clinical trials. This is partly because clinical trials have yet to show compelling evidence in favor of a particular treatment approach but also because approaches that have shown promise (e.g., the structured psychological treatments discussed above) require considerable resources to implement and/or face logistical problems with their implementation. These approaches have been implemented in an ad hoc way, even in countries that have devoted considerable resources to tackling ATS use through treatment. Far more resources will need to be devoted both to the trialing of various treatment approaches and also to their implementation before we see treatment for ATS use that can be lauded as effective.

In the meantime, most treatment provided for ATS is provided through the same types of treatment facilities that are used to manage other drug and alcohol problems. These approaches to drug treatment were designed primarily with opioids or alcohol in mind and their utility for ATS use is not well understood. Evaluations of the effect of treatment on ATS use (primarily for methamphetamine dependence) are positive, showing that reductions in methamphetamine use and crime occur while ATS users are engaged in drug treatment.[110, 111] However, outcomes seem to vary depending on the type of treatment provided, while the ability of these treatments to produce lasting changes in ATS use (i.e., beyond the period that the person is in treatment) is questionable.[112] Treatment options provided within the community include managing withdrawal symptoms (i.e., detoxification, as discussed above), providing outpatient counseling to help patients manage their ATS use and associated lifestyle issues, while other services operate within a residential setting (e.g., therapeutic communities), as described below.

Residential Rehabilitation

Providing residential programs for drug users (e.g., therapeutic communities) is commonplace in most parts of the world. Residential rehabilitation typically involves long stays (weeks to months) in a drug-free residential setting, where clients engage in structured activities within the facility, and may also engage in specific treatment activities (e.g., group or individual counseling sessions). Residential services are very expensive compared to outpatient services, due to the low number of people who can be treated at a given time, the longstays often required in treatment, and simply that they are residential.[113]

The limited available evidence on the effectiveness of residential rehabilitation for ATS use is based on methamphetamine users attending these types of services in Australia. It suggests that residential rehabilitation may produce short-term gains in reducing ATS use levels and related health problems (including psychotic symptoms that are associated with the drug's use). The greatest gains were seen in terms of instating abstinence during and soon after treatment (e.g., three months after starting treatment), which is in keeping with most of these programs being drug-free and lasting several weeks to months. However, the number of people who benefited from these treatments in the longterm (e.g., one to three years after treatment) was limited.[114] By this time, methamphetamine users had long left the residential facility, and their levels of drug use were largely similar to people who had not received treatment.

Counseling

In many contexts, outpatient counseling is provided to help ATS user reduce their use and/or cope with related lifestyle issues. Positive outcomes have been observed among people who receive outpatient counseling.[115, 116] Specific psychological therapies that have been shown to reduce ATS use (e.g., cognitive behavioral therapy and contingency management, as described earlier) can also be implemented within the framework of outpatient counseling services. The low cost of providing treatment in an outpatient setting makes it appealing against the high costs and infrastructure required to provide residential treatment. However, counseling attracts ATS users with less severe/entrenched patterns of ATS use, and who tend to have less complex needs (vis-à-vis comorbid health problems) than clients attending residential rehabilitation services. Residential services may still be necessary in cases where people need a stable environment to initiate changes in their drug use, for example, if they do not have stable housing or are residing with people who are continuing to use drugs.

Specialized Treatment Services for ATS

Specialized treatment approaches for ATS use have been developed to attract stimulant users into treatment and provide tailored care. One such approach adopted in the United States, the MATRIX program, involved a sixteen-week outpatient program for methamphetamine users. An evaluation of the MATRIX study found decreased levels of methamphetamine use during the treatment regime against the "treatment as usual" control condition but no benefit over treatment as usual once clients had left the program.[117] A similar specialized treatment approach has been trialed in Australia (the Stimulant Treatment Program).[118] This treatment program catered primarily to methamphetamine users and involved outpatient counseling with a harm-minimization philosophy. Approximately half of the clients entering the service showed recovery from methamphetamine dependence six months after starting treatment.[119] However, this was an uncontrolled trial, so it was not clear how much of the reductions in methamphetamine use seen after treatment were due to natural remission from the drug.

While these services appear to be beneficial in attracting stimulant users into treatment, they have little benefit over other standard forms of drug treatment used within the community in terms of reducing drug use after treatment has been completed.[120] A further caution with the implementation of specialized treatment approaches is that a previous evaluation of one such service found that it did not reduce concurrent polydrug use (i.e., concurrent levels of cannabis and alcohol use),[121] whereas more generic drug treatment approaches appear to do so.[122] Given that dependence on ATS goes hand in hand with polydrug use, the adoption of specialized treatment approaches needs to consider carefully the potential benefits of such services over conventional treatment services. These benefits are likely to be not so much in terms of superior performance in reducing ATS or other drug use but in terms of attracting ATS users into treatment and honing the skills of clinicians to deal with stimulant specific problems (e.g., sexual risk behavior related to ATS use, psychiatric complications from the use of these drugs).

Improving Treatment Coverage for ATS Use

Treatment coverage for ATS dependence is quite low in comparison with opioid use. This problem is likely to reflect the lack of low-threshold interventions, such as pharmacotherapies. But it also reflects that many people who use ATS prefer to self-manage their drug use rather than attend a formal drug treatment program, while others are concerned about confidentiality, or they feel that the available treatment options are not suitable for ATS use. [123, 124] This situation has led to the development of specialized treatment options for ATS use, as described above, in an attempt to better market treatment to people using ATS. Other approaches include the use of internet interventions, phone counseling and the provision of self-help style resources on ATS-related health problems to engage with users who are not seeking treatment. Some of the more recent developments in this area are discussed below.

Providing Treatment via the Internet

Currently an online intervention is being developed for people who use ATS. [125] The purpose of this intervention is to attract ATS users who would not otherwise go to treatment and encourage them to reflect on their ATS use patterns, the relationship between their ATS use, and other aspects of their life, and increase their motivation to reduce their ATS use and seek further treatment. The benefit of online interventions is that they can incorporate the principles used in structured psychological therapies that have been found to be effective in reducing ATS use. While some people argue that providing psychological interventions via the internet lack the flexibility and sophistication that is possible in a face-to-face consultation with a clinician, online psychological interventions have been proven to work for other conditions (e.g., depression, see Christensen et al. 2004), [126] and they provide an opportunity for people to access treatment anonymously, which can be incredibly valuable in situations where drug use is stigmatized, and in smaller tight-knit communities where anonymity is unlikely to be possible. They also reduce the need to up-skill clinicians to be able to deliver complex structured psychological interventions, which is often not practical or attainable within the resource constraints of less developed countries.

Providing a Flexible Approach to Treatment

Focusing treatment on the harms associated with use (e.g., related mental health problems or financial and social problems), and doing this within a harm reduction framework, appears to be successful in attracting ATS users into treatment. Indeed, a "stepped care" approach has been strongly promoted within this realm,[127] whereby the focus and intensity of the treatment intervention is tailored to the needs of the client in order to make treatment more appealing and helpful from their viewpoint. This approach is also particularly helpful in allowing the duration, intensity, and content of the treatment to be modified to deal with comorbid problems (e.g., clinical levels of depression which commonly co-occur with stimulant dependence).

Recent Developments in Southeast Asia

Specialized community-based treatments are being developed within East and Southeast Asia to cater for the growing use of ATS. Because of the limited treatment infrastructure in some parts of East and Southeast Asia, and because most existing treatment approaches are geared toward opioid dependence, development assistance has been provided to countries in the Mekong subregion to assist with the establishment of community-based treatment programs that are more suitable for ATS use. The development of these programs is occurring in Myanmar, Vietnam, and Cambodia (Juana Tomas-Rosello, August 1, 2012, *pers. comm.*). A hospital-based drug treatment facility, which primarily caters for methamphetamine use, has also been established in Vientiane, the capital of Lao PDR.[128] Specialized treatment programs have also been developed in Thailand. Indeed, these developments are very positive in light of the historical trends to place ATS users, and other illicit drug users alike, in detention-like facilities.

Summary

In summary, current evidence is that intensive application of psychological interventions such as cognitive-behavioral therapy and/or contingency management can reduce ATS use in people who are dependent and seeking treatment. However, these treatments are rarely implemented in practice, mainly because considerable skill is required to undertake these treatments, and this capacity does not exist in most drug treatment settings. However, the development of online interventions that incorporate principles of CBT may overcome skill shortages and increase the accessibility of these types of treatments. Pharmacotherapy for ATS dependence, which could prove to be a more scalable treatment option, has not been developed to the point where it has been approved for use in clinical practice.

In the interim, most people who use ATS receive care from the same drug and alcohol treatment services that service other drugs (e.g., opioid use, alcohol dependence). Attending certain types of generic drug treatment services, for example, residential rehabilitation or structured outpatient programs for stimulant use, appears to be associated with time-limited reductions in ATS use. Specialized treatment services for ATS use may have utility where there is a need to increase the number of people who access ATS treatment or develop the skill base required to manage ATS. However, the provision of specialized services needs to be balanced against the need to treat other patterns of drug use, including polydrug use among ATS users.

Finally, much of the evidence around the effectiveness of treatment for ATS use has arisen from the United States and to a lesser extent from Australia and the United Kingdom. It might not apply to treatment services in East and Southeast Asia. Many treatment options also require considerable investment both in terms of infrastructure and technical capacity to implement them successful and achieve sufficient coverage to reduce problematic ATS use.

PREVENTION

Preventing the uptake of ATS use is a key strategy in reducing harms from use. Preventing use can not only reduce acute harms from using ATS but, more importantly, it reduces the pool of people who are at risk of developing dependent ATS use and related problems. In particular, early onset drug use is linked to an increased risk of drug dependence later in life and can also have negative consequences for educational achievement and subsequent vocational opportunities because of its impact on school attendance.[129] Early cannabis use and alcohol use are important antecedents of ATS use and dependence,[130, 131] and, therefore, prevention efforts should target the early onset of a broad range of drugs and alcohol in order to reduce ATS consumption.

Conveniently, effective strategies to prevent drug use are generic to all drug types. They typically target teens and adolescents, this being the age when people are first exposed to drugs. Most prevention efforts take place in schools because this provides a captive audience of teenagers. In this context, providing information on drug use alone can increase students' knowledge about drugs, but it does not reduce their use of drugs.[132] However, programs that develop individual social skills among adolescents have been found to successfully prevent early drug use. They have been found to reduce the risk of marijuana use to 80 percent of that seen among children who do not receive such an intervention, this figure being 50 percent for heroin use.[133] There is little data on whether or how they work for ATS use, but one study from the United States found that the "Iowa Strengthening Families Program" coupled with life-skills training significantly reduced the uptake of methamphetamine use.[134]

Increasingly prevention programs are being developed through electronic media (e.g., CD-ROM).[135] These interventions have the potential to be accessible to a broader group of students at low cost. Randomized trials have found that these types of intervention can reduce alcohol use and related harms.[136] CD-ROM interventions have since been tailored to address ATS use specifically.[137] While such interventions would need to be tailored to the local social context, because much of their content is based on social influence models, online prevention interventions could provide a cost-effective scalable alternative to conventional drug prevention programs.

While school-based programs that focus on improving social skills among adolescents can reduce early drug use, adolescents who are most at risk of drug use are often those not attending school. Unfortunately fewer programs to prevent drug use among out-of-school youth have been developed or evaluated. An approach that is often used in this situation is to target out-of-school youth who are at high risk of using drugs or already known to be using drugs. Providing these groups with information on the harms associated with using ATS, and how to minimize these harms, can help alleviate problems that arise from ATS use, such as the risk of sexually transmitted diseases (including HIV), overdose and drug-related mental health problems. In this context, information on drug use patterns and their consequences can be conveyed openly because there is little risk that it will entice or normalize drug use among people who are already engaged in using drugs or who are associating with peers who are using drugs.

In less developed countries within the region, it may be more appropriate to focus on preventing vulnerabilities to developing drug problems, rather than solely implementing programs that attempt to dissuade drug use among adolescents. Alleviating poverty and providing education may increase the potential of individuals to engage in gainful employment and reduce the risk that they will become involved in ATS supply chains or work industries that are affected by high rates of drug use (e.g., the sex trade). Focusing on vulnerable segments of the community, such as minority ethnic groups and displaced people, to ensure that they are not disenfranchised from society is also likely to increase resilience against drug use. Finally, it is inevitable that drug use will occur within vulnerable communities, and this is borne out in many parts of East and Southeast Asia. These groups are the least likely to have access to health care and social support and are at high risk of becoming dependent on drugs. Therefore targeted interventions (e.g., outreach) are needed to ensure that harm reduction strategies are made available to reduce the adverse consequences of using ATS among marginalized segments of the population.

ENFORCEMENT OF NON-DRUG USING BEHAVIOR
THROUGH DRUG TESTING

In countries where nonmedical use of scheduled drugs is a criminal offense or violation of workplace ethics, drug testing has become a routine practice. Specimens for drug testing can be urine, hair, sweat or saliva, but urine is most commonly used. Among the amphetamine-type stimulants (ATS), amphetamine, methamphetamine, and MDMA are frequently monitored by urine tests, which generally consist of immunoassays for screening and analyses with gas chromatography/mass spectrometry (GC/MS) for confirmation.[138]

Administration of some commonly prescribed medications, such as brompheniramine, bupropion, trazodone, chlorpromazine, promethazine, and ranitidine, could result in false-positive results of urine drug screens for amphetamine/methamphetamine. Therefore, confirmation tests are imperative to avoid misjudgment.[139] However, some "precursor" drugs, such as amphetaminil, deprenyl, famprofazone, and fenethylline, can be metabolized *in vivo* to amphetamine and/or methamphetamine, thereby leading to positive results of amphetamines.[140] In other words, the urine of people who take these "precursor" drugs will show positive results of amphetamine and/or methamphetamine even though one does not take amphetamine or methamphetamine.

To protect innocent people from being charged with illicit drug use, medical/prescription records should be well kept for reference. But for over-the-counter drugs that do not need prescription, the availability without the endorsement of medical or pharmacy professions could be a threat to an innocent patient. Famprofazone, one of such an OTC "precursor" drug,[141] was therefore removed from the market in Korea.[142] However, it is available as an OTC drug in Taiwan and misinterpretation as methamphetamine abuse could possibly occur.[143]

A further issue to consider is how people who return drug-positive urines are handled by the government system and the consequences of this handling for the individual and society. In the event that these individuals receive a criminal record, this is going to have a lasting detrimental impact on the person's vocational and educational opportunities, which may decrease their capacity to contribute to society and increase their risk of developing subsequent drug problems. Sending these individuals to drug treatment, as done in some settings, may be problematic for two reasons. First, the individuals may not be experiencing dependence on drugs (as toxicology tests do not distinguish between recreational ATS use and ATS dependence), and therefore drug treatment may not be an inappropriate option. This approach would waste scarce treatment resources that would be better directed toward people who need treatment. Second, in many contexts, evidence-based treatments may not be available, and therefore mandatory treatment presents an ethical dilemma, whereby individuals are subjected to treatment regimes that may not have any beneficial impact on the individual or their drug use.

In some circumstances mandatory drug testing is used among arrestees to identify individuals who would benefit from drug treatment. Indeed, referral of people arrested for drug use into treatment has proved to be a worthwhile strategy in reducing drug-related crime. However, using drug testing even within this constrained environment has problems. An evaluation of a pilot program used in Scotland to identify drug-taking arrestees found that few additional drug users ended up receiving treatment as a result of being identified through mandatory testing. The program was also less cost-effective than their standard system to refer arrestees into drug treatment.[144] In fact, because of the narrow window period to detect drugs in urine, the mandatory drug-testing procedure was missing many arrestees who had serious drug problems and would have benefited from drug treatment.

A further potential rationale behind the use of mandatory drug testing is that it acts as a deterrent from using drugs. While random testing in some contexts can reduce the risk of intoxication in specific contexts (e.g., roadside alcohol testing), and this can in turn reduce the risk of accidents and other problems from drug/alcohol use, there is little evidence that targeted drug-testing procedures can be used successfully to reduce the overall number of people who use drugs. One study in the United States found that schools that administered random drug tests did not have lower levels of drug use than those that did not use these drug-testing procedures.[145] Another study had more positive results but only slightly decreased the self-reported use of drugs that were being tested for and did not alter overall levels of substance use.[146] There is also little evidence in support of using other policing strategies to deter people from using drugs. For example, attempts to police drug use in dance venues using drug detector dogs appears to have little deterrent effect on regular drug users and merely shift the way in which people carry drugs and when they choose to use them.[147]

The consequences of detecting an illicit drug in a minor also needs to be considered: whether this would result in the young person having a criminal record, being expelled from school, or receiving mandatory detention—all of which could adversely affect the student's life prospects and unintentionally increase their risk of becoming dependent on drugs by creating vulnerabilities for drug dependence (e.g., unemployment, family problems). Therefore appropriate follow-up and prevention or treatment options need to be available for those people who are believed to be using drugs.[148] It also needs to be appreciated that testing for illicit drug use would miss people who would benefit from help for legal drugs, including alcohol and prescription medications, which are far more common than illicit drugs, and an increasingly abused in many countries. The high cost of illicit drug testing would also draw resources away from providing these more effective drug prevention and treatment programs. [149]

In essence, mandatory drug testing procedures are costly, yield limited return on detecting people who use drugs, miss the majority of people at risk of drug or alcohol problems, and have limited benefit in deterring drug use more generally. They have significant consequences for governments in taking responsibility for the consequences imposed on people who test positive (e.g., job loss, imprisonment) and the costs that this will translate into for society (e.g., providing additional mandatory drug treatment or detention). The responses that are provided (e.g., mandatory drug treatment) may not be appropriate in all cases, and may waste scarce resources. In some situations, these responses may reduce a person's capacity to contribute effectively to society (e.g., in the event that they lose their job). Arguably the most critical concern is the moral problem of placing individuals in detention or treatment because they have received a false-positive reading on a toxicology test, which will inevitably occur in a proportion of cases because these tests are not 100 percent accurate.

SUMMARY AND CONCLUSION

ATS use has substantially increased in East and Southeast Asia over the past two decades and now presents a significant concern for many countries in the region. Methamphetamine is the primary ATS used in the region, although ATS are often available in the form of pills that contain various types of synthetic drugs. The market for ecstasy, while smaller than that for methamphetamine, is also growing. East and Southeast Asia has also become home to large-scale ATS manufacture, which has impacted on local drug-use levels, particularly in trafficking regions along the Mekong Delta.

East and Southeast Asia is a region traditionally dominated by opioid use, and the advent of ATS use presents significant new challenges. Patterns of use, and the types of people who use ATS, are more varied than traditionally seen with opioid drugs, extending from recreational use among youth in the nightclub/entertainment scene, occupational/functional use in the labor force, to daily dependent use of methamphetamine. Existing treatment facilities have been developed with opioids in mind, and treatment facilities that cater to ATS users are scarce. [150] Not all ATS use patterns warrant treatment, and it is likely that prevention and harm reduction will play a much greater role. In this context, the more widespread use and acceptability of ATS is likely to have implications for whether conventional drug prevention programs are effective for ATS use, and consideration needs to be given as to whether the purpose of these programs is to prevent harms from using these drugs (e.g., overdose, the progression to dependent use) compared to preventing use altogether.

Pragmatic considerations need to play in to the equation, such as what types of ATS use patterns are driving the greatest problems from these drugs (e.g., heavy methamphetamine use vs. recreational ecstasy use). When resources are scarce, it is critical to consider which interventions are likely to be most effective in decreasing the adverse consequences that ATS use has on individuals and society. The evidence base for what works to reduce ATS use and related harms is weak. However, there are some key points that can be used to guide practice in responding to the ATS situation.

First, prevention programs can be implemented to reduce the uptake of ATS use. The programs should also cover various drugs and alcohol use as these are antecedents to ATS use. For targeted prevention interventions to be effective, high-risk groups and their risk behaviors should be identified by epidemiological approaches for the development of individual social skills on risk populations, especially among adolescents. Similar to treatments for ATS use, prevention programs are now being developed so that they can be delivered in an online environment, or through electronic media (e.g., CD-ROMs) to improve their portability. Within resource-poor settings greater emphasis should be placed on reducing risk factors for dependence on drugs (and increasing resilience) among vulnerable communities by addressing more basic needs (e.g., education).

Second, treatment for dependence on ATS use can reduce levels of use and related harms. Evidence around what treatments are most effective is limited, but current evidence indicates that structured psychological treatments can been effective when applied intensively (e.g., one to two sessions per week over several months). The principles underpinning these types of treatments are now being incorporated into internet-based interventions to increase treatment access and these types of internet interventions could be adapted to work within various social/cultural contexts.

Third, reducing the supply of ATS through regulating chemicals used in synthetic drug manufacture has the potential to reduce the purity and availability of ATS and consequent ATS-related problems. These interventions specifically target manufacture of illicit ATS and therefore avoid criminal consequences for people who use ATS.

On the other hand, approaches that involve policing drug use through mandatory testing or other detection procedures have been less effective in deterring use, and even in cases where they can deter use (e.g., among school children) the benefits of this deterrent risk need to be weighed against the cost of criminalizing a population of drug-using youth, including the inevitable consequence of criminalizing innocent people because toxicology tests are not 100 percent accurate. Because of the widespread use of ATS use among today's youth, and that many of these young people will not go on to develop dependence on ATS (unlike the situation with opioid/heroin use), it is likely that high criminal penalties for using ATS will have a more lasting and detrimental effect both on the people using these drugs, and on society, than will their actual use.

NOTES

1. BSc(Psychol)Hons. PhD, fellow, Centre for Research on Ageing Health and Well-being, The Australian National University, Australia.
Correspondence:
Rebecca McKetinFellow
Centre for Research on Ageing, Health and Well-being
ANU College of Medicine, Biology and Environment
Building 63, Eggleston Road
The Australian National University
Canberra ACT 0200 Australia
T: +61 2 61258407
F: +61 2 61250733
W: http://cmhr
2. PhD, professor and dean, College of Pharmacy, Kaohsiung Medical University, Taiwan.
3. UNODC (United Nations Office on Drugs and Crime), *2010 World Drug Report* (Vienna: UNODC, 2010).
4. Sara Grant, Philip Burgess, Meredith Harris, Gin Malhi, and Harvey Whiteford, "Stimulant Use and Stimulant Disorders in Australia: Findings from the National Survey of Mental Health and Wellbeing," *Medical Journal of Australia* 195 (2011): 607–10.
5. Nancy Nicosia, Rosalie Pacula Liccardo, Beau Kilmer, Russell Lundberg, and James Chiesa, "The Economic Cost of Methamphetamine Use in the United States, 2005," RAND Drug Policy Research Center, Rand Corporation, Los Angeles, California, 2009.
6. Louisa Degenhardt, Bruno Raimondo, and Libby Topp, "Is Ecstasy a Drug of Dependence?" *Drug and Alcohol Dependence* 107 (2010): 1–10.
7. Chen Chuan-Yu and Lin Keh-Ming, "Health Consequences of Illegal Drug Use," *Current Opinion in Psychiatry* 22 (2009): 287–92.
8. Euphrosyne Gouzoulis-Mayfrank and Joerg Daumann, "Neurotoxicity of Methylenedioxyamphetamines (MDMA; Ecstasy) in Humans: How Strong is the Evidence for Persistent Brain Damage?" *Addiction* 101 (2006): 348–61.
9. Sharlene Kaye, Shane Darke., and Joe Duflou, "Methylenedioxymethamphetamine (MDMA)-related Fatalities in Australia: Demographics, Circumstances, Toxicology and Major Organ Pathology," *Drug and Alcohol Dependence* 104 (2009): 254–61.
10. Grant Colfax, Glenn-Milo Santos, Priscilla Chu, Eric Vittinghoff, Andreas Pluddemann, Suresh Kumar, and Carl Hart, "Amphetamine-Group Substances and HIV," *Lancet* 376 (2010): 458–74.
11. Rebecca McKetin, Erin Kelly, and Jennifer McLaren, "The Relationship between Crystalline Methamphetamine Use and Methamphetamine Dependence," *Drug and Alcohol Dependence* 85 (2006): 198–204.
12. Rebecca McKetin, Nicholas Kozel, Jeremy Douglas, Robert Ali, Balasingam Vicknasingam, Johannes Lund, and Jih-Heng Li, "The Rise of Methamphetamine in Southeast and East Asia," *Drug and Alcohol Review* 27 (2008): 220–28.
13. Toshihiko Matsumoto, Atsushi Kamijo, Tomohiro Miyakawa, Keiko Endo, Tatsuo Yabana, Hideji Kishimoto, Kenichi Okudaira, Eizo Iseki, Takeshi Sakai, and Kenji Kosaka, "Methamphetamine in Japan: The Consequences of Methamphetamine Abuse as a Function of Route of Administration," *Addiction* 97 (2002): 809–17.
14. Wayne Hall and Julie Hando, "Route of Administration and Adverse Effects of Amphetamine Use among Young Adults in Sydney, Australia," *Drug and Alcohol Review* 13 (1994): 277–84.

15. Shane Darke, Julie Cohen, Joanne Ross, Julie Hando, and Wayne Hall, "Transitions between Routes of Administration of Regular Amphetamine Users," *Addiction* 89 (1994): 1077–83.

16. Arthur K. Cho, "Ice: A New Dosage Form of an Old Drug." *Science* 249 (4969) (1990): 631–34.

17. Kelly McKetin and McLaren, *The Sydney Methamphetamine Market.*

18. Darke et al., *Transitions between Routes*, 1077–83.

19. Amanda Baker, Frances Kay-Lambkin, Nicole K Lee, Melissa Claire, and Linda Jenner, "A Brief Cognitive Behavioural Intervention for Regular Amphetamine Users." Australian Government Department of Health and Ageing, Canberra, 2003. Accessed October 14, 2012. www.health.gov.au/internet/main/publishing.nsf/Content/health-pubhlth-publicat-document-cognitive_intervention-cnt.htm.

20. Darke et al., *Transitions between Routes*, 1077–83.

21. Baker et al., *A Brief Cognitive Behavioural Intervention.*

22. Rebecca McKetin, Dan I. Lubman, Amanda L. Baker, Sharon Dawe, and Robert Ali, "Psychotic Symptoms are Dose-related in Chronic Methamphetamine Users: Evidence from a Prospective Longitudinal Study," *JAMA Psychiatry* (2013): 1–6. DOI:10.1001/jamapsychiatry.2013.283.

23. Everitt H. Ellinwood, "Assault and Homicide Associated with Amphetamine Abuse," *American Journal of Psychiatry* 127 (1971): 90–95.

24. UNODC (United Nations Office on Drugs and Crime), *2012 World Drug Report* (Vienna: UNODC, 2012).

25. Fred E. Shick, "Stimulant Abuse And Dependence," *Pusat Penyelidikan Dadah Dan Ubat-Ubatan, Review Papers Series No.1* (Penang: Universiti Sains Malaysia, 1997).

26. Shick, *Stimulant Abuse.*

27. Hiroshi Suwaki, "Methamphetamine Abuse in Japan," in *Methamphetamine Abuse, Epidemiologic Issues and Implications, NIDA Research Monograph 115*, ed. Marissa A. Miller and Nicholas Kozel (Washington, DC: U.S. Government Printing Office, 1991).

28. Shick, *Stimulant Abuse.*

29. Suwaki, *Methamphetamine Abuse.*

30. Japanese Ministry of Health and Welfare, *Brief Account of Drug Abuse and Countermeasures in Japan* (Tokyo: Japanese Ministry of Health and Welfare, 1993).

31. Suwaki, *Methamphetamine Abuse.*

32. Japanese Ministry of Health and Welfare, *Brief Account.*

33. Japanese Ministry of Health and Welfare, *Brief Account.*

34. Byung-In Cho, "Trends and Patterns of Methamphetamine Abuse in the Republic of Korea," in *Methamphetamine Abuse, Epidemiologic Issues and Implications*, ed. by Marissa A. Miller and Nicholas Kozel, 99–106 (Rockville, MD: NIDA Research Monograph, 1991).

35. Cho, *Trends and Patterns.*

36. Jih-Heng Li, Shu-Fen, and Wen-Jing Yu, "Patterns and Trends of Drug Abuse in Taiwan: A Brief History and Report from 2000 through 2004," in *Epidemiologic Trends in Drug Abuse, Volume II , Proceedings of the Community Epidemiology Work Group*, ed. by Moira P. O'Brien (Washington, DC: U.S. Department of Health and Human Services, National Institutes of Health, 2005).

37. Rebecca McKetin, Joanne Ross, Erin Kelly, Amanda Baker, Nicole Lee, Daniel I. Lubman, and Richard Mattick, "Characteristics and Harms Associated with Injecting Versus Smoking Methamphetamine among Methamphetamine Treatment Entrants," *Drug and Alcohol Review* 27 (2008): 277–85.

38. McKetin et al., *Characteristics and Harms*, 277–85.

39. Byung-Inz Cho, "Drug Control Policy in Korea." International Centre for Criminal Law Reform and Criminal Justice Policy, Vancouver, British Columbia, 2004. Accessed October 14, 2012. www.icclr.law.ubc.ca/Publications/Reports/Dr.Chos%20paper%20Drug%20Control%20Policy.pdf.

40. Cho, *Drug Control Policy.*

41. Shu-Fen Li and Wen-Jing Yu, *Patterns and Trends of Drug Abuse in Taiwan.*

42. Kit-Sang Leung, Jih-Heng Li, Wen-Ing Tsay, Catina Callahan, Shu-Fen Liu, Jui Hsu, Lee Hoffer, and Linda B. Cottler, "Dinosaur Girls, Candy Girls, and Trinity: Voices of Taiwanese Club Drug Users," *Journal of Ethnicity in Substance Abuse* 7 (2008): 237–57.

43. Jih-Heng Li, Balasingam Vicknasingam, Yuet-Wah Cheung, Wang Zhou, Adhi Wibowo Nurhidayat, Don C. Des Jarlais, and Richard Schottenfeld, "To Use or Not to Use: An Update on Licit and Illicit Ketamine Use," *Substance Abuse and Rehabilitation* 2 (2011): 11–20.

44. Ko-Lin Chin, *The Golden Triangle: Inside Southeast Asia's Drug Trade* (Ithaca: Cornell University Press, 2009).

45. UNODC (United National Office of Drugs and Crime), *Patterns and Trends of Amphetamine-Type Stimulants (ATS) and Other Drugs of Abuse in East Asia and the Pacific 2005* (Bangkok: United Nations Office on Drugs and Crime Regional Centre for East Asia and the Pacific, 2006).

46. US Department of State. Bureau for International Narcotics and Law Enforcement Affairs, *International Narcotics Control Strategy (INCS) Report: Volume I. Drug and chemical Control* (Washington, DC: Government Printing Office, 2007). Accessed October 14, 2012. www.state.gov/documents/organization/81446.pdf.

47. Madonna Devaney, Gary Reid, and Simon Baldwin, *Situational Analysis of Illicit Drug Issues and Responses in the Asia-Pacific Region* (Canberra: Australian National Council on Drugs, 2006).

48. Jonathan Cohen, "Thailand—Not Enough Graves: the War on Drugs, HIV/AIDS, and Violations of Human Rights," *Human Rights Watch* 16, no. 8C (2007): 1–58. Accessed December 18, 2007. http://hrw.org/reports/2004/thailand0704/thailand0704.pdf.

49. Tassanai Vongchak, Surinda Kawichai, Susan Sherman, David D. Celentano, Thira Sirisanthana, Carl Latkin, Kanokporn Wiboonnatakul, Namtip Srirak, Jaroon Jittiwutikarn, and Apinun Aramrattana, "The Influence of Thailand's 2003 'War on Drugs' Policy on Self-Reported Drug Use among Injection Drug Users in Chiang Mai, Thailand," *International Journal of Drug Policy* 16 (2005): 115–21.

50. McKetin et al., *Characteristics and Harms*, 277–85.

51. UNODC (United Nations Office on Drugs and Crime), *Patterns and Trends in Amphetamine-Type Stimulants in East Asia and the Pacific 2006* (Bangkok: United Nations Office on Drugs and Crime Regional Centre for East Asia and the Pacific, 2007).

52. UNODC, *2012 World Drug Report.*

53. UNODC, *2010 World Drug Report.*

54. UNODC (United Nations Office on Drugs and Crime), *2009 Patterns and trends of Amphetamine-Type Stimulants and other Drugs in East and Southeast Asia (and Neighbouring Regions)* (Bangkok: United Nations Office on Drugs and Crime Regional Centre for East Asia and the Pacific, 2009).

55. UNODC, *2010 World Drug Report.*

56. UNODC, *2009 Patterns and Trends.*

57. John Marsden, Robert Ali, Moruf Adelekan, Usaneya Perngparn, Tieqiao Liu, Agueda Sunga, Michael Farrell, and Maristela Monteiro, *WHO Multi-Site Project on Functional/Instrumental Use of Amphetamine-Type Stimulants: Study Protocol and Instrumentation* (Geneva: World Health Organization, 2000).

58. Dan Werb, Kanna Hayashi, Nadia Fairbairn, Karyn Kaplan, Paisan Suwannawong, Calvin Lai, and Thomas Kerr, "Drug Use Patterns among Thai Illicit Drug Injectors amidst Increased Police Presence," *Substance Abuse Treatment Prevention and Policy* 4 (2009): 16.

59. McKetin et al., *Characteristics and Harms*, 277–85.

60. Chin, *The Golden Triangle.*

61. UNODC, *2009 Patterns and Trends.*

62. UNODC, *2009 Patterns and Trends.*

63. Mark E. Barrett, "Nature and Scope of Substance Use among Survivors of Exploitation in Cambodia: an Assessment," (The Asia Foundation, Phnom Penh, Cambodia, 2006).

64. Barrett, *Nature and Scope.*

65. UNODC (United Nations Office on Drugs and Crime), *Assessment Report: Drug Abuse among Disco Clients in Vientiane* (Bangkok: UNODC, 2002).

66. UNODC (United Nations Office on Drugs and Crime), *Drug Abuse among Service Girls in Vientiane: Assessment Report* (Bangkok: UNODC, 2002).

67. Christopher Beyrer, Myat H. Razak, Khomdon Lisam, Jie Chen, Weic Lui, and Xiao-Fang Yu, "Overland Heroin Trafficking Routes and HIV-1 Spread in South and South-east Asia," *AIDS* 7 (2000): 75–83.

68. McKetin et al., *The Rise of Methamphetamine*, 220–28.

69. Werb et al, *Drug Use Patterns*, 16.

70. Colfax, *Amphetamine-Group Substances*, 458–74.

71. United Nations, *Convention on Psychotropic Substances, 1971* (Vienna: United Nations, 1971).

72. United Nations, *United Nations Convention against Illicit Traffic in Narcotic Drugs and Psychotropic Substances, 1988* (Vienna: United Nations, 1988).

73. Rebecca McKetin, Rachel Sutherland, David A. Bright, and Melissa M. Norberg, "A Systematic Review of Methamphetamine Precursor Regulations," *Addiction* 106 (2011): 1911–24.

74. James K. Cunningham and Lon-Mu Liu, "Impacts of Federal Ephedrine and Pseudoephedrine Regulations on Methamphetamine-related Hospital Admissions," *Addiction* 98 (2003): 1229–37.

75. James K. Cunningham and Lon-Mu Liu, "Impacts of Federal Precursor Chemical Regulations on Methamphetamine Arrests," *Addiction* 100 (2005): 479–88.

76. James K. Cunningham, Lon-Mu Liu, Russell Callaghan, "Impact of US and Canadian precursor regulation on methamphetamine purity in the United States," *Addiction* 104 (2009): 441–53.

77. Liu Cunningham and Callaghan, *Impact of US and Canadian Precursor Regulation*, 441–53.

78. James K. Cunningham, Ietza Bojorquez, Octavio Campollo, Lon-Mu Liu, Jane C. Maxwell, "Mexico's Methamphetamine Precursor Chemical Interventions: Impacts on Drug Treatment Admissions," *Addiction* 105 (2010): 1973–83.

79. Cunningham et al., *Mexico's Methamphetamine*, 1973–83.

80. Carlos Dobkin and Nancy Nicosia, "The War on Drugs: Methamphetamine, Public Health, and Crime," *American Economic Review* 99 (2009): 324–49.

81. Cunningham et al., *Mexico's Methamphetamine*, 1973–83.

82. McKetin et al., *A Systematic Review*, 1911–24.

83. McKetin, Kelly, and McLaren, *The Sydney Methamphetamine Market*.

84. Nicosia et al., *The Economic Cost*.

85. Srisurapanont Manit, Ngamwong Jarusuraisin, and Phunnapa Kittirattanapaiboon, "Treatment for Amphetamine Dependence and Abuse," *Cochrane Database of Systematic Reviews* 4 (2001): *CD003022*. DOI: 10.1002/14651858.CD003022.

86. Steven J. Shoptaw, Uyen Kao, Keith Heinzerling, and Walter Ling, "Treatment for Amphetamine Withdrawal," *Cochrane Database Systematic Review Issue* 2 (2009): CD003021.

87. Colfax et al., *Amphetamine-Group Substances*, 458–74.

88. Ahmed Elkashef, Frank Vocci, Glen Hanson, Jason White, Wendy Wickes, and Jari Tiihonen, "Pharmacotherapy of Methamphetamine Addiction: An Update." *Substance Abuse* 29 (2008): 31–49.

89. James Shearer, John Sherman, Alex Wodak, and Ingrid van Beek, "Substitution Therapy for Amphetamine Users," *Drug and Alcohol Review* 21 (2002): 179–85.

90. Srisurapanont, Jarusuraisin, and Kittirattanapaiboon, *Treatment*.

91. Srisurapanont, Jarusuraisin, and Kittirattanapaiboon, *Treatment*.

92. Srisurapanont, Jarusuraisin, and Kittirattanapaiboon, *Treatment*.

93. Steve Shoptaw, Alice Huber, James Peck, Xiawei Yang, Juanmei Liu, Jeff Dang, John Roll, Benjamin Shapiro, Erin Rotheram-Fuller, and Walter Ling, "Randomized, Placebo-controlled Trial of Sertraline and Contingency Management for the Treatment of Methamphetamine Dependence," *Drug and Alcohol Dependence* 85 (2006): 12–18.

94. Nitya Jayaram-Lindstrom, Anders Hammarberg, Olof Beck, and Johan Franck, "Naltrexone for the Treatment of Amphetamine Dependence: a Randomized, Placebo-Controlled Trial," *American Journal of Psychiatry* 165 (2008): 1442–48.

95. Jari Tiihonen, Evgeny Krupitsky, Elena Verbitskaya, Elena Blokhina, Olga Mamontova, Jaana Fohr, Pekka Tuomola, Kimmo Kuoppasalmi, Vesa Kiviniemi, and Edwin Zwartau, "Naltrexone Implant for the Treatment of Polydrug Dependence: a Randomized Controlled Trial," *American Journal of Psychiatry* 169 (2012): 531–36.

96. Jari Tiihonen, Kimmo Kuoppasalmi, Jaana Föhr, Pekka Tuomola, Outi Kuikanmäki, Helena Vorma, Petteri Sokero, Jari Haukka, and Esa Meririnne, "A Comparison of Aripiprazole, Methylphenidate, and Placebo for Amphetamine Dependence," *American Journal of Psychiatry* 164 (2007): 160–62.

97. Elkashef et al., *Pharmacotherapy*, 31–49.

98. Richard P. Mattick and Shane Darke, "Drug Replacement Treatments: is Amphetamine Substitution a Horse of a Different Colour?" *Drug and Alcohol Review* 14 (1995): 389–94.

99. Catherine McGregor, Manit Srisurapanont, Jaroon Jittiwutikarn, Suchart Laobhripatr, Thirawat Wongtan, and Jason M. White, "The Nature, Time Course and Severity of Methamphetamine Withdrawal," *Addiction* 100 (2005): 1320–29.

100. Shoptaw et al, *Treatment for Amphetamine Withdrawal*.

101. Rebecca McKetin, Jake M. Najman, Amanda Baker, Daniel I. Lubman, Sharon Dawe, Robert Ali, Nicole K. Lee, Richard Mattick, and Abdullah Mamun, "Evaluating the Impact of Community-based Treatment Options on Methamphetamine Use: Findings from the Methamphetamine Treatment Evaluation Study (MATES)," *Addiction* 107, no. 11 (2012): 1998 – 2008.

102. Richard A. Rawson, M. J. McCann, Frank Flammino, Steven Shoptaw, Karen Miotto, Chris Reiber, and Walter Ling, "A Comparison of Contingency Management and Cognitive-Behavioral Approaches for Stimulant-Dependent Individuals," *Addiction* 101 (2006): 267–74.

103. Colfax et al., *Amphetamine-Group Substances*, 458-74.

104. Baker et al., *A Brief Cognitive Behavioural Intervention*.

105. Steven Shoptaw, Cathy J. Reback, James A. Peck, Xiaowei Yang, Erin Rotheram-Fuller, Sherry Larkins, Rosemary C. Veniegas, Thomas E. Freese, and Christopher Hucks-Ortiz, "Behavioral Treatment Approaches for Methamphetamine Dependence and HIV-Related Sexual Risk Behaviors among Urban Gay and Bisexual Men," *Drug and Alcohol Dependence* 78 (2005): 125–34.

106. Rawson et al., *A Comparison*, 267–74.

107. Rawson et al., *A Comparison*, 267–74.

108. Colfax et al., *Amphetamine-Group Substances*, 458–74.

109. Colfax et al., *Amphetamine-Group Substances*, 458–74.

110. Yih-Ing Hser, David Huang, Chih-Ping Chou, Cheryl Teruya, and Douglas M. Anglin, "Longitudinal Patterns of Treatment Utilization and Outcomes among Methamphetamine Abusers: a Growth Curve Modeling Approach," *Journal of Drug Issues* 33 (2003): 921–38.

111. Yih-Ing Hser, Elizabeth Evans, and Yu-Chuang Huang, "Treatment outcomes among women and men methamphetamine abusers in California," *Journal of Substance Abuse Treatment* 28 (2005): 77–85.

112. McKetin et al., *Evaluating the Impact*, 1998 – 2008 .

113. Patrick M. Flynn, Patricia L. Kristiansen, James V. Porto, and Robert L. Hubbard, "Costs and Benefits of Treatment for Cocaine Addiction in DATOS," *Drug and Alcohol Dependence* 57 (1999): 167–74.

114. McKetin et al., *Evaluating the Impact*, 1998 – 2008 .

115. McKetin et al., *Treatment Outcomes*.

116. Richard A. Rawson, Alice Huber, Paul Brethen, Jeanne Obert, Vikas Gulati, Steven Shoptaw, and Walter Ling, "Status of Methamphetamine Users 2–5 Years after Outpatient Treatment," *Journal of Addictive Diseases* 21 (2002): 107–19.

117. Richard A. Rawson, Patricia Marinelli-Casey, Douglas M. Anglin, Alic Dickow, Yvonne Frazier, Cheryl Gallagher, Gantt P. Galloway, James Herrell, Alice Huber, Michael J. McCann, Jeanne Obert, Susan Pennell, Chris Reiber, Denna Vandersloot, Joan Zweben, and Methamphetamine Treatment Project Corporate Authors. "A Multi-Site Comparison of

Psychosocial Approaches for the Treatment of Methamphetamine Dependence," *Addiction* 99 (2004): 708–17.

118. McKetin et al., *Treatment Outcomes*.

119. McKetin et al., *Treatment Outcomes*.

120. Rawson et al., *A Multi-site Comparison*, 708–17.

121. McKetin et al., *Treatment Outcomes*.

122. McKetin et al., *Evaluating the Impact*, 1998 – 2008 .

123. Julie Hando, Libby Topp, and Wayne Hall, "Amphetamine-Related Harms and Treatment Preferences of Regular Amphetamine Users in Sydney, Australia," *Drug and Alcohol Dependence* 46 (1997): 105–13.

124. Cate Wallace, Tony Galloway, Rebecca McKetin, Erin Kelly, and John Leary, "Methamphetamine Use, Dependence and Treatment Access in Rural and Regional North Coast New South Wales, Australia," *Drug and Alcohol Review* 28 (2009): 592–99.

125. Robert J. Tait, Rebecca McKetin, Frances Kay-Lambkin, Kylie Bennett, Ada Tam, Jenny Geddes, Adam Garrick, Helen Christensen, and Kathy M. Griffiths, "Breaking the Ice: A Protocol for a Randomised Controlled Trial of an Internet-Based Intervention Addressing Amphetamine-type Stimulant Use," *BMC Psychiatry* 12 (2012) 67–75.

126. Christensen, Helen, Kathleen Griffiths, and Anthony Jorm, "Delivering Interventions for Depression by Using the Internet: Randomised Controlled Trial," *British Medical Journal* 328 (2004): 265.

127. Frances J. Kay-Lambkin, Amanda L. Baker, Rebecca McKetin, and Nicole Lee, "Stepping through Treatment: Reflections on an Adaptive Treatment Strategy among Methamphetamine Users with Depression," *Drug and Alcohol Review* 29 (2010): 475–82.

128. UNODC, *2006 Patterns and Trends of Amphetamine-Type Stimulants*.

129. John L. Horwood, David M. Fergusson, Mohammad R. Hayatbakhsh, Jake M. Najman, Carolyn Coffey, George C. Patton, Edmund Silins, and Delyse M Hutchinson, "Cannabis use and Educational Achievement: Findings from Three Australasian Cohort Studies," *Drug and Alcohol Dependence* 110 (2010): 247–53.

130. Joseph M. Boden, David M. Fergusson, and John L. Horwood, "Illicit Drug Use and Dependence in a New Zealand Birth Cohort," *Australian & New Zealand Journal of Psychiatry* 40 (2006): 156–63.

131. David M. Fergusson, Joseph M. Boden, and John L. Horwood, "The Developmental Antecedents of Illicit Drug Use: Evidence from a 25-year Longitudinal Study,"*Drug and Alcohol Dependence* 96 (2008): 165–77.

132. Fabrizio Faggiano, Federica D. Vigna-Taglianti, Elisabetta Versino, Alessio Zambon, Alberto Borraccino, and Patrizia Lemma, "School-Based Prevention for Illicit Drugs' Use," *Cochrane Database of Systematic Reviews* Issue 2. (2005): Art. No. CD003020. doi: 10.1002/14651858.CD003020.pub2.

133. Faggiano et al., *School-based Prevention*.

134. Spoth, Richard L., Scott Clair, Chungyeol Shin, Cleve Redmond. "Long-term Effects of Universal Preventive Interventions on Methamphetamine Use among Adolescents," *Archives of Pediatrics and Adolescent Medicine* 160 (2006): 876–82.

135. Simon Gates, Jim McCambridge, Lesley A. Smith, and David Foxcroft, "Interventions for Prevention of Drug Use by Young People Delivered in Non-school Settings," *Cochrane Database of Systematic Reviews* Issue 1 (2006): Art. No. CD005030. DOI: 10.1002/14651858.CD005030.pub2.

136. Nicky C. Newton, Gavin Andrews, Maree Teesson, and Laura E. Vogl, "Delivering Prevention for Alcohol and Cannabis using the Internet: a Cluster Randomised Controlled Trial," *Preventive Medicine* 48 (2009): 579–84.

137. Laura Vogl, Nicola Newton, Maree Teesson, Wendy Swift, Aspasia Karageorge, Catherine Deans, Rebecca McKetin, Bronwyn Steadman, Jennifer Jones, Paul Dillon, Alys Havard, and Gavin Andrews, "Climate Schools: Universal Computer-Based Programs to Prevent Alcohol and other Drug Use in Adolescence," Technical Report No. 321, National Drug and Alcohol Centre (Sydney: University of New South Wales, 2012).

138. Nancy C. Brahm, Lynn L. Yeager, Mark D. Fox, Kevin C. Farmer, and Tony A. Palmer, "Commonly Prescribed Medications and Potential False-Positive Urine Drug Screens," *American Journal of Health-System Pharmacy* 67 (2010): 1344–50.

139. Brahm et al., *Commonly Prescribed Medications*, 1344–50.

140. John T. Cody, " Precursor Medications as a Source of Methamphetamine and/or Amphetamine Positive Drug Testing Results, " *Journal of Occupational and Environmental Medicine* 44 (2002): 435 – 50.

141. John T. Cody, " Enantiomeric Composition of Amphetamine and Methamphetamine Derived from the Precursor Compound Famprofazone, " *Forensic Science International* 80 (1996): 189-199.

142. E. S. Oh, S. K. Hong, G. I. Kang, "Plasma and Urinary Concentrations of Methamphetamine after Oral Administration of Famprofazone to Man," *Xenobiotica* 22 (1992): 377–84.

143. Kuei-Hui Chan , Mei-Chich Hsu, Chen-Yu Tseng, and Wei-Lan Chu, "Famprofazone Use can be Misinterpreted as Methamphetamine Abuse," *Journal of Analytical Toxicology* 34 (2010): 347–53.

144. Kate Orr Skellington, Shirley McCoard, and Paul McCartney, "Evaluation of the Mandatory Drug Testing of Arrestees Pilot" (Edinburgh: The Scottish Government, Queens Printers of Scotland, 2009). www.scotland.gov.uk/socialresearch.

145. Yamaguchi Ryoko, Lloyd D. Johnston, and Patrick M. O'Malley, "Relationship Between Student Illicit Drug Use and School Drug-Testing Policies," *Journal of School Health* 73 (2003): 159–64.

146. Susanne James-Burdumy, Brian Goesling, John Deke, and Eric Einspruch, "The Effectiveness of Mandatory-Random Student Drug Testing: a Cluster Randomized Trial," *Journal of Adolescent Health* 50 (2012): 172–78.

147. Matthew Dunn and Louisa Degenhardt, "The Use of Drug Detection Dogs in Sydney, Australia," *Drug and Alcohol Review* 28 (2009): 658–62.

148. Woody Caan, "Random Drug Testing in Schools Fails Screening Criteria," *British Medical Journal* 328 (2004): 641.

149. Clare Gerada and Eilish Gilvarry, "Random Drug Testing in Schools," *British Journal of General Practice* 55 (2005): 499–501.

150. UNODC, *Patterns and Trends of Amphetamine-Type Stimulants.*

BIBLIOGRAPHY

Baker, Amanda, Frances Kay-Lambkin, Nicole K. Lee, Melissa Claire, and Linda Jenner, "A Brief Cognitive Behavioural Intervention for Regular Amphetamine Users." Australian Government Department of Health and Ageing, Canberra, 2003. Accessed October 14, 2012. www.health.gov.au/internet/main/publishing.nsf/Content/health-pubhlth-publicat-document-cognitive_intervention-cnt.htm.

Barrett, Mark E. "Nature and Scope of Substance Use among Survivors of Exploitation in Cambodia: an Assessment." The Asia Foundation, Phnom Penh, Cambodia, 2006.

Beyrer, Christopher, Myat H. Razak, Khomdon Lisam, Jie Chen, Weic Lui, and Xiao-Fang Yu, "Overland Heroin Trafficking Routes and HIV-1 Spread in South and South-east Asia," *AIDS* 7 (2000): 75–83.

Boden, Joseph M., David M. Fergusson, and John L. Horwood, "Illicit Drug Use and Dependence in a New Zealand Birth Cohort," *Australian & New Zealand Journal of Psychiatry* 40 (2006): 156–63.

Brahm, Nancy C., Lynn L. Yeager, Mark D. Fox, Kevin C. Farmer, and Tony A. Palmer, "Commonly Prescribed Medications and Potential False-Positive Urine Drug Screens, " *American Journal of Health-System Pharmacy* 67 (2010): 1344–50.

Caan, Woody. "Random Drug Testing in Schools Fails Screening Criteria." *British Medical Journal* 328 (2004): 641.

Chan, Kuei-Hui , Mei-Chich Hsu, Chen-Yu Tseng, and Wei-Lan Chu, "Famprofazone Use can be Misinterpreted as Methamphetamine Abuse," *Journal of Analytical Toxicology* 34 (2010): 347–53.

Chen Chuan-Yu and Lin Keh-Ming. "Health Consequences of Illegal Drug Use." *Current Opinion in Psychiatry* 22 (2009): 287–92.

Chin, Ko-Lin. *The Golden Triangle: Inside Southeast Asia's Drug Trade.* Ithaca: Cornell University Press, 2009.

Cho, Arthur K. "Ice: A New Dosage Form of an Old Drug." *Science* 249, no. 4969 (1990): 631–34.

Cho, Byung-In. "Trends and Patterns of Methamphetamine Abuse in the Republic of Korea." In *Methamphetamine Abuse, Epidemiologic Issues and Implications,* edited by Marissa A. Miller and Nicholas Kozel, 99–106. Rockville, MD: NIDA Research Monograph, 1991.

Cho, Byung-In. "Drug Control Policy in Korea." International Centre for Criminal Law Reform and Criminal Justice Policy, Vancouver, British Columbia, 2004. Accessed October 14, 2012. www.icclr.law.ubc.ca/Publications/Reports/Dr.Chos%20paper%20Drug%20Control-%20Policy.pdf.

Christensen, Helen, Kathleen Griffiths, and Anthony Jorm. "Delivering Interventions for Depression by Using the Internet: Randomised Controlled Trial." *British Medical Journal* 328 (2004): 265.

Cody, John T. "Enantiomeric Composition of Amphetamine and Methamphetamine Derived from the Precursor Compound Famprofazone," *Forensic Science International* 80 (1996): 189–99.

Cody, John T. "Precursor Medications as a Source of Methamphetamine and/or Amphetamine Positive Drug Testing Results." *Journal of Occupational and Environmental Medicine* 44 (2002): 435–50.

Cohen, Jonathan. "Thailand—Not Enough Graves: The War on Drugs, HIV/AIDS, and Violations of Human Rights." *Human Rights Watch* 16, no. 8C (2007): 1–58. Accessed December 18, 2007. http://hrw.org/reports/2004/thailand0704/thailand0704.pdf.

Colfax, Grant, Glenn-Milo Santos, Priscilla Chu, Eric Vittinghoff, Andreas Pluddemann, Suresh Kumar, and Carl Hart. "Amphetamine-Group Substances and HIV." *Lancet* 376 (2010): 458–74.

Cunningham, James K., Ietza Bojorquez, Octavio Campollo, Lon-Mu Liu, and Jane C. Maxwell, "Mexico's Methamphetamine Precursor Chemical Interventions: Impacts on Drug Treatment Admissions." *Addiction* 105 (2010): 1973–83.

Cunningham James K. and Lon-Mu Liu, "Impacts of Federal Ephedrine and Pseudoephedrine Regulations on Methamphetamine-related Hospital Admissions." *Addiction* 98 (2003): 1229–37.

Cunningham, James K. and Lon-Mu Liu, "Impacts of Federal Precursor Chemical Regulations on Methamphetamine Arrests." *Addiction* 100 (2005): 479–88.

Cunningham, James K., Lon-Mu Liu, Russell Callaghan, "Impact of US and Canadian precursor regulation on methamphetamine purity in the United States." *Addiction* 104 (2009): 441–53.

Darke, Shane, Julie Cohen, Joanne Ross, Julie Hando, and Wayne Hall, "Transitions between Routes of Administration of Regular Amphetamine Users." *Addiction* 89 (1994): 1077–83.

Degenhardt, Louisa, Bruno Raimondo, and Libby Topp, "Is Ecstasy a Drug of Dependence?" *Drug and Alcohol Dependence* 107 (2010): 1–10.

Devaney, Madonna, Gary Reid, and Simon Baldwin. *Situational Analysis of Illicit Drug Issues and Responses in the Asia-Pacific Region.* Canberra: Australian National Council on Drugs, 2006.

Dobkin, Carlos and Nancy Nicosia. "The War on Drugs: Methamphetamine, Public Health, and Crime." *American Economic Review* 99 (2009): 324–49.

Dunn, Matthew and Louisa Degenhardt. "The Use of Drug Detection Dogs in Sydney, Australia." *Drug and Alcohol Review* 28 (2009): 658–62.

Elkashef, Ahmed, Frank Vocci, Glen Hanson, Jason White, Wendy Wickes, and Jari Tiihonen. "Pharmacotherapy of Methamphetamine Addiction: an Update." *Substance Abuse* 29 (2008): 31–49.

Ellinwood, Everitt H. "Assault and Homicide Associated with Amphetamine Abuse." *American Journal of Psychiatry* 127 (1971): 90–95.

Faggiano, Fabrizio, Federica D. Vigna-Taglianti, Elisabetta Versino, Alessio Zambon, Alberto Borraccino, and Patrizia Lemma. "School-based Prevention for Illicit Drugs' Use." *Cochrane Database of Systematic Reviews* Issue 2 (2005): Art. No. CD003020. DOI: 10.1002/14651858.CD003020.pub2.

Fergusson, David M., Joseph M. Boden, and John L. Horwood, "The Developmental Antecedents of Illicit Drug Use: Evidence from a 25-Year Longitudinal Study." *Drug and Alcohol Dependence* 96 (2008): 165–77.

Flynn, Patrick M., Patricia L. Kristiansen, James V. Porto, and Robert L. Hubbard. "Costs and Benefits of Treatment for Cocaine Addiction in DATOS." *Drug and Alcohol Dependence* 57 (1999): 167–74.

Gates, Simon, Jim McCambridge, Lesley A. Smith, and David Foxcroft. "Interventions for Prevention of Drug Use by Young People Delivered in Non-school Settings." *Cochrane Database of Systematic Reviews* Issue 1 (2006): Art. No. CD005030. DOI: 10.1002/14651858.CD005030.pub2.

Gerada, Clare and Eilish Gilvarry. "Random Drug Testing in Schools." *British Journal of General Practice* 55 (2005): 499–501.

Gouzoulis-Mayfrank, Euphrosyne and Joerg Daumann. "Neurotoxicity of Methylenedioxyamphetamines (MDMA; Ecstasy) in Humans: How Strong is the Evidence for Persistent Brain Damage?" *Addiction* 101 (2006): 348–61.

Grant, Sara, Philip Burgess, Meredith Harris, Gin Malhi, and Harvey Whiteford. "Stimulant Use and Stimulant Disorders in Australia: Findings from the National Survey of Mental Health and Wellbeing." *Medical Journal of Australia* 195 (2011): 607–10.

Hall, Wayne and Julie Hando. "Route of Administration and Adverse Effects of Amphetamine Use among Young Adults in Sydney, Australia." *Drug and Alcohol Review* 13 (1994): 277–84.

Hando, Julie, Libby Topp, and Wayne Hall, "Amphetamine-related Harms and Treatment Preferences of Regular Amphetamine Users in Sydney, Australia." *Drug and Alcohol Dependence* 46 (1997): 10–13.

Horwood, John L., David M. Fergusson, Mohammad R. Hayatbakhsh, Jake M. Najman, Carolyn Coffey, George C. Patton, Edmund Silins, and Delyse M Hutchinson, "Cannabis Use and Educational Achievement: Findings from Three Australasian Cohort Studies." *Drug and Alcohol Dependence* 110 (2010): 247–53.

Hser, Yih-Ing, Elizabeth Evans, and Yu-Chuang Huang. "Treatment Outcomes among Women and Men Methamphetamine Abusers in California," *Journal of Substance Abuse Treatment* 28 (2005): 77–85.

Hser, Yih-Ing, David Huang, Chih-Ping Chou, Cheryl Teruya, and Douglas M. Anglin. "Longitudinal Patterns of Treatment Utilization and Outcomes among Methamphetamine Abusers: A Growth Curve Modeling Approach." *Journal of Drug Issues* 33 (2003): 921–38.

James-Burdumy, Susanne, Brian Goesling, John Deke, and Eric Einspruch. "The Effectiveness of Mandatory-Random Student Drug Testing: A Cluster Randomized Trial." *Journal of Adolescent Health* 50 (2012): 172–78.

Japanese Ministry of Health and Welfare. *Brief Account of Drug Abuse and Countermeasures in Japan.* Tokyo: Japanese Ministry of Health and Welfare, 1993.

Jayaram-Lindstrom, Nitya, Anders Hammarberg, Olof Beck, and Johan Franck. "Naltrexone for the Treatment of Amphetamine Dependence: A Randomized, Placebo-Controlled Trial." *American Journal of Psychiatry* 165 (2008): 1442–48.

Kay-Lambkin, Frances J., Amanda L. Baker, Rebecca McKetin, and Nicole Lee. "Stepping through Treatment: Reflections on an Adaptive Treatment Strategy among Methamphetamine Users with Depression." *Drug and Alcohol Review* 29 (2010): 475–82.

Kaye, Sharlene, Shane Darke, and Joe Duflou. "Methylenedioxymethamphetamine (MDMA)-related Fatalities in Australia: Demographics, Circumstances, Toxicology and Major Organ Pathology." *Drug and Alcohol Dependence* 104 (2009): 254–61.

Leung, Kit-Sang, Jih-Heng Li, Wen-Ing Tsay, Catina Callahan, Shu-Fen Liu, Jui Hsu, Lee Hoffer, and Linda B. Cottler. "Dinosaur Girls, Candy Girls, and Trinity: Voices of Taiwanese Club Drug Users." *Journal of Ethnicity in Substance Abuse* 7 (2008): 237–57.

Li, Jih-Heng, Shu-Fen, and Wen-Jing Yu. "Patterns and Trends of Drug Abuse in Taiwan: A Brief history and Report from 2000 through 2004." In *Epidemiologic Trends in Drug Abuse, Volume II , Proceedings of the Community Epidemiology Work Group,* edited by Moira P. O'Brien. US Department of Health and Human Services. Washington DC: National Institutes of Health, 2005.

Li, Jih-Heng, Balasingam Vicknasingam, Yuet-Wah Cheung, Wang Zhou, Adhi Wibowo Nurhidayat, Don C. Des Jarlais, and Richard Schottenfeld. "To Use or Not to Use: an Update on Licit and Illicit Ketamine Use." *Substance Abuse and Rehabilitation* 2 (2011): 11–20.

Marsden, John, Robert Ali, Moruf Adelekan, Usaneya Perngparn, Tieqiao Liu, Agueda Sunga, Michael Farrell, and Maristela Monteiro. *WHO Multi-Site Project on Functional/Instrumental Use of Amphetamine-Type Stimulants: Study Protocol and Instrumentation.* Geneva: World Health Organization, 2000.

Matsumoto, Toshihiko, Atsushi Kamijo, Tomohiro Miyakawa, Keiko Endo, Tatsuo Yabana, Hideji Kishimoto, Kenichi Okudaira, Eizo Iseki, Takeshi Sakai, and Kenji Kosaka. "Methamphetamine in Japan: The Consequences of Methamphetamine Abuse as a Function of Route of Administration." *Addiction* 97 (2002): 809–17.

Mattick, Richard P. and Shane Darke. "Drug Replacement Treatments: is Amphetamine Substitution a Horse of a Different Colour?" *Drug and Alcohol Review* 14 (1995): 389–94.

McGregor, Catherine, Manit Srisurapanont, Jaroon Jittiwutikarn, Suchart Laobhripatr, Thirawat Wongtan, and Jason M. White. "The Nature, Time Course and Severity of Methamphetamine Withdrawal." *Addiction* 100 (2005): 1320–29.

McKetin, Rebecca, Erin Kelly, and Jennifer McLaren. "The Relationship between Crystalline Methamphetamine Use and Methamphetamine Dependence." *Drug and Alcohol Dependence* 85 (2006): 198–204.

McKetin, Rebecca, Erin Kelly, and Jennifer McLaren. "The Sydney Methamphetamine Market: Patterns of Supply, Use, Personal Harms and Social Consequences." National Drug Law Enforcement Research Fund Monograph Series No. 13, Australasian Centre for Policing Research, Adelaide, Commonwealth of Australia, 2005.

McKetin, Rebecca, Nicholas Kozel, Jeremy Douglas, Robert Ali, Balasingam Vicknasingam, Johannes Lund, and Jih-Heng Li, "The Rise of Methamphetamine in Southeast and East Asia." *Drug and Alcohol Review* 27 (2008): 220–28.

McKetin, Rebecca, Dan I. Lubman, Amanda L. Baker, Sharon Dawe, and Robert Ali. "Psychotic Symptoms are Dose-related in Chronic Methamphetamine Users: Evidence from a Prospective Longitudinal Study." *JAMA Psychiatry* (2013): 1–6. DOI: 10.1001/jamapsychiatry.2013.283.

McKetin, Rebecca, Jake M. Najman, Amanda Baker, Daniel I. Lubman, Sharon Dawe, Robert Ali, Nicole K. Lee, Richard Mattick, and Abdullah Mamun. "Evaluating the Impact of Community-based Treatment Options on Methamphetamine Use: Findings from the Methamphetamine Treatment Evaluation Study (MATES)." *Addiction* 107, no. 11 (2012): 1998–2008.

McKetin, Rebecca, Joanne Ross, Erin Kelly, Amanda Baker, Nicole Lee, Daniel I. Lubman, and Richard Mattick. "Characteristics and Harms Associated with Injecting Versus Smoking Methamphetamine among Methamphetamine Treatment Entrants." *Drug and Alcohol Review* 27 (2008): 277–85.

McKetin, Rebecca, Rachel Sutherland, David A. Bright, and Melissa M. Norberg. "A Systematic Review of Methamphetamine Precursor Regulations," *Addiction* 106 (2011): 1911–24.

Newton, Nicky C., Gavin Andrews, Maree Teesson, and Laura E. Vogl. "Delivering Prevention for Alcohol and Cannabis using the Internet: a Cluster Randomised Controlled Trial." *Preventive Medicine* 48 (2009): 579–84.

Nicosia, Nancy, Rosalie Pacula Liccardo, Beau Kilmer, Russell Lundberg, and James Chiesa. "The Economic Cost of Methamphetamine Use in the United States, 2005." RAND Drug Policy Research Center, Rand Corporation, Los Angeles, California, 2009.

Oh, E. S., Hong, S. K., Kang, G. I. "Plasma and Urinary Concentrations of Methamphetamine after Oral Administration of Famprofazone to Man." *Xenobiotica* 22 (1992): 377–84.

Rawson, Richard A., Alice Huber, Paul Brethen, Jeanne Obert, Vikas Gulati, Steven Shoptaw, and Walter Ling. "Status of Methamphetamine Users 2–5 years after Outpatient Treatment." *Journal of Addictive Diseases* 21 (2002): 107–19.

Rawson, Richard A., Patricia Marinelli-Casey, Douglas M. Anglin, Alice Dickow, Yvonne Frazier, Cheryl Gallagher, Gantt P. Galloway, James Herrell, Alice Huber, Michael J. McCann, Jeanne Obert, Susan Pennell, Chris Reiber, and Denna Vandersloot, "Joan Zweben and Methamphetamine Treatment Project Corporate Authors. "A Multi-Site Comparison of Psychosocial Approaches for the Treatment of Methamphetamine Dependence." *Addiction* 99 (2004): 708–17.

Rawson, Richard A., M. J. McCann, Frank Flammino, Steven Shoptaw, Karen Miotto, Chris Reiber, and Walter Ling. "A Comparison of Contingency Management and Cognitive-Behavioral Approaches for Stimulant-Dependent Individuals." *Addiction* 101 (2006): 267–74.

Ryoko, Yamaguchi, Lloyd D. Johnston, and Patrick M. O'Malley. "Relationship Between Student Illicit Drug Use and School Drug-Testing Policies." *Journal of School Health* 73 (2003): 159–64.

Shearer, James, John Sherman, Alex Wodak, and Ingrid van Beek. "Substitution Therapy for Amphetamine Users." *Drug and Alcohol Review* 21 (2002): 179–85.

Shoptaw, Steven, Alice Huber, James Peck, Xiawei Yang, Juanmei Liu, Jeff Dang, John Roll, Benjamin Shapiro, Erin Rotheram-Fuller, and Walter Ling. "Randomized, Placebo-controlled Trial of Sertraline and Contingency Management for the Treatment of Methamphetamine Dependence." *Drug and Alcohol Dependence* 85 (2006): 12–18.

Shoptaw, Steven J., Uyen Kao, Keith Heinzerling, and Walter Ling. "Treatment for Amphetamine Withdrawal." *Cochrane Database Systematic Review Issue* 2 (2009): CD003021.

Shoptaw, Steven, Cathy J. Reback, James A. Peck, Xiaowei Yang, Erin Rotheram-Fuller, Sherry Larkins, Rosemary C. Veniegas, Thomas E. Freese, and Christopher Hucks-Ortiz. "Behavioral Treatment Approaches for Methamphetamine Dependence and HIV-related Sexual Risk Behaviors among Urban Gay and Bisexual Men." *Drug and Alcohol Dependence* 78 (2005): 125–34.

Skellington, Kate Orr, Shirley McCoard, and Paul McCartney. "Evaluation of the Mandatory Drug Testing of Arrestees Pilot." Edinburgh: The Scottish Government, Queens Printers of Scotland, 2009. www.scotland.gov.uk/socialresearch.

Spoth, Richard L., Scott Clair, Chungyeol Shin, Cleve Redmond. "Long-term Effects of Universal Preventive Interventions on Methamphetamine Use among Adolescents." *Archives of Pediatrics and Adolescent Medicine* 160 (2006): 876–82.

Srisurapanont Manit, Ngamwong Jarusuraisin, and Phunnapa Kittirattanapaiboon. "Treatment for Amphetamine Dependence and Abuse." *Cochrane Database of Systematic Reviews* 4 (2001): *CD003022*. DOI: 10.1002/14651858.CD003022.

Suwaki, Hiroshi. "Methamphetamine Abuse in Japan," In *Methamphetamine Abuse, Epidemiologic Issues and Implications, NIDA Research Monograph 115,* edited by Marissa A. Miller and Nicholas Kozel. Washington, DC: US Government Printing Office, 1991.

Tait, Robert J., Rebecca McKetin, Frances Kay-Lambkin, Kylie Bennett, Ada Tam, Jenny Geddes, Adam Garrick, Helen Christensen, and Kathy M. Griffiths, "Breaking the Ice: A Protocol for a Randomised Controlled Trial of an Internet-Based Intervention Addressing Amphetamine-type Stimulant Use." *BMC Psychiatry* 12 (2012): 67–75.

Tiihonen, Jari, Evgeny Krupitsky, Elena Verbitskaya, Elena Blokhina, Olga Mamontova, Jaana Fohr, Pekka Tuomola, Kimmo Kuoppasalmi, Vesa Kiviniemi, and Edwin Zwartau. "Naltrexone Implant for the Treatment of Polydrug Dependence: A Randomized Controlled Trial." *American Journal of Psychiatry* 169 (2012): 531–36.

Tiihonen, Jari, Kimmo Kuoppasalmi, Jaana Föhr, Pekka Tuomola, Outi Kuikanmäki, Helena Vorma, Petteri Sokero, Jari Haukka, and Esa Meririnne. "A Comparison of Aripiprazole, Methylphenidate, and Placebo for Amphetamine Dependence." *American Journal of Psychiatry* 164 (2007): 160–62.

United Nations. *Convention on Psychotropic Substances, 1971.* Vienna: United Nations, 1971.

United Nations. *United Nations Convention against Illicit Traffic in Narcotic Drugs and Psychotropic Substances, 1988.* Vienna: United Nations, 1988.

UNODC (United Nations Office on Drugs and Crime). *Assessment Report: Drug Abuse among Disco Clients in Vientiane.* Bangkok: UNODC, 2002.

UNODC (United Nations Office on Drugs and Crime). *Drug Abuse among Service Girls in Vientiane: Assessment Report.* Bangkok: UNODC, 2002.

UNODC (United National Office of Drugs and Crime). *Patterns and Trends of Amphetamine-Type Stimulants (ATS) and other Drugs of Abuse in East Asia and the Pacific 2005.* Bangkok: United Nations Office on Drugs and Crime Regional Centre for East Asia and the Pacific, 2006.

UNODC (United Nations Office on Drugs and Crime). *Patterns and Trends in Amphetamine-Type Stimulants in East Asia and the Pacific 2006.* Bangkok: United Nations Office on Drugs and Crime Regional Centre for East Asia and the Pacific, 2007.

UNODC (United Nations Office on Drugs and Crime). *Patterns and trends of Amphetamine-Type Stimulants and other Drugs in East and Southeast Asia (and Neighbouring Regions).* Bangkok: United Nations Office on Drugs and Crime Regional Centre for East Asia and the Pacific, 2009.

UNODC (United Nations Office on Drugs and Crime). *2010 World Drug Report.* Vienna: UNODC, 2010.

UNODC (United Nations Office on Drugs and Crime). *2012 World Drug Report.* Vienna: UNODC, 2012.

US Department of State. Bureau for International Narcotics and Law Enforcement Affairs. 2007. *International Narcotics Control Strategy (INCS) Report: Volume I. Drug and chemical Control.* Washington, D.C.: Government Printing Office. Accessed October 14, 2012. www.state.gov/documents/organization/81446.pdf.

Vogl, Laura, Nicola Newton, Maree Teesson, Wendy Swift, Aspasia Karageorge, Catherine Deans, Rebecca McKetin, Bronwyn Steadman, Jennifer Jones, Paul Dillon, Alys Havard, and Gavin Andrews. "Climate Schools: Universal Computer-Based Programs to Prevent Alcohol and other Drug Use in Adolescence." Technical Report No. 321, National Drug and Alcohol Centre, University of New South Wales, Sydney, 2012.

Vongchak, Tassanai, Surinda Kawichai, Susan Sherman, David D. Celentano, Thira Sirisanthana, Carl Latkin, Kanokporn Wiboonnatakul, Namtip Srirak, Jaroon Jittiwutikarn, and Apinun Aramrattana. "The Influence of Thailand's 2003 'War on Drugs' Policy on Self-Reported Drug Use among Injection Drug Users in Chiang Mai, Thailand." *International Journal of Drug Policy* 16 (2005): 115–21.

Wallace, Cate, Tony Galloway, Rebecca McKetin, Erin Kelly, and John Leary. "Methamphetamine Use, Dependence and Treatment Access in Rural and Regional North Coast New South Wales, Australia." *Drug and Alcohol Review* 28 (2009): 592–99.

Werb, Dan, Kanna Hayashi, Nadia Fairbairn, Karyn Kaplan, Paisan Suwannawong, Calvin Lai, and Thomas Kerr. "Drug Use Patterns among Thai Illicit Drug Injectors amidst Increased Police Presence." *Substance Abuse Treatment Prevention and Policy* 4 (2009): 16.

Chapter Twelve

One Step Forward, Two Steps Back

Consequences of Thailand's Failure to Adopt Evidence-Based Drug Policy

Karyn Kaplan and Pascal Tanguay

On December 10, International Human Rights Day, in 2002, dozens of people who inject drugs attended a meeting at the Royal Hotel in Bangkok. They listened to a report from a human rights documentation project conducted by their peer, HIV-positive drug user activist Paisan Suwannawong, then chairman of the Thai Network of People Living with HIV/AIDS (TNP+). Paisan and his partner, US-based HIV and Human Rights Program Officer Karyn Kaplan of the International Gay and Lesbian Human Rights Commission (IGLHRC), had traveled across the country to interview thirty-three men and women who inject drugs about their experiences accessing healthcare and interfacing with the criminal justice system in Northern, Southern, and Central Thailand. Many of the people in the room had been interviewed for the project, but had little knowledge about the experiences of other injecting drug users in different parts of the country. (Karyn Kaplan, *pers. comm.)*

After Paisan and Karyn summarized the project's origins, methodology, and results, a lively discussion ensued. There was a palpable energy in the room. "This cannot go on," said one person. "We have to do something. We cannot sit still anymore," said another. They were responding to the litany of human rights violations that had been documented, from arbitrary arrests, drug planting, forced confessions, and beatings by the police and border military, to mandatory HIV testing, the denial of HIV treatment, and other forms of healthcare-setting-based discrimination. Homogeneity of drug user experiences across the three regions, despite the geographic, cultural, linguistic, and other differences, formed a strong bond between them.

At the end of the day, borne of a need to form a collective in order to more effectively take action against these injustices, the Thai Drug Users' Network (TDN) was founded. Despite their illegal status, as drug consumption and possession are criminally sanctioned in Thailand, this initial group of approximately seventy people vowed to put the human rights of people who use drugs on the national agenda and ensure access to essential services and the realization of rights for their community.

Ten years later, in 2012, Thailand continues to criminalize people who use drugs, deny them access to essential services, and violate their rights with impunity. HIV and viral hepatitis rates remain astronomically high due to lack of evidence-based approaches to prevention, treatment, and care. While TDN and allies made great strides in promoting awareness of the negative consequences of legal and social marginalization and criminalization on the health and quality of life of people who use drugs, their families, and communities, including securing a ground-breaking harm reduction grant to people who use drugs from the Global Fund to Fight AIDS, TB and Malaria (GFATM) in Round 3, the Thai government continues to shirk its human rights obligations vis-à-vis people who inject drugs, who are disproportionately imprisoned, HIV- and hepatitis-C infected, and economically and socially marginalized.[1] This article will review the legal and political barriers that perpetuate this injustice and analyze the reasons that Thailand, a former leader in the global response to HIV prevention, is one of the only countries in the region to fail to adopt evidence-based approaches to health and justice for people who use drugs.

THE SITUATION OF DRUGS IN THAILAND

Thailand is part of the region known as the Golden Triangle, which includes Burma, Vietnam, Laos, and Yunnan province in the People's Republic of China. Seventy percent of the world's opium was once grown in this area, and Southeast Asia continues to be a major source of the world's opium and heroin. Though opium was legalized in Thailand in 1851, by 1959 opium smoking and selling was banned, and all opium users had to be registered.[2] Over a twenty-five-year period, Thailand saw a shift from predominantly opium smoking, to smoking of heroin ("chasing the dragon"), to injection of heroin. There have been numerous attributions for these shifts, including: increased drug production and trade in the Golden Triangle and the subsequent availability of injectable-grade heroin,[3] increased drug prices and reduced availability fueled by increases in law enforcement approaches to drug control, promoting the need for quicker and more efficient routes of administration such as injecting, changing and expanding trafficking routes in the face of increased crackdowns, individual preference and economizing, and so on.

Today, though a relatively small percentage of drug users are estimated to be opiate injectors, overshadowed by the millions who report oral ingestion or smoking of methamphetamine pills,[4] there remain at least 40,000 people who inject drugs,[5] and blood-borne viruses including HIV and hepatitis C have still not been adequately addressed. In addition, the dominant government response, favoring criminal justice approaches under the umbrella campaign of a "war on drugs," has led to increases in drug-related harm and no documented reductions in drug use.[6] Widespread human rights violations are associated with the government's approach, which in 2003 under then Prime Minister Thaksin Shinawatra's watch, tens of thousands of people were arbitrarily arrested and forced into drug "treatment" camps run by the military, and over 2,800 alleged drug users and traffickers were extra-judicially executed.[7] Despite an internal government investigation showing more than half of those killed had no connection whatsoever to drugs, none of the perpetrators were ever held accountable. Subsequent anti-drugs campaigns including under the present administration of PM Yingluck Shinawatra, Thaksin's sister, rely on similar approaches that eschew human rights protections, giving broad powers and discretion in the campaign's implementation to the police and military in the name of promoting "national security."

Several conflicting laws dictate penalties and punishments, from prison to compulsory drug detention and "treatment," for drug consumption, possession, selling and trafficking in Thailand. These will be discussed below.

HIV/AIDS

Thailand has experienced one of the worst HIV/AIDS epidemics in Asia, with an estimated 530,000 people living with HIV/AIDS[8] and more than half a million dead, ranking thirteenth highest in global HIV mortality.[9] National HIV prevalence stands at 1.3 percent in 2011, but most at-risk populations (MARPs) experience much higher rates and have done so since the early years of the epidemic, beginning in 1984 when the first HIV case was discovered. Men who have sex with men (MSM), identified in Thailand's first wave of infections, today suffer at least 30 percent HIV prevalence. People who inject drugs (PWID) experienced over two decades of 50 percent HIV prevalence starting in 1987, when prevalence leapt from 2 to 43 percent within a year among incarcerated injectors;[10] commercial sex workers, undocumented citizens, and migrants also experience rates above the national average.[11] However, data on MARPs is necessarily conservative in light of their criminalized status, social stigma, linguistic barriers, and other factors obstructing access to government services where national-level data is collected. [12, 13]

Though Thailand has received well-deserved recognition for radically reducing new infections in the 1990s through aggressive condom promotion campaigns primarily targeting direct female commercial sex workers, who represented 80 percent of the epidemic in those days, the equivalent evidence-based approach to injectors, who suffered decades of 50 percent HIV prevalence since the 1980s, was not applied. Political will concerning HIV among sex workers ushered in progressive awareness campaigns and public health policies that led to a dramatic reduction in annual new sexually transmitted infections, which dropped six-fold within a single decade, from 143,000 in 1990 to 23,676 in 2002. [14]

Thailand acknowledged in its 2010 UNGASS report on HIV/AIDS to the UN General Assembly there were "warning signs that an increasing trend can return." [15] The government also acknowledged its own failures to adequately address the HIV needs of certain populations, like IDU, and committed to improve its universal access goals. Dr. Petchsri Sririnund, director of the National Aids Management Centre at the Ministry of Public Health and a supporter of harm reduction, acknowledged in 2011 the urgent need for the expansion of such programs. Dr. Petchsri stated that health authorities "faced difficulties in implementing the project [a Global Fund-funded harm reduction program run by Population Services International in partnership with Thai NGOs] as the Council of State considered providing syringes to be illegal, in accordance with the 1979 Narcotics Act." [16]

DRUG LAW BARRIERS TO UNIVERSAL ACCESS

Legislation governing drug use in Thailand criminalizes consumption, possession, and sale, among other acts related to the production and trafficking of a number of controlled substances. Key legislation include the Psychotropic Substances Act (1975), setting out a list of controlled psychotropic drugs, the Narcotics Act (1979), which lists controlled narcotic substances, and the Narcotics Control Act (1976), the basis for the criminalization of controlled narcotics. [17] In 2002, the Narcotic Addict Rehabilitation Act (2002) came into force, in the context of prison overcrowding, and diverts some people arrested for drug use from incarceration to compulsory drug treatment facilities. Those eligible include first-time drug consumption offenders, those arrested for consumption and possession, consumption and possession for disposal, and drug consumption and disposal. However, the co-existence of the aforementioned acts are also applicable to drug-related offenses and are enforced.

Civil society advocates for harm reduction have been calling for a review of the laws and policies criminalizing people who use drugs. They find the conflict among the laws unacceptable, as the government claims on the one hand that people who use drugs are "patients, not criminals" but on the other, continuing to arrest and incarcerate tens of thousands of people for drug-related offenses. More than 60 percent of men in prison and a higher percentage of women are held on drug-related offenses.

Authorities in the Ministry of Public Health plan to discuss these issues with legal experts on the National AIDS Committee, over which PM Yingluck Shinawatra presides.

DRUG TREATMENT?

In early September 2012, the Office of the Narcotics Control Board (ONCB) publicly announced the success of the war on drugs with over 500,000 drug users having been sent to compulsory rehabilitation over a twelve-month period.[18] The numbers are significant given that Thailand estimates a total of 1.2 million drug users nationwide. In addition, during the 2003–2004 war on drugs, approximately 150,000 drug users were ushered into these same centers. The government's approach to one-size-fits-all treatment does not distinguish recreational drug use from drug dependence and those testing positive on a urine test are sent to any of the 1,200 so-called treatment centers.[19] To add insult to injury, the Thai government has systematically failed to conduct any assessment of effectiveness or cost-effectiveness of such centers which are generally operated by military personnel without any medical training.[20] "Treatment" thus generally implies military type exercise drills, forced labor, physical and psychological abuse and/or traditional herbal saunas.[21]

CONCLUSION

Thai civil society groups, in particular the member organizations of "12-D," a network of twelve non-government organizations working in harm reduction, are currently involved in promoting and providing evidence-based approaches to reducing harms from drug use, such as clean injecting equipment and linkages to HIV testing and treatment among people who inject drugs. In the absence of government-funded projects, these groups are providing Thailand's only comprehensive HIV prevention programs for injectors, through a Round 8 GFATM grant to principal recipient, PSI-Thailand. Yet these programs are limited in their effect by the lack of legal grounding that jeopardizes their existence, sustainability, and potential for expansion. Without an enabling legal and policy environment, harm reduction programs cannot achieve significant coverage or generate a meaningful impact on the country's epidemic.

Government approaches to reduce drug use in Thailand have failed to achieve their goal, rather creating conditions that perpetuate the problems they purport to solve. A 2011 study showed no reduction in drug use among a cohort of 252 Bangkok injectors, despite increased perceived police presence. Of those who had been through government-mandated drug treatment (32 percent), 96 percent reported injecting in the past week. During the 2003 drug war, Bangkok Metropolitan Authority's methadone programs saw a 50 percent decrease in client attendance due to users being driven underground. The public health crisis of HIV and hepatitis C, and even the epidemic of over-incarceration, have failed to move policymakers away from punitive, law enforcement approaches to drugs and toward adopting, for example, internationally recognized interventions, such as the nine "key interventions" endorsed by WHO, UNODC, and UNAIDS as essential to reducing HIV in people who inject drugs. [22]

Also disappointing for Thai harm reduction advocates, a rights-based draft National Harm Reduction Policy they were fighting for was abandoned under former Prime Minister Abhisit Vejjajiva due to a technicality over language and the legality of needle and syringe programs (NSP), while actual programs providing clean injecting equipment under the GFATM Round 8 project are operating without adequate government support. Many of the GFATM-supported CHAMPION-IDU peer outreach workers are routinely arrested and harassed by police and other law enforcement agencies despite the Country Coordinating Mechanism (CCM) having approved the project, including the needle and syringe distribution. [23] Not a single clean needle was provided to injectors by the Thai government since the beginning of the well-documented epidemic in the late 1980s.

People who use drugs in Thailand continue to experience high rates of HIV, hepatitis C, overdose, and ill health, as well as social exclusion and constant arrest and police harassment. The Thai government stubbornly refuses to respect, protect, and fulfill the rights of people who use drugs, including in prisons, despite their obligations under international law. At the height of the war on drugs under PM Thaksin Shinawatra, when confronted by a reporter about the high rates of killings and concern expressed by the international community over alleged rights violations in the name of drug control, the PM retorted, "the UN is not my father!" This arrogance and ignorance is dangerous, and likely informs the lack of a supportive legal and policy environment for implementing evidence-based approaches to HIV among people who inject drugs. While countries across the region, from China to Malaysia, have made great strides in embracing programs proven to work, Thailand lags criminally behind.

NOTES

1. Thomas Kerr, Karyn Kaplan, Paisan Suwannawong, and Evan Wood, "Getting Global Funds to Those Most in Need: The Thai Drug Users' Network," *Health and Human Rights* 8, no. 2 (2005): 170–86.

2. APMG (AIDS Projects Management Group), *A Review of Recent Research Findings and other Literature on Injecting Drug Use and Related HIV Risk and Infection in Kingdom of Thailand and Lao Democratic People's Republic* (Australia: APMG, 2005). Accessed October 8, 2011 at www.aidsprojects.com/wp-content/uploads/2011/05/APMG-Thai-Lao-Literature-Review.pdf.

3. Gerry Stimson and Kachit Choopanya, "Global Perspectives on Drug Injecting," in Drug Injecting and HIV Infection, ed. Gerry Stimson, Don C. Des Jarlais, and Andrew Ball, pp. 1–21 (London: UCL Press, 1998).

4. UNODC (United Nations Office of Drugs and Crime), *Patterns and Trends of Amphetamine-Type Stimulants and other Drugs: Asia and the Pacific* (Vienna: UNODC, 2011), 133.www.unodc.org/documents/eastasiaandpacific//2011/11/ats-2011/2011_Patterns_and_Trends_of_ATS_and_Other_Drugs.pdf.

5. Ministry of Public Health, Thailand, *Integrated Bio-Behavioral Surveillance* (Bangkok: MPH, 2010).

6. UHRI/TTAG (Urban Health Research Initiative/Thai AIDS Treatment Action Group), *Reducing Drug-related Harm in Thailand: Evidence and Recommendations from the Mitsampan Community Research Project* (Bangkok: UHRI/TTAG, 2012). http://ttag.info/pdf/MSCRP_en.pdf.

7. HRW (Human Rights Watch), *Not Enough Graves: The War on Drugs, HIV/AIDS and Violations of Human Rights (Thailand)* (New York: HRW, 2004).

8. UNICEF (United Nations Children's Fund). "Thailand Statistics." Accessed October 5, 2010.www.unicef.org/infobycountry/Thailand_statistics.html.

9. CIA (Central Intelligence Agency). "The World Factbook: Thailand." Accessed October 5, 2011. www.cia.gov/library/publications/the-world-factbook/geos/th.html .

10. WHO/UNODC/UNAIDS (World Health Organization/United Nations Office of Drugs and Crime/Joint United Nations Programme on HIV/AIDS), *Effectiveness of Interventions to Address HIV in Prisons*. Evidence for Action Technical Papers (Geneva: WHO, 2007). Accessed October 8, 2011.www.who.int/hiv/idu/OMS_E4Acomprehensive_WEB.pdf.

11. National AIDS Management Center, Ministry of Public Health, "National Monitoring and Evaluation Plan for HIV Prevention Targeting Most-at-risk Populations and Migrant Workers 2010–2011." National AIDS Management Center (Bangkok, Thailand, 2010).

12. Christopher S. Walsh, "Expanding HIV prevention programmes at Mplus+: Researching sexual practice to produce animations for HIV prevention and outreach to men that have sex with men and male sex workers in Chiang Mai Thailand." Accessed October 8, 2011.www.aare.edu.au/08pap/wal08123.pdf.

13. HRW, *Not Enough Graves.*

14. Ana Revenga, Mead Over, Emiko Masaki, Wiwat Peerapatanapokin, Julian Gold, Viroj Tangcharoensathien, and Sombat Thanprasertsuk, "The Economics of Effective AIDS Treatment: Evaluating Policy Options for Thailand" (Washington, DC: The World Bank, Health, Population and Nutrition Series, 2006).

15. UNGASS Country Progress Report: Thailand: Reporting Period January 2008–December 2009, National AIDS Prevention and Alleviation Committee.

16. Apiradee Treerutkuarkul, "HIV Rate among Drug Users Sparks Concern." *Bangkok Post*, September 7, 2011. www.bangkokpost.com/lite/news/255329/hiv-rate-among-drug-users-sparks-concern.

17. Canadian HIV/AIDS Legal Network, Thailand: Outline of Legal and Policy Framework (2012). On file with author.

18. ONCB Press Release. "The Directorate Center for Overcoming Drug Problem in Thailand's National Success in Sending 500,000 Drug Users and addicts to Drug Treatment." September 12, 2012.

19. Richard Pearshouse, "Compulsory Drug Treatment in Thailand: Observations on the Narcotic Addict Rehabilitation Act B.E. 2545 (2002)," Canadian HIV/AIDS Legal Network, Toronto, 2009.www.aidslaw.ca/publications/interfaces/downloadFile.php?ref=1429.

20. Pearshouse, *Compulsory Drug Treatment in Thailand.*

21. Nick Thomson, "Detention as Treatment: Detention of Methamphetamine Users in Cambodia, Laos, and Thailand." Open Society Institute (OSI), NY, 2010. Accessed October 4, 2012. www.unhcr.org/refworld/docid/4cbd342f2.html.

22. WHO/UNODC/UNAIDS (World Health Organization/United Nations Office of Drugs and Crime/Joint United Nations Programme on HIV/AIDS), *Technical Guide for Countries to Set Targets for Universal Access to HIV Prevention, Treatment and Care for Injecting Drug Users* (Geneva: WHO, 2009). Accessed October 4, 2012.

23. HRI (Harm Reduction International), *The Global State of Harm Reduction* (London: HRI, 2012).

BIBLIOGRAPHY

APMG (AIDS Projects Management Group), *A Review of Recent Research Findings and other Literature on Injecting Drug Use and Related HIV Risk and Infection in Kingdom of Thailand and Lao Democratic People's Republic.* Australia: APMG, 2005. Accessed October 8, 2011 at www.aidsprojects.com/wp-content/uploads/2011/05/APMG-Thai-Lao-Literature-Review.pdf.

Canadian HIV/AIDS Legal Network, Thailand: Outline of Legal and Policy Framework, 2012. On file with author.

CIA (Central Intelligence Agency). "The World Factbook: Thailand." Accessed October 5, 2011. www.cia.gov/library/publications/the-world-factbook/geos/th.html.

HRI (Harm Reduction International). *The Global State of Harm Reduction.* London: HRI, 2012.

HRW (Human Rights Watch). *Not Enough Graves: The War on Drugs, HIV/AIDS and Violations of Human Rights (Thailand).* New York: HRW, 2004.

Kerr, Thomas, Karyn Kaplan, Paisan Suwannawong, and Evan Wood. "Getting Global Funds to Those Most in Need: The Thai Drug Users' Network." *Health and Human Rights* 8, no. 2 (2005): 170–86.

Ministry of Public Health, Thailand. *Integrated Bio-Behavioral Surveillance.* Bangkok: MPH, 2010.

National AIDS Management Center, Ministry of Public Health. "National Monitoring and Evaluation Plan for HIV Prevention Targeting Most-at-risk Populations and Migrant Workers 2010–2011." National AIDS Management Center, Bangkok, Thailand, 2010.

ONCB Press Release. "The Directorate Center for Overcoming Drug Problem in Thailand's National Success in Sending 500,000 Drug Users and addicts to Drug Treatment." September 12, 2012.

Pearshouse, Richard. "Compulsory Drug Treatment in Thailand: Observations on the Narcotic Addict Rehabilitation Act B.E. 2545 (2002)." Canadian HIV/AIDS Legal Network, Toronto, 2009. www.aidslaw.ca/publications/interfaces/downloadFile.php?ref=1429.

Revenga, Ana, Mead Over, Emiko Masaki, Wiwat Peerapatanapokin, Julian Gold, Viroj Tangcharoensathien, and Sombat Thanprasertsuk. "The Economics of Effective AIDS Treatment: Evaluating Policy Options for Thailand." Washington, DC: The World Bank, Health, Population and Nutrition Series, 2006.

Stimson, Gerry and Kachit Choopanya. "Global Perspectives on Drug Injecting." In Drug Injecting and HIV Infection, edited by Gerry Stimson, Don C. Des Jarlais, and Andrew Ball, pp. 1–21, London: UCL Press, 1998.

Thomson, Nick. "Detention as Treatment: Detention of Methamphetamine Users in Cambodia, Laos, and Thailand." Open Society Institute (OSI), NY, 2010. Accessed October 4, 2012. www.unhcr.org/refworld/docid/4cbd342f2.html.

Treerutkuarkul, Apiradee. "HIV Rate among Drug Users Sparks Concern." *Bangkok Post*, September 7, 2011. www.bangkokpost.com/lite/news/255329/hiv-rate-among-drug-users-sparks-concern.

UHRI/TTAG (Urban Health Research Initiative/Thai AIDS Treatment Action Group). 2012. *Reducing Drug-related Harm in Thailand: Evidence and Recommendations from the Mitsampan Community Research Project*. Bangkok: UHRI/TTAG. http://ttag.info/pdf/MSCRP_en.pdf.

UNGASS Country Progress Report: Thailand: Reporting Period January 2008–December 2009, National AIDS Prevention and Alleviation Committee.

UNICEF (United Nations Children's Fund). "Thailand Statistics." Accessed October 5, 2010. www.unicef.org/infobycountry/Thailand_statistics.html.

UNODC (United Nations Office of Drugs and Crime). *Patterns and Trends of Amphetamine-Type Stimulants and other Drugs: Asia and the Pacific*. Vienna: UNODC, 2011, 133. www.unodc.org/documents/eastasiaandpacific//2011/11/ats-2011/2011_Patterns_and_Trends_of_ATS_and_Other_Drugs.pdf.

Walsh, Christopher S. "Expanding HIV prevention programmes at Mplus+: Researching sexual practice to produce animations for HIV prevention and outreach to men that have sex with men and male sex workers in Chiang Mai Thailand." Accessed October 8, 2011. www.aare.edu.au/08pap/wal08123.pdf.

WHO/UNODC/UNAIDS (World Health Organization/United Nations Office of Drugs and Crime/Joint United Nations Programme on HIV/AIDS). *Effectiveness of Interventions to Address HIV in Prisons*. Evidence for Action Technical Papers, Geneva: WHO, 2007. Accessed October 8, 2011. www.who.int/hiv/idu/OMS_E4Acomprehensive_WEB.pdf.

WHO/UNODC/UNAIDS (World Health Organization/United Nations Office of Drugs and Crime/Joint United Nations Programme on HIV/AIDS). *Technical Guide for Countries to Set Targets for Universal Access to HIV Prevention, Treatment and Care for Injecting Drug Users*. Geneva: WHO, 2009. Accessed October 4, 2012.

Chapter Thirteen

From Gradual Prohibition to Harm Reduction

The Experience of Drug Policy and Law Reform in Taiwan

Jih-Heng Li

With history as the mirror, the rise or fall of a dynasty can be learned.
—Emperor Tang Tai Chung, China

THE PROLOGUE: ORIGIN OF DRUG USE IN TAIWAN

Taiwan, located in the West Pacific Rim, is one of the major connecting hubs between East Asia and Southeast Asia. Because of its geo-strategic position for global commerce and shipping logistics, Taiwan has been occupied by one historical power after another since the Great Navigations. Opium was thus introduced into Taiwan via the Dutch opium trade in the late Ming Dynasty of China, in the seventeenth century.[1] During the reign of the Kang-xi Emperor in the Qing Dynasty, there were already commercial opium dens in Taiwan, providing an opium-smoking service. In 1827, the British began trading opium in exchange for silver and camphor in China, resulting in a situation of revenue deficit and a prevailing problem of opium dependency.[2] Although Chinese high-ranking officials, especially Lin Zexu, endeavored to eliminate opium-smoking problem with tough measures,[3] the Qing Dynasty eventually succumbed to Britain by opening "treaty ports" for more opium trade and legalizing the use of opium, after losing the two Opium Wars.[4] As a free-trade commodity, opium became even more accessible to the general public, and opium smoking gradually evolved into pervasive social and health problems, in the Qing Dynasty in the late nineteenth century. Taiwan, still under the reign of Qing Dynasty at that time, suffered from the same problem. After the Qing Dynasty was defeated by Japan in the first Sino-Japanese War, Taiwan was ceded to Japan in 1895 and became a Japanese colony for fifty years.[5] Without the opium trade, recent history between China and Taiwan might be totally different. Nevertheless, Taiwan has since witnessed three waves of drug epidemics. Each wave involved different types of drugs that caused different types of harm. In response to these different drug problems, differential policies with pragmatic approaches were adopted to tackle individual drug issues.

FIRST WAVE OF DRUG EPIDEMIC: OPIUM SMOKING AND GRADUAL PROHIBITION POLICY IN THE JAPANESE COLONIAL PERIOD

When the Japanese took over Taiwan in 1895, opium smoking had already become an epidemic. Opium smoking was a prohibited behavior according to the drug-related statutes in Japan, and the colonial government rapidly banned opium smoking on the island in September 1895. In November they announced that any soldier or civilian would be sentenced to death if he or she smoked opium.[6] However, the colonial administration soon realized how serious the opium smoking situation was. It was estimated that if total abstinence policy were to be implemented in Taiwan immediately, at least two divisions of army would be needed to repress the social unrest.[7] Goto Shinpei, the head of civilian affairs in the colonial government, therefore proposed the so-called "gradual prohibition" policy instead. After a policy debate, the colonial administration adopted the concept of gradual prohibition in February 1896 and formally implemented the policy on January 21, 1897.[8]

The Gradual Prohibition Policy and Opium Licensing System at the Initial Stage

Under the "gradual prohibition" policy, opium smoking was acknowledged as a "bad social habit" that was contained by providing opium to licensed opium users. An opium user who was diagnosed by a public physician with a dependency problem would be eligible for issuance of a license for an opium quota.[9] The opium license system, which provided pharmaceutical-grade opium to opium users through a government monopoly, was similar to today's methadone maintenance program and could be called the first harm reduction measure in the world. The opium license was further classified into three grades: red (superior), green (second), and yellow (third). Unfortunately, the classification was not based on the doses of opium required for treating different levels of addiction (dependence) but rather on the amounts of tax that the licensees paid for the purity of opium.[10] The gradual prohibition policy eventually ameliorated the situation of opium smoking. According to license issuance records, the number of opium licensees decreased steadily from some 169,000 (or approximately 6.3 percent of the total population) in 1900 to 23,237 (0.5 percent) in 1930.[11] At the same time, the opium monopoly also brought a fortune for the colonial government.[12] For instance, in 1898 the revenue from opium monopoly was 3,467,339 yen, which accounted for 46.3 percent of the total revenue (7,493,650 yen) for the year.[13]

Detoxification Program with Morphine Tapering Off at the Late Stage

In July 1927, the Taiwan People's Party (TPP), Taiwan's first political party led by Dr. Weishui Chiang, publicly denounced the Japanese colonial government as having no intention of stopping selling opium even though the number of opium users was in decline.[14] In 1929, the TPP petitioned the League of Nations to investigate the continuous sale of opium by the Japanese colonial government which created new opium users. In response, the League of Nations dispatched an investigation team to look into the issue. Facing the accusation, the colonial government declared a new policy that swung back to strict abstinence for opium addiction in January 1930.[15] As a result, professor Tsung-Ming Tu, the first Taiwanese MD/PhD in pharmacology and founder of Taiwan's first private medical school, Kaohsiung Medical College (now Kaohsiung Medical University), was appointed in the same year as the medical director of the newly established Taiwan Rehabilitation Center at the Government Center Hospital, to take charge of the treatment program for opium users.[16] In the initial phase of treatment, Dr. Tu applied small amounts of morphine together with a variety of preparations, such as scopolamine extract (a parasympatholytic agent) and sedatives, to alleviate the withdrawal symptoms of the opium users.[17] Later, the amounts of morphine were gradually tapered off. Urine tests were also performed on the patients to ensure their compliance. By such a treatment regimen, the habit of opium smoking was eliminated in a few weeks with an abstinence rate of 46 percent.[18] Thereafter, from 1930 till the end of World War II, the number of opium smokers gradually decreased to several thousand in Taiwan. In addition to Dr. Tu's efforts, the endeavors of other physicians are also worthy of mention. Dr. Ching-yue Lin, who worked at the Red Cross Hospital in Taipei, substituted opium with tapering doses of heroin and obtained a high abstinence rate of 80 percent.[19]

When the gradual prohibition policy was implemented by the Japanese colonial government on Taiwan, it was clearly not intended to be a treatment program for the opium addicts. Nevertheless, the opium licensing system for opium quota turned out very similar to today's methadone maintenance treatment program. The policy steadily reduced the number of opium users from about 169,000 (6.3 percent of the total population) in 1900 to 23,237 (0.5 percent) in 1930,[20] indicating its effectiveness.

SECOND WAVE OF DRUG EPIDEMIC: METHAMPHETAMINE USE AND DRUG LAW REFORM IN THE 1990S

Only 2,000 opium users remained when the Republic of China reclaimed Taiwan after World War II. However, due to the Civil War, Chiang Kai-Shek and his Nationalist Government retreated to Taiwan and imposed martial law on the island from 1949 to 1987. In the 1950s, Taiwan was practically a drug-free society. From the 1960s on, substance use cases were reported occasionally. They include glue-sniffing in the 1960s, pentazocine in the 1970s, and sedatives-hypnotics (mainly secobarbital, amobarbital, and methaqualone) in the early 1980s. Thus, drug use was not a major problem until the methamphetamine epidemic occurred in the early 1990s.[21]

Methamphetamine Use and Law Reform

The raising of martial law in 1987 and the flourishing economy fostered a liberal aura in the late 1980s. However, in the early 1990s, about 5000 illicit methamphetamine users were identified per month, according to the results of urine tests for court referrals.[22] The seizures of illicit methamphetamine were 2381, 1791, 2569, 1368 and 1621 kg, from 1992 through 1996, respectively.[23] On the one hand, the huge amounts of methamphetamine seizure demonstrated the efforts of law enforcement agencies from the supply side. On the other hand, it also implied the methamphetamine use was indeed a serious problem.[24]

Owing to the long-term isolation from the international community because of martial law and deprivation of United Nations membership since 1971, Taiwan was ignorant of the UN Convention on Psychotropic Substances that was enacted in 1971 and the subsequent UN Convention against Illicit Traffic in Narcotic Drugs and Psychotropic Substances in 1988.[25] As a result, the drug-related legislation stagnated at the obsolete "Act for Eradication of Illicit Narcotics" (for illicit narcotic control) and "Narcotics Control Act" (for medical narcotics control), which only abided by the 1961 Single Convention of Narcotic Drugs with a cold war ideology of preventing the "intoxicating" effect of narcotics smuggled into Taiwan from the Communist China. Facing the worsening methamphetamine use situation, Ma Ying-Jeou, then Minister of Justice (and later President of Taiwan, ROC in 2008), led an inter-ministerial task force in 1994 to tackle this drug issue. As a result, a new "Act for Prevention and Control of Illicit Drug Hazard" was enacted in 1998.

The new Act for Prevention and Control of Illicit Drug Hazard, encompassing the spirit of all three UN anti-drug conventions and stressing both supply and demand sides, stated that smuggling, transportation, manufacturing, and "illicit" use of Schedule I (such as opium, heroin, and cocaine) and II drugs (such as amphetamines and cannabis) were all criminal offenses. For illicit use of Schedule I and II drugs, the penalties can be imprisonment for six months to five years and one to three years, respectively. However, it is noteworthy that in this act the status of an illicit drug user changed from a simple law offender to a "diseased offender." This means an illicit drug user who proactively seeks treatment in the government-designated hospitals now does not have to worry about being reported or indicted. But if a person is caught using an illicit schedule I or II drug outside a medical setting and diagnosed as having "an addiction tendency" by two psychiatrists, he or she will still be sentenced to jail for coercive treatment. This new act also rules that if one who uses an illicit drug is diagnosed as being without "an addiction tendency," he or she may be released without being indicted for coerced treatment.[26]

As a complementary law to the Act for Prevention and Control of Illicit Drug Hazard, the Narcotics Control Act was also revised as the Controlled Drugs Act in 1999 to provide and control the controlled drugs for medical and scientific use. The National Bureau of Controlled Drugs (NBCD) under the Department of Health was thereby established in 1999. In addition to providing licit, controlled drugs, the NBCD was also the coordinative platform for inter-ministerial drug-related issues. The author (Jih-Heng Li), who served as the founding director-general of NBCD, was dedicated to constructing some major counterdrug infrastructures, which included establishment of the management system of scheduled drugs for medical and scientific purposes, control of precursors from diversion, construction of an epidemiology network to monitor drug use trend and pattern,[27] collaboration with the Ministry of Education to implement proactive drug educational program,[28] and implementation of the national laboratory certification program for urine drug testing.[29] From the aspects of prevention for drug misuse and abuse, these infrastructures and measures turned out to be very crucial.[30]

Drug Education and Psychosocial Therapy for Methamphetamine Dependency

In less than a decade, the methamphetamine issue was brought under control in Taiwan after the epidemic was first observed in 1990.[31] At this stage, harm reduction measures were limited to drug education programs for general public and the youth, and psychosocial interventions for methamphetamine users who developed psychosis, because there was no well-established substitution therapy for methamphetamine dependence. Control of precursors such as ephedrine and pseudoephedrine was also regarded as a very crucial measure because of the easy access of precursors for clandestine methamphetamine manufacturing.

THIRD WAVE OF DRUG EPIDEMIC: HIV SPREAD AMONG HEROIN INTRAVENOUS DRUG USERS (IDUS) AND HARM REDUCTION POLICY

In the early 2000s, despite a steady decrease in the proportion of methamphetamine users observed in psychiatric admissions and urine drug testing for court referral,[32] another wave of drug epidemics appeared, and the incidence of HIV/AIDS began to escalate due to needle/syringe sharing among IDUs, mainly heroin users. The percentage of IDUs among all addiction treatment admissions increased from 34.7 percent in 2000 to 63.9 percent in 2004, and the percentage of IDUs sharing needles increased from 4.0 percent in 2000 to 15 percent in 2004.[33] In this wave, use of club drugs such as MDMA, ketamine, and flunitrazepam (Rohypnol, also known as FM2 in Taiwan) has also become popular in local rave parties and dance clubs.[34, 35, 36]

Early Detection of HIV/AIDS Spread among IDUs

To promote the concept of harm reduction, Pat O'Hare, executive director of International Harm Reduction Association (IHRA), was invited by J-H. Li, head of the NBCD, to participate in an international conference organized in 2001.[37] The NBCD then became the first institutional member of the International Harm Reduction Association (IHRA) in Taiwan in 2003. Afterward, upon analyzing the data from the epidemiology network for monitoring drug use trends and patterns, and quickly sensing the seriousness of the HIV situation that was associated with needle/syringe sharing among IDUs, J-H. Li, on behalf of the NBCD, presented the first alarming report on the brink of an HIV outbreak due to needle-sharing among IDUs at the weekly meeting of the Department of Health on June 30, 2004.[38] After a thorough discussion, the Health Minister mandated Taiwan Centers for Disease Control (TCDC), the incumbent agency for the control of HIV/AIDS, to take appropriate action on the issue.[39] Subsequently Gerry Stimson, Alex Wodex, and other harm reduction experts were invited to provide advice in order to prevent the spread of HIV/AIDS and drug-related problems.[40]

National Pilot Harm Reduction Program and Control of HIV Situation

In August 2005, after the approval of the Executive Yuan (the Cabinet), the TCDC in collaboration with other incumbent agencies initiated a national pilot harm reduction program (PHRP), with measures including mainly a needle/syringe exchange program, a methadone maintenance treatment program, and HIV education and counseling, on four of twenty-five administrative areas in Taiwan.[41] One year after the PHRP, the TCDC reported a dramatic 10 percent decrease in all new HIV seropositive cases, and a nationwide harm reduction program was subsequently implemented.[42]

In addition to the harm reduction policy, other measures including HIV education programs and HIV testing of drug users could also contribute to the effective control of HIV spread.[43]

Implementation of National Harm Reduction Program

The National Harm Reduction Program, an expansion of the PHRP to all cities/counties, has been in place since 2006. This was indeed quite different from many other countries' harm reduction movements that were usually promoted from NGOs. In Taiwan, the harm reduction policy and programs were initiated by the NBCD, launched by TCDC and all local health departments, and even coordinated at the level of the Executive Yuan (Cabinet). For example, the NBCD helped the manufacturing and distribution of methadone preparations and all local health departments helped distributing free clean needles/syringes. The Ministry of Justice enacted a regulation which suspended prosecution of illicit heroin users so that they could be treated in the methadone maintenance program. With the assistance of harm reduction experts from the international community, such a high-profile harm reduction policies, resulting from the concerted efforts of all levels of government agencies, could well explain why the HIV/AIDS situation has been stabilized ever since.

Recently, club drug use is on the rise in Taiwan. Epidemiological studies suggest that club drugs may play a role in increasing sexual risk behavior, and some studies have shown an association between use of certain club drugs and HIV infection.[44] With a similar harm reduction strategy, it would be necessary to conduct an epidemiological approach to identify the populations at risk of HIV infection and associated risk factors so that practical measures can be taken to prevent HIV spread from unprotected sex due to club drug use.

CONCLUSION

Problems resulting from drug use are a global issue. Drug use, once it becomes a compulsive behavior, will turn the pleasure of use into misery no matter how resilient and strong a person is. Although conventional wisdom treats this millennium-old problem as a moral issue, addiction (or dependence) cannot be solved simply by providing moral advice or lip service. In real life, the drug-use-related issue is not only the problem of an individual but also a public health and social concern, which should be tackled with medical expertise, humanity, and practicability. The three waves of drug epidemics in Taiwan which have been successfully brought into manageable situations each required differential policies and measures. Each individual drug provided a unique problem that needed to be countered with a practical approach. While drug-related issues are deemed to persist in the foreseeable future, the Taiwan case study has clearly shown that the harm reduction policy, which elaborates public-health-oriented and pragmatic efforts, is the key to managing drug problems cost-effectively. With history as a mirror, the success or failure of a drug policy may actually be in our own hands.

In the future, it will be a priority to further revise the drug-related laws in order that drug users with dependence problems can be granted the status of patients, thereby enabling them to receive more humane and accessible treatments.

NOTES

1. John M. Jennings, *The Opium Empire: Japanese Imperialism and Drug Trafficking in Asia, 1895–1945* (Westport: Praeger, 1997).
2. Weisheng Lin, "Smoking Opium." *Encyclopedia of Taiwan*. Accessed September 27, 2012. http://taiwanpedia.culture.tw/en/content?ID=3662.
3. Harrison Evans Salisbury, *China: 100 Years of Revolution* (London: Andre Deutsch, 1983).
4. Patricia B. Ebrey, Anne Walthall, and James B. Palais, *East Asia: A Cultura l, Social and Political History* (Boston: Houghton Mifflin, 2006).
5. Hideo Naito, *Taiwan: A Unique Colonial Record* (Tokyo: Kokusai Nippon Kyokai, 1938).
6. Seinosuke Fujisaki, *History of Taiwan and Admiral Kabayama Sukenori* (Tokyo: Japanese Association for National History Publication, 1926).
7. Min-Sheu Liu, *Taiwan Governance and the Problem of Opium* (Taipei: Avanguard Publishing House, 1983).
8. Liu, *Taiwan Governance*.
9. Liu, *Taiwan Governance*.
10. Liu, *Taiwan Governance*.
11. Liu, *Taiwan Governance*.
12. Y.-H Chen, *History of Taiwan Medical Development* (Taipei: Ye-Dan, 1997).
13. Liu, *Taiwan Governance*.
14. Coral Lee, *A Light in the Political Darkness: Nationalist Pioneer Chiang Wei-Shui* (Taipei: Taiwan Panorama, 2003).
15. Lee, *A Light in the Political Darkness.*

16. Chi-Min Cheng, *Study on Tsungming Tu and Taiwan Medical History* (Taipei: National Research Institute of Chinese Medicine, 2005).

17. Cheng, *Study on Tsungming Tu.*

18. Nai-Shin Chu, "Eradication of Opium Smoking in Taiwan during the Japanese Colonial Period (1895–1945)," *Acta Neurologica Taiwanica* 17, no. 1 (2008): 66–73.

19. Chu, *Eradication of Opium Smoking,* 66–73.

20. Liu, *Taiwan Governance.*

21. Jih-Heng Li, "Drug Abuse Situation and Anti-Drug Programs in Taiwan, R.O.C." Report of the Asian Multicity Epidemiology Workgroup, Universiti Sains Malaysia International Monograph Series (Penang, Malaysia, 1997).

22. Li, *Drug Abuse Situation and Anti-Drug Programs in Taiwan.*

23. Li, *Drug Abuse Situation and Anti-Drug Programs in Taiwan.*

24. Li, *Drug Abuse Situation and Anti-Drug Programs in Taiwan.*

25. Convention against Illicit Traffic in Narcotic Drugs and Psychotropic Substances: United Nations, 1988.

26. Jih-Heng Li, "In Celebration of the 6th Anniversary of the National Bureau of Controlled Drugs." Communications of Controlled Drugs, July 1, 2005.

27. Shu-Fen Liu, Ping-Chu Lee, Ming-Ing Lu, Wen-Ing Tsay, and Jih-Heng Li, "A Survey on Substance Abuse in the Greater Taipei area. *Taiwan Journal of Public Health* 25 (2006): 274–82.

28. C.-C. Lee, J.-C. Chu, D.-N. Chen, J.-S. Lai, and Jih-Heng Li, "Awareness of Illegal Drug Use in Senior and Vocational High School Students that Participated in the Anti-drug Ambassador Campaign," *Taiwan Journal of Public Health* 24 (2005): 224–29.

29. Chiareiy Liu, Wen-Ing Tsay, and Jih-Heng Li, "Taiwan Conducts Urine Tests as Part of War on Drugs." *Clinical & Forensic Toxicology News,* June 7, 2001.

30. Jih-Heng Li, "In Celebration of the 6th Anniversary of the National Bureau of Controlled Drugs," Communications of Controlled Drugs, July 1, 2005.

31. Rebecca McKetin, Nicholas Kozel, Jeremy Douglas, Robert Ali, Balasingam Vicknasingam, Johaness Lund, and Jih-Heng Li, "The Rise of Methamphetamine in Southeast and East Asia," *Drug and Alcohol Review* 27, no. 3 2008: 220–74.

32. Jih-Heng Li, Shu-Fen Liu, and Wen-Jing Yu, "Patterns and Trends of Drug Abuse in Taiwan: A Brief History and Report from 2000 through 2004," in *Epidemiologic Trends in Drug Abuse, Volume II* (Maryland: US Department of Health and Human Services, 2005).

33. Hsin-Ya Lee, Yi-Hsin Yang, Wen-Jing Yu, Lien-Wen Su, Tsang-Yaw Lin, Hsien-Jane Chiu, Hsin-Pei Tang, Chien-Yang Lin, Ryh-Nan Pan, and Jih-Heng Li, "Essentiality of HIV Testing and Education for Effective HIV Control in the National Pilot Harm Reduction Program: the Taiwan Experience," *Kaohsiung Journal of Medical Science* 28, no. 2 (2012): 79–85.

34. Kit-Sang Leung, Jih-Heng Li, Wen-Ing Tsay, Catina Callahan, Shu-Fen Liu, Jui Hsu, Lee Hoffer, and Linda B. Cottler, "Dinosaur Girls, Candy Girls, and Trinity: Voices of Taiwanese Club Drug Users," *Journal of Ethnicity in Substance Abuse* 7, no. 3 (2008): 237–57.

35. Jih-Heng Li, Balasingam Vicknasingam, Yuet-Wah Cheung, Wang Zhou, Adhi Wibowo Nurhidayat, Don C. Des Jarlais, and Richard Schottenfeld, "To Use or Not to Use: an Update on Licit and Illicit Ketamine Use," *Substance Abuse and Rehabilitation* 2 (2011): 11–20.

36. Chiareiy Liu, Jih-Heng, Li, Wen-Ing Tsay, and Jui Hsu, "Drug Use and Profile of Individuals Arrested on Drug-Related Charges in Taiwan," *Journal of Food and Drug Analysis* 13 (2005): 3–8.

37. Pat O'Hare, "The Concept of Harm Reduction," *2001 International Conference on Drug Abuse* (Taipei: National Bureau of Controlled Drugs, Taiwan, 2001).

38. Jih-Heng Li, " Drug Abuse Situation and Preparative Pharmacotherapy for Heroin Addicts," *Weekly Meeting of Department of Health, Taiwan, R.O.C.* Taipei, 2004.

39. Li, *Drug Abuse Situation and Preparative Pharmacotherapy.*

40. Yi-Ming Arthur Chen and Steve Hsu-Sung Kuo, "HIV-1 in Taiwan," *Lancet* 369, no. 9562 (2007): 623–25.

41. Hsin-Ya Lee, Yi-Hsin Yang, Wen-Jing Yu, Lien-Wen Su, Tsang-Yaw Lin, Hsien-Jane Chiu, Hsin-Pei Tang, Chien-Yang Lin, Ryh-Nan Pan, and Jih-Heng Li, "Essentiality of HIV Testing and Education for Effective HIV Control in the National Pilot Harm Reduction Pro-

gram: The Taiwan Experience," *Kaohsiung Journal of Medical Science* 28, no. 2 (2012): 79–85.
   42. Chen and Kuo, *HIV-1 in Taiwan*, 623–25.
   43. Hsin-Ya Lee et al., "Essentiality of HIV Testing," 79–85.
   44. Grant Colfax and Robert Guzman, "Club Drugs and HIV Infection: A Review," *Clinical Infectious Diseases* 42, no. 10 (2006): 1463–69.

BIBLIOGRAPHY

Chen, Y.-H. *History of Taiwan Medical Development*. Taipei: Ye-Dan, 1997.
Chen, Yi-Ming Arthur and Steve Hsu-Sung Kuo. "HIV-1 in Taiwan." *Lancet* 369, no. 9562 (2007): 623–25.
Cheng, Chi-Min. *Study on Tsungming Tu and Taiwan Medical History*. Taipei: National Research, 2005.
Chu, Nai-Shin. "Eradication of Opium Smoking in Taiwan during the Japanese Colonial Period (1895–1945)." *Acta Neurologica Taiwanica* 17, no. 1 (2008): 66–73.
Colfax, Grant and Robert Guzman. "Club Drugs and HIV Infection: A Review." *Clinical Infectious Diseases* 42, no. 10 (2006): 1463–69.
Institute of Chinese Medicine, 2005.
Ebrey, Patricia B., Anne Walthall, and James B. Palais. *East Asia: A Cultural, Social and Political History*. Boston: Houghton Mifflin, 2006.
Fujisaki, Seinosuke. *History of Taiwan and Admiral Kabayama Sukenori*. Tokyo: Japanese Association for National History Publication, 1926.
Jennings, John M. *The Opium Empire: Japanese Imperialism and Drug Trafficking in Asia, 1895–1945*. Westport: Praeger, 1997.
Lee, Coral. *A Light in the Political Darkness: Nationalist Pioneer Chiang Wei-Shui*. Taipei: Taiwan Panorama, 2003.
Lee, C.-C., J.-C. Chu, D.-N. Chen, J.-S. Lai, and Jih-Heng Li. "Awareness of Illegal Drug Use in Senior and Vocational High School Students that Participated in the Anti-drug Ambassador Campaign." *Taiwan Journal of Public Health* 24 (2005): 224–29.
Lee, Hsin-Ya, Yi-Hsin Yang, Wen-Jing Yu, Lien-Wen Su, Tsang-Yaw Lin, Hsien-Jane Chiu, Hsin-Pei Tang, Chien-Yang Lin, Ryh-Nan Pan, and Jih-Heng Li. "Essentiality of HIV Testing and Education for Effective HIV Control in the National Pilot Harm Reduction Program: the Taiwan Experience." *Kaohsiung Journal of Medical Science* 28, no. 2 (2012): 79–85.
Leung, Kit-Sang, Jih-Heng Li, Wen-Ing Tsay, Catina Callahan, Shu-Fen Liu, Jui Hsu, Lee Hoffer, and Linda B. Cottler. "Dinosaur Girls, Candy Girls, and Trinity: Voices of Taiwanese Club Drug Users." *Journal of Ethnicity in Substance Abuse* 7, no. 3 (2008): 237–57.
Li, Jih-Heng. "Drug Abuse Situation and Anti-Drug Programs in Taiwan, R.O.C." Report of the Asian Multicity Epidemiology Workgroup, Universiti Sains Malaysia International Monograph Series, Penang, Malaysia, 1997.
———. Drug Abuse Situation and Preparative Pharmacotherapy for Heroin Addicts. In *the Weekly Meeting of Department of Health, Taiwan, R.O.C.* Taipei, 2004.
———. "In Celebration of the 6th Anniversary of the National Bureau of Controlled Drugs." Communications of Controlled Drugs, July 1, 2005.
Li, Jih-Heng, Balasingam Vicknasingam, Yuet-Wah Cheung, Wang Zhou, Adhi Wibowo Nurhidayat, Don C. Des Jarlais, and Richard Schottenfeld. "To Use or Not to Use: an Update on Licit and Illicit Ketamine Use." *Substance Abuse and Rehabilitation* 2 (2011): 11–20.
Li, Jih-Heng, Shu-Fen Liu, and Wen-Jing Yu. "Patterns and Trends of Drug Abuse in Taiwan: A Brief History and Report from 2000 through 2004." In *Epidemiologic Trends in Drug Abuse, Volume II*, Maryland: US Department of Health and Human Services, 2005.
Lin, Weisheng. "Smoking Opium." Encyclopedia of Taiwan. Accessed September 27, 2012. http://taiwanpedia.culture.tw/en/content?ID=3662.

Liu, Chiareiy, Jih-Heng, Li, Wen-Ing Tsay, and Jui Hsu. "Drug Use and Profile of Individuals Arrested on Drug-Related Charges in Taiwan." *Journal of Food and Drug Analysis* 13 (2005): 3–8.

Liu, Chiareiy, Wen-Ing Tsay, and Jih-Heng Li. "Taiwan Conducts Urine Tests as Part of War on Drugs." *Clinical & Forensic Toxicology News*, June 7, 2001.

Liu, Min-Sheu. *Taiwan Governance and the Problem of Opium*. Taipei: Avanguard Publishing House, 1983.

Liu, Shu-Fen, Ping-Chu Lee, Ming-Ing Lu, Wen-Ing Tsay, and Jih-Heng Li. "A Survey on Substance Abuse in the Greater Taipei Area. *Taiwan Journal of Public Health* 25 (2006): 274–82.

Mcketin, Rebecca, Nicholas Kozel, Jeremy Douglas, Robert Ali, Balasingam Vicknasingam, Johaness Lund, and Jih-Heng Li. "The Rise of Methamphetamine in Southeast and East Asia." *Drug and Alcohol Review* 27, no. 3 (2008): 220–28.

Naito, Hideo. *Taiwan: A Unique Colonial Record*. Tokyo: Kokusai Nippon Kyokai, 1938.

O'Hare, Pat. "The Concept of Harm Reduction." In *2001 International Conference on Drug Abuse*. Taipei: National Bureau of Controlled Drugs, Taiwan, 2001.

Salisbury, Harrison Evans. *China: 100 Years of Revolution*. London: Andre Deutsch, 1983.

United Nations: Convention against Illicit Traffic in Narcotic Drugs and Psychotropic Substances: United Nations, 1988.

Chapter Fourteen

Emerging from a Black Box

Drug Policymaking in Vietnam

Simon Baldwin and Thu Vuong

Historically, in post-colonial times, Vietnam has responded to drug use by administering harsh punishment on drug users and has attempted to limit supply though local crop-eradication programs.[1, 2] The strong emphasis on supply reduction has led to significant reductions in domestic opium cultivation, from 12,199 hectares in 1992 to 32 hectares in 2004.[3] However, despite a substantial decline in opium cultivation, since Vietnam's economy opened in 1984 the use and availability of heroin and amphetamines have increased dramatically.[4] The Ministry of Labour, Invalids and Social Affairs (MOLISA), the government body responsible for managing drug users, estimates that in 2009 there were about 150,000 people nationwide using illicit drugs, including heroin, opium, synthetic drugs, and cannabis.[5] MOLISA's figure probably underestimates the size of the population, especially if non-injecting drug users are included; other estimates suggest that there could be as many as five hundred thousand people who use illicit drugs in Vietnam.[6]

Like most countries in Southeast Asia, from the mid-1990s, Vietnam's drug policy has been strongly influenced by the broad ideological campaign against "social evils." During this time, the government adopted a wide range of regulations to control activities including sex work, drug use, and the influence of foreign culture.[7] In addition to these legislations, the government's endorsement of the UN International Drug Conventions of 1961, 1971, and 1988 (which occurred in 1997) has also shaped Vietnam's drug policy. Vietnam has adopted an overly restrictive interpretation of these conventions, which has in turn resulted in a drug policy focused on harsh punishments for producing, distributing or using drugs and targeted eradication of opium crops.[8, 9, 10]

Largely driven by the rapid spread of HIV among people who inject drugs, Vietnam's response to drug use has undergone a degree of transformation in the past decade.[11] These recent changes, however, have resulted in considerable philosophical, political, and practical divisions between the three key ministries responsible for managing drugs in Vietnam. The Ministry of Health (MoH) emphasizes a public health approach to drug use and focuses on services that reduce health and social harms, while both MoLISA and the Ministry of Public Security (MoPS) pursue a more punitive framework focused on coerced detoxification, compulsory detention in rehabilitation centers and the punishment of drug users.[12]

KEY INSTITUTIONS AND POLICYMAKING PROCESSES

In Vietnam, as in other countries with a long history of single-party governments, it is often unclear how policy has been formulated, who has been involved, what relationships exist between different actors, and the effects that different policies have on each other.[13] Policymaking in Vietnam has traditionally been the preserve of the political elite and not open to scrutiny from those outside the Communist Party.[14]

There are three key institutions in the policymaking process in Vietnam (figure 14.1). These are the Communist Party of Vietnam, the National Assembly, and the government. The Communist Party of Vietnam is the highest political organ and executes the constitution through issuing resolutions and directives. The Party provides policy direction for all aspects of national life.[15]

According to the Constitution, the National Assembly is the highest representative body of the people and the only organization with legislative powers. The National Assembly has authority over lawmaking but is still subject to Communist Party direction.[16] The National Assembly is made up of 493 deputies who are nominated and elected by party members for five-year terms. The National Assembly is increasingly regarded as playing a more active and independent role in Vietnam's political life.[17]

The government is the executive branch of the National Assembly. It carries out overall management of the fulfillment of the political, economic, cultural, social, defense, security, and external duties of the state. The government ensures the effectiveness of the state apparatus from the central government to the grassroots and enforces respect for and implementation of the Constitution and the laws.[18]

In 2000, the government of Vietnam established the National Committee on HIV/AIDS, Drugs and Prostitution Prevention and Control (NCADP), which was tasked with coordination of programs for the prevention and control of HIV, drug use, and prostitution. The NCADP, chaired by one

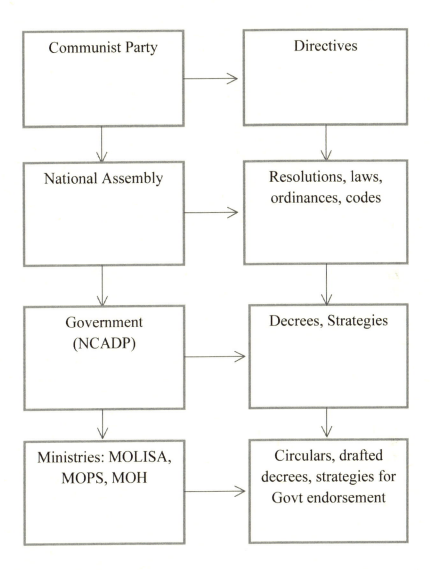

Figure 14.1.   Key Political Figures in Vietnam

deputy prime minister, is in charge of social affairs and consists of eighteen members from government agencies, some sociopolitical (mass organizations like Women's Union) and professional organizations, and centrally run government agencies. Since 2008, the NCADP has been playing an active role in ensuring the introduction and rapid expansion of methadone maintenance treatment in Vietnam.

The MoH, MoLISA, and MoPS are responsible for drafting legal documents relating to their particular interests with regard to drug policy, which are submitted to the government and/or national assembly for endorsement. The ministries are also in charge of developing specific circulars for the operationalization of the government's decrees.

Despite a history of policymaking behind closed doors, the National Assembly is increasingly seeking guidance from technical experts and civil society—for example, the passage of the 2006 HIV Law involved open dialogue with stakeholders, including people living with HIV, international organizations, and NGOs.[19] In addition, in response to concerns raised by the international community related to the detention of sex workers and illicit drug users in 2005 and 2006 centers, the Ministry of Justice and the National Assembly have led a multi-ministry discussion with the international community to get inputs on, and insights into how, the Ordinance on Administrative Violations could be amended.

KEY LEGAL DOCUMENTS

The highest legal document in Vietnam is the Constitution. Directives, orders, laws, and ordinance and codes, descending in order of importance, follow this. The operationalization of these documents is prescribed in decrees, strategies, and circulars.[20]

Four key laws form the backbone of the legal and policy response to drugs in Vietnam. These are the Penal Code (2009), the Law on Drug Control (2008), the Law on Administrative Violations (2012), and the HIV Law (2006). Other documents, such as the Methadone Guidelines (2009) and the Post Detox Management Decree (2010), are also important. Together these documents outline sanctions for drug use, production, and trafficking as well as the responsibilities of government agencies, organizations, and individuals in drug control and HIV prevention.

In an attempt to focus criminal sanctions on drug production and trafficking Vietnam made a series of revisions to the Law on Drug Control and the Penal Code in 2008 and 2009 which downgraded drug possession from a criminal offence to an administrative one.

The revised Law on Drug Control (2008) acknowledges that drug use is a social problem and that drug users should be provided treatment not punishment. In theory the revised law is a marked divergence from the 1999 Penal Code that defined illicit drug use as a criminal activity.[21]

However, the prevailing model, made up of a series of Ordinances and Decrees, maintains an overly punitive approach toward people who use drugs. For example, the National Assembly Ordinance on Administrative Violations which prescribes sanctions for a range of infringements against security, social order and the interests of the Vietnamese state includes Articles 23 and 26 that contain measures allowing for the compulsory treatment of people who use drugs, either in the community (Article 23) or in closed settings for up to two years (Article 26).

In response to criticisms about administrative detention, the National Assembly revised the Ordinance on Administrative Violations in July 2012, upgrading it to the Law on Handling Administrative Offences. The new law makes considerable changes toward the management of sex workers, removing all provisions that support their compulsory rehabilitation. While the same move was considered for drug users it was not passed. The new law, however, moves the authority for sentencing to compulsory rehabilitation from the Chairman of the People's Committee to the district court. This move is considered to be an attempt to provide a judicial oversight of sentencing. However, as discussed in the chapter on compulsory detention (Baldwin and Thomson, in this book), this maneuver does little to address either the ethical or the efficacy problems associated with this practice.

In 2009, the Decree on Post Detoxification was issued under the Drug Law. The decree mandates a series of provisions for "post rehabilitation management" for an additional period of up to two years for "drug users who are at high risk of relapse." Post-detoxification management decision-making power is delegated to the district people's committee.[22]

The other law relevant to drug policy is the HIV Law (2006), which provides a framework that supports interventions such as the provision of sterile injecting equipment, protection of peer outreach workers and the provision of methadone maintenance therapy to people dependent on opiates. While many have argued that the HIV Law supports "harm reduction,"[23, 24, 25] it is the opinion of this author that the HIV Law offers support for interventions that reduce HIV transmission among drug users but does little in the way of addressing the compulsory rehabilitation of drug users or challenging the "tough on drugs" sentiment embedded in the Drug Law.

A recent paper[26] outlines several of the key inconsistencies between the HIV Law and the Drug Law. The authors argue that persistent inconsistencies and the resultant conflation of punishment and treatment cause major impediments to the provision of effective services to drug users in the community.

KEY PLANS AND STRATEGIES

Two key strategies broadly outline Vietnam's approach to drug use and how drug users are treated. These are the National Strategy on Drug Prevention and Control until 2020 with a Vision to 2030 and the National Strategy on HIV/AIDS Prevention and Control that was approved in 2004 and is current until 2010 with a vision until 2020. A new HIV action plan/AIDS strategy is currently in its fifth draft and is nearing completion.

In June 2011, the government of Vietnam issued an updated drug strategy drafted by the Ministry of Public Security. The objectives of the strategy are:

1. To enhance the accountability of individuals, families and the broader society to prevent and eliminate drug use; and
2. To reduce the number of drug users by 30 to 40 percent with 70 percent of communes free of drug use.

The general objective of the new National Strategy on HIV/AIDS Prevention and Control is to control the HIV prevalence and reduce HIV transmission among the general population to reach below 0.3 percent by 2020. The National Strategy also aims at a reduction of 50 percent of new HIV infections by 2015 and by 80 percent by 2020 among people who inject drugs.

WHERE ARE THINGS HEADING IN THE FUTURE?

The battle waged by the Vietnamese government against illicit drug use is beginning to be questioned due to its limited success. Many Vietnamese policymakers are realizing that the massive law enforcement effort combined with preventive education and compulsory detainment will not eliminate the country's drug problems. In questioning the current approach, it is legitimate to ask how the government's future commitments should be balanced and prioritized. Thus far, harm reduction intervention coverage is low.[27, 28] Moreover, many national, provincial, and local authorities continue to oppose harm reduction approaches, preferring to maintain the strong emphasis on law enforcement and compulsory rehabilitation.[29] The ongoing political commitment to compulsory treatment centers in Vietnam has been further strengthened in the new Law on Administrative Violations.

However, some feel that change is in the air.[30] Vietnam is increasingly committed to scaling up access to methadone maintenance therapy and from the initial pilot studies conducted in the mid-2000s, the government has plans to scale up in to reach 80,000 drug users by 2015.[31] This is of course only of use for opiate-dependent people, when the emerging problems are synthetics.

By September 2011, MMT services were provided in nine provinces/cities with thirty clinics with 4,904 patients enrolled. A cohort study conducted by MOH found extremely positive results after nine months of treatment[32] in terms of reduced HIV risk, improved social and health status, and crime reduction.[33]

Having recognized the criticism of the international community toward the Vietnamese compulsory treatment system, many key leaders of Vietnam have been proactive in seeking alternative solutions. In a speech given earlier in 2012, the new deputy prime minister announced a review of the compulsory treatment in the country and stated that no more new centers will be built and half of the existing centers must be converted to "open centers" for voluntary treatment by 2015.

In June 2012, about thirty senior government officials visited Malaysia to study the voluntary "Cure and Care" model in Malaysia and the government's transition away from compulsory rehabilitation toward an open and voluntary system. Following this, MOLISA has been requested to develop a "renovation plan" in line with the deputy prime minister's announcement. Opinion about the impact of the plan or what it will recommend remains divided among the international community. Some are worried that simply opening a few centers and making them voluntary will achieve little under a backdrop that remains involuntary. Others suggest optimistically that change is nigh.

NOTES

1. Hammett, Theodore M., Zunyou Wu, Tran Tien Duc, David Stephens, Sheena Sullivan, Wei Liu, Yi Chen, Doan Ngu, and Don C. Des Jarlais, "'Social evils' and Harm Reduction: the Evolving Policy Environment for Human Immunodeficiency Virus Prevention among Injection Drug Users in China and Vietnam." *Addiction* 103(1) (2008): 137–145.
2. Gary Reid, Madonna L. Devaney, and Simon Baldwin, "Drug Production, Trafficking and Trade in Asia and Pacific Island Countries," *Drug & Alcohol Review* 25, no. 6 (2006): 647–50.
3. UNODC (United Nations Office of Drugs and Crime), Vietnam Country Profile (Hanoi, Vietnam: United Nations Office on Drug and Crime (UNODC) Country Office Vietnam, 2005).
4. Van T. Nguyen and Maria Scannapieco, "Drug Abuse in Vietnam: A Critical Review of the Literature and Implications for Future Research," *Addiction* 103, no. 4 (2008): 535–43.
5. MOLISA (Ministry of Labor Invalids and Social Affairs of Vietnam), *Tong Quan Ve Tac Dong Cua Chinh Sach Dieu Tri Cai Nghien Ma Tuy Doi Voi Cong Tac Trien Khai Thuc Hien o Vietnam. (Overview of the impact of policies on drug rehabilitation treatment on its implementation in Vietnam.)* (Hanoi: MOLISA, 2010).
6. DEA (Drug Enforcement Agency—Drug Enforcement Administration Intelligence Division), *Drug Intelligence Brief: Vietnam Country Brief* (Washington, DC: DEA, 2003).
7. HRW (Human Rights Watch), *The Rehab Archipelago: Forced Labor and Other Abuses in Drug Detention Centers in Southern Vietnam* (New York: HRW, 2011) www.hrw.org/sites/default/files/reports/vietnam0911ToPost.pdf.
8. Devaney, Reid, and Baldwin, *Drug Production, Trafficking*, 647–50.
9. Hammett et al., "Social Evils," 137–45.
10. The Beckley Foundation, "Recalibrating the Regime: the Need for a Human Rights-Based Approach to International Drug Policy." Report 13, The Beckley Foundation Drug Policy Programme, London, 2008. www.beckleyfoundation.org/pdf/report_13.pdf.
11. Thu Vuong, Robert Ali, Simon Baldwin, and Stephen Mills, "Drug Policy in Vietnam: a Decade of Change?" *International Journal of Drug Policy* 23, no. 4 (2012): 319–26.
12. Vuong et al., *Drug Policy in Vietnam*, 319–26.
13. Thi Hai Oanh Khuat, "HIV/AIDS Policy in Vietnam: A Civil Society Perspective" (New York: Open Society Institute, 2007).

14. Ha Pham Nguyen, Anastasia Pharris, Nguyen Thanh Huong, Nguyen Thi Kim Chuc, Ruairi Brugha, and Anna Thorson, "The Evolution of HIV policy in Vietnam: from Punitive Control Measures to a More Rights-Based Approach," *Global Health Action* 3 (2010): 4625–34.

15. Nguyen et al., *The Evolution of HIV Policy*, 4625–34.

16. US Department of State, "US Relations with Vietnam." Accessed September 13, 2012. www.state.gov/r/pa/ei/bgn/4130.htm.

17. Sonia Palmieri, "Representation from the Top: Ethnic Minorities in the National Assembly of Viet Nam," IPU and UNDP Case Study, Inter-Parliamentary Union, Geneva and United Nations Development Programme, NY, 2010. www.ipu.org/splz-e/chiapas10/vietnam.pdf.

18. Embassy of the Socialist Republic of Vietnam, "Government Structure," Accessed June 10, 2010. http://vietnamembassy-usa.org/vietnam/politics/government-structure.

19. Hammett et al., "Social Evils," 137–45.

20. Vuong et al., *Drug Policy in Vietnam*, 319–26.

21. National Assembly of Vietnam, Resolution 06/CP on Strengthening Drug Control and Prevention, 1993.

22. HRW, *The Rehab Archipelago*.

23. Hammett et al., "Social Evils," 137–45.

24. Nguyen et al., *The Evolution of HIV P olicy*, 4625–34

25. Vuong et al., *Drug Policy in Vietnam*, 319–26.

26. Vuong et al., *Drug Policy in Vietnam*, 319–26.

27. Bradley M. Mathers, Louisa Degenhardt, Benjamin Phillips, Lucas Wiessing, Matthew Hickman, Steffanie A. Strathdee, Alex Wodak, Samiran Panda, Mark Tyndall, Abdalla Toufik, and Richard P. Mattick, "Global Epidemiology of Injecting Drug Use and HIV among People Who Inject Drugs: A Systematic Review," *Lancet* 372, no. 9651 (2008): 1733–45.

28. World Bank, "Evaluation of Epidemiological Impact of Harm Reduction Programs on HIV in Vietnam." Accessed October 19, 2012. http://documents.worldbank.org/curated/en/2010/01/16417792/vietnam-evaluation-epidemiological-impact-harm-reduction-programs-hiv-rates-vietnam-evaluation-epidemiological-impact-harm-reduction-programs-hiv-rates.

29. Hammett et al., "Social Evils," 137–45.

30. Vuong et al., *Drug Policy in Vietnam*, 319–26.

31. MOH (Ministry of Health Vietnam), *Summary Report on HIV/AIDS in 2009 and Key Missions* (Hanoi: MOH, 2010).

32. MOH (Ministry of Health Vietnam), *Report on Progress of Methadone Maintenance Treatment Pilot Program 2009* (Hanoi: MOH, 2010).

33. MOH, *Summary Report on HIV/AIDS.*

BIBLIOGRAPHY

DEA (Drug Enforcement Agency—Drug Enforcement Administration Intelligence Division). *Drug Intelligence Brief: Vietnam Country Brief.* Washington, DC: DEA, 2003.

Embassy of the Socialist Republic of Vietnam. "Government Structure." Accessed June 10, 2010. http://vietnamembassy-usa.org/vietnam/politics/government-structure.

Hammett, Theodore M., Zunyou Wu, Tran Tien Duc, David Stephens, Sheena Sullivan, Wei Liu, Yi Chen, Doan Ngu, and Don C. Des Jarlais. "'Social Evils' and Harm Reduction: the Evolving Policy Environment for Human Immunodeficiency Virus Prevention among Injection Drug Users in China and Vietnam." *Addiction* 103, no. 1 (2008): 137–45.

HRW (Human Rights Watch). *The Rehab Archipelago: Forced Labor and Other Abuses in Drug Detention Centers in Southern Vietnam.* New York: HRW, 2011. www.hrw.org/sites/default/files/reports/vietnam0911ToPost.pdf.

Khuat, Thi Hai Oanh. "HIV/AIDS Policy in Vietnam: a Civil Society Perspective." Open Society Institute, New York, 2007.

Mathers, Bradley M., Louisa Degenhardt, Benjamin Phillips, Lucas Wiessing, Matthew Hickman, Steffanie A. Strathdee, Alex Wodak, Samiran Panda, Mark Tyndall, Abdalla Toufik, and Richard P. Mattick. "Global Epidemiology of Injecting Drug Use and HIV among

People Who Inject Drugs: A Systematic Review." *The Lancet* 372, no. 9651 (2008): 1733–45.

MOH (Ministry of Health Vietnam). *Report on Progress of Methadone Maintenance Treatment Pilot Program 2009.* Hanoi: MOH, 2010a.

MOH (Ministry of Health Vietnam). *Summary Report on HIV/AIDS in 2009 and Key Missions.* Hanoi: MOH, 2010b.

MOLISA (Ministry of Labor Invalids and Social Affairs of Vietnam) *Tong Quan Ve Tac Dong Cua Chinh Sach Dieu Tri Cai Nghien Ma Tuy Doi Voi Cong Tac Trien Khai Thuc Hien o Vietnam. (Overview of the impact of policies on drug rehabilitation treatment on its implementation in Vietnam.)* Hanoi: MOLISA, 2010.

National Assembly of Vietnam. Resolution 06/CP on Strengthening Drug Control and Prevention, 1993.

Nguyen, Ha Pham, Anastasia Pharris, Nguyen Thanh Huong, Nguyen Thi Kim Chuc, Ruairi Brugha, and Anna Thorson. "The Evolution of HIV policy in Vietnam: from Punitive Control Measures to a More Rights-Based Approach." *Global Health Action* 3 (2010): 4625–34.

Nguyen, Van T. and Maria Scannapieco. "Drug Abuse in Vietnam: A Critical Review of the Literature and Implications for Future Research." *Addiction* 103, no. 4 (2008): 535–43.

Palmieri, Sonia. "Representation from the Top: Ethnic Minorities in the National Assembly of Viet Nam." IPU and UNDP Case Study, Inter-Parliamentary Union, Geneva and United Nations Development Programme, NY, 2010. www.ipu.org/splz-e/chiapas10/vietnam.pdf.

Reid, Gary, Madonna L. Devaney, and Simon Baldwin. "Drug Production, Trafficking and Trade in Asia and Pacific Island countries." *Drug & Alcohol Review* 25, no. 6 (2006): 647–50.

Reid, Gary, Madonna L. Devaney, and Simon Baldwin. "Drug Production, Trafficking and Trade in Asia and Pacific Island countries." *Drug & Alcohol Review* 25, no. 6 (2006): 647–50.

The Beckley Foundation. "Recalibrating the Regime: the Need for a Human Rights-Based Approach to International Drug Policy." Report 13, The Beckley Foundation Drug Policy Programme, London, 2008. www.beckleyfoundation.org/pdf/report_13.pdf.

UNODC (United Nations Office of Drugs and Crime). Vietnam Country Profile. Hanoi, Vietnam: United Nations Office on Drug and Crime (UNODC) Country Office Vietnam, 2005.

US Department of State. "US Relations with Vietnam." Accessed September 13, 2012. www.state.gov/r/pa/ei/bgn/4130.htm.

Vuong, Thu, Robert Ali, Simon Baldwin, and Stephen Mills. "Drug Policy in Vietnam: a Decade of Change?" *International Journal of Drug Policy* 23, no. 4 (2012): 319–26.

World Bank. "Evaluation of Epidemiological Impact of Harm Reduction Programs on HIV in Vietnam." Accessed October 19, 2012. http://documents.worldbank.org/curated/en/2010/01/16417792/vietnam-evaluation-epidemiological-impact-harm-reduction-programs-hiv-rates-vietnam-evaluation-epidemiological-impact-harm-reduction-programs-hiv-rates.

Chapter Fifteen

Drug Policy in China

Susan Trevaskes

The Peoples' Republic of China (PRC) government recognizes that China has a problem with serious drug crime. There are over 1.5 million registered drug users, over 70 percent of whom are heroin users, although the real number is thought to be millions more. China's production of synthetic drugs increases exponentially each year. Therefore, China, like the West, declared a war on drugs in 2005.

There are global dimensions to China's drug crime. Over the past decade, China has become a major regional transit and production center for illicit synthetic drugs including amphetamine-type stimulants (ATS) and precursors. The UN Office on Drugs and Crime (UNODC) Report on ATS patterns and trends for 2006 estimated that Asia produces one-half of the world supply of ATS; China produces 50 percent and Burma 43 percent of the supply. [1] Five years later, the UNODC Asia and the Pacific report for 2011 noted that of the 136 million methamphetamine pills seized in the region that year, 58.4 million were found in China. [2] Furthermore, the majority of Burma's ATS and heroin is smuggled into international markets in Europe and North America through China. Heroin production in Burma has slowed in recent years, but heroin coming into China from the Golden Crescent region of Afghanistan has increased significantly in the past five years. [3] Most of the heroin coming into the transit route of China via air, sea, and overland is destined for international markets through ports in northern and southern China. In short, China's drug crime is both a national and international issue which impacts of China's social and economic development and human security.

China's policing and judicial response to drug crime has changed under the umbrella of a "People's War on Drugs." Since 2006, the Ministry of Public Security's reliance on Mao-style shock-and-awe policing tactics has declined. Nowadays, the modus operandi favors greater intra-agency and inter-agency cooperation and an "all round" approach to policing drug crime, coupled with a relatively more lenient approach to punishing drug mules. This chapter surveys drug control and punishment in China today.

THE NATIONAL IMPERATIVE TO CONTROL DRUG CONSUMPTION AND TRAFFICKING

China has a tragic and complex history with illicit drugs. Opium trade and use in the nineteenth century was tied inextricably to China's national development and image as a victim of western imperialism. The contemporary history of drug prohibition and control began in the post-Mao period of the late 1980s and 1990s when Golden Triangle heroin trade was at its peak. China's 4,000 kilometer shared border with the Golden Triangle nations of Burma, Thailand, and Laos attracted major traffickers to its porous national borders during these decades. The notorious drug lord Tan Xiaolin, for instance, trafficked over 100 metric tones of heroin into China from Burma over a ten-year period.[4]

In response, China's counter-narcotics authorities relied strongly on the shock-and-awe value of anti-crime campaigns and "expressive" policing activities; widely publicized policing operations and stings concentrated in China's southern drug capital of Yunnan province. These practices persisted until around the mid-2000s. Since then, China's drug policy relating to drug control and punishment has developed in sophistication and complexity. Importantly, both drug control and punishment policies are always linked to generic national political narratives. These key narratives—encapsulated in catchcries such as "class struggle" in the Mao era and in the post-Mao period, "protecting social order," "maintaining social stability," "building a harmonious society," and more recently, "social management"—relate to drug control and punishment as they provide the legitimizing context for police action.

In the social stability obsession of the post-Mao era in the 1980s, 1990s, and early twenty-first century, managing social stability involved a "strike hard" (*yanda*) criminal justice policy against social order crimes in general and drug crime in particular. Drug crime involving both drug trafficking and transporting incurred "severe and swift punishment" (*congzhong congkuai*).[5, 6] During the two decades of anti-crime campaigns from the early 1980s to the mid-2000s, authorities placed particular deterrence value on expressive punishment rituals such as mass sentencing rallies where dozens of drug offenders convicted of drug trafficking and transporting would be publicly sentenced to death at public stadiums with thousands in attendance.[7, 8]

In the early 1990s, the authority to review and approve death sentences for drug crimes in China's major drug provinces was delegated from the Supreme People's Court (SPC) to the provincial courts.[9] This shift supposedly enabled "severe and swift" punishment policy, and provincial courts, encouraged by provincial communist party bosses who were bent on cracking down on drug crime, to approve thousands of executions. Thus, more robust legal scrutiny of drug cases bypassed central authorities in Beijing's SPC.

From the mid-2000s, further changes to national policy on drug punishment reflected Hu Jintao's "harmonious society" doctrine. Thus, a new criminal justice policy of "balancing leniency and severity," linked to the "harmonious society" narrative, overtook "strike hard" as the dominant judicial response to drug and other serious crime. In 2007, the SPC regained its exclusive authority to review and approve all death sentences in China. These two changes—"balancing leniency and severity" and the return of authority to the SPC—have ushered in a new era of "killing fewer" (*shaosha*) drug offenders in China.

Within the framework of protecting the social order, China's counter-narcotics policies and strategies have nevertheless grown progressively more complex in response to the increasingly sophisticated and prolific nature of organized drug crime. In recent years a new narrative of "social management" (*shehui guanli*) emerged within senior ranks of the Communist Party.[10] Many of the draconian ingredients of anti-drug crime campaigns are no longer in operation and the more bureaucratic-rationalist framework of social management has overtaken the anti-crime campaign template as the dominant framework of drug control policy. Hence, while the "People's War on Drugs" still operates, it is no longer referred to as a campaign.

Counter-narcotics policy, which focuses on both supply and demand, is formulated and implemented through the Bureau of Counter Narcotics and its subsidiary, the National Narcotics Control Commission (NNCC). The NNCC involves twenty-five government agencies including the Ministry of Public Security, the General Customs Administration agency and the Ministry of Health. While a multi-agency presence in NNCC has long been part of the drug policy agenda, intra-agency and inter-agency cooperation is nowadays the central modus operandi of China's drug policy.

THE "ALL-ROUND" APPROACH

Large-scale, generic anti-crime campaigns vanished from the policing landscape after 2003, but "specialized campaigns" aimed at one type of crime remained in operation. The Bureau of Counter-Narcotics began a specialized campaign called the "People's War on Drugs" in 2005. This war was launched with all the paraphernalia of a standard anti-crime campaign marked by publicity-focused policing stings and other operations such as mass drug burn-offs and mass sentencing rallies. But within the first year of the campaign, the People's War began marrying the campaign-style approach to a "comprehensive management of public order" (CMPO) approach to crime control, which emphasized interagency cooperation and crime prevention.[11] Over the last six years, the CMPO has been reinterpreted to include more community-based and governmental programs to address the growing drug problem. Combining comprehensive management and community-governmental programs is now referred to in policing circles as "social management innovation" (*shehui guanli chuangxin*).[12]

The year following the start of the War on Drugs marked a significant change in counter-narcotics strategy in twenty-first-century China, thus making 2006 a landmark period for the development of counter-narcotics policing policy. With the traditional "strike hard" campaign shell gradually removed, the Bureau of Narcotics Control institutionalized a comprehensive "all-round" approach. In previous campaigns (including the start of the 2005 campaign) the main strategy was for border police, criminal investigators, customs police and transport and railways police to act relatively independently of each other.[13] The post-2006 strategy encouraged these agencies to work together, focusing inter-agency and intra-agency cooperation on five different fronts which policing authorities called the five anti-crime campaign "battles" or "offensives" (*zhanyi*). These battles are:

1. The offensive on drug control and prevention
2. The offensive on drug treatment and rehabilitation
3. The offensive on strengthening drug control administration
4. The offensive on blocking the source and interdiction of drugs
5. The offensive on fighting serious drug crime and targeting new drug types

This five-pronged approach, together with developments in promoting international cooperation, remains the bedrock of anti-drug policing policy in China today, although the term "campaign offensives" has been replaced by "tasks."

1. Drug Control and Prevention

The first task entails education and propaganda drives targeting four at-risk groups in the community: youth, rural workers, unemployed urban residents, and people in the entertainment and club industry including the prostitution industry. Prevention work incorporates routine policing tasks—for example, inspections of crime-prone places such as clubs and other entertainment venues, hotels, ports, and markets—and regular street patrols of crime areas.

Within the first year of the People's War on Drugs, more than ten thousand entertainment venues were asked to participate in the war by pledging to "fight against drugs with self-discipline, and not to permit any drug-related activities in their venues."[14] The prevention task also includes monitoring non-police activities such as establishing safe environments through CCTV surveillance technology. By the end of 2006, 90 percent of entertainment venues in Beijing had installed CCTV cameras.[15]

The education task involving promotional activities is funded by the NNCC, the Ministry of Education and local public security agencies. In 2011, promotional activities were across all social media; over two hundred anti-drug television and radio programs were produced by the major media outlets in China during the anti-drug promotion month in 2011. Over fifty newspaper articles on drug prevention were published as special editions of major newspapers. There were also around forty thousand news articles relating to anti-drug promotions published on the internet. Weibo, China's version of Twitter, has also entered the propaganda war along with anti-drug promotions featuring numerous movie stars and sports stars.[16]

2. Drug Treatment and Rehabilitation

While drug dependency is not a crime, it is an illegal behavior and is dealt with through administrative punishment.[17] Hence, the second task—drug treatment and rehabilitation—is run out of the Ministry of Public Security and the Ministry of Justice rather than the Ministry of Health, making the control, treatment and rehabilitation process a decidedly "police-centric" affair.[18] Rehabilitation comes in the form of two- to three-year detention and compulsory drug treatment for drug users identified and arrested by police. The number of detainees sent to compulsory rehabilitation centers reached 171,000 in 2011. China has around 250 compulsory treatment centers treating mainly heroin addicts (see Biddulph's chapter in this volume for a detailed account of this aspect of drug policy).

3. Drug Control Administration

The third task primarily focuses on improving the enforcement of laws and regulations that administer the manufacture and distribution of licit drugs and chemicals that can find their way into the illicit ATS narcotics manufacturing industry. This task has become increasingly important due to the explosion of ATS manufacturing bases in China and Burma. In 2011, 529 synthetic drug manufacturing cases were solved in China, 192 of which originated in Guangdong province, a 20 percent increase from the previous year. 2011 also saw 414 cases of illegal manufacturing of precursor chemicals and 339 large-scale cases of illegal selling of precursor chemicals.[19] Two State Council regulations which strengthen the ability of customs, food and drug agencies, and the public security bureau in their fight against the diversion of illegal chemicals have been in force since 2005. The State Council's *Regulations on the Administration of Narcotics Drugs and Psychotropic Substances* and the *Regulations on the Administration of Precursor Chemicals* have tightened control over the manufacture and exporting of licit chemicals. China's Drug Prohibition Law (2008) also fortifies the state's commitment to more stringent administration of chemicals that can be diverted to illegal drug markets.

4. Blocking the Source and Interdiction of Drugs

Over the last decade, the fourth main task has focused on three main border areas: the southwest Golden Triangle region,[20, 21] the northwest Golden Crescent region,[22] and the northeast region at the North Korean border.[23, 24] This fourth task concentrates efforts on establishing more comprehensive and effective border control operations to stop the flow of drugs at key highway, railway, shipping and postal points. In recent years, the volumes of heroin and opium flowing into China from Afghanistan and Pakistan have increased substantially.[25] Nowadays, nearly one-third of heroin seized in China comes from the Golden Crescent region.[26, 27] However, the China-Burma border remains the main entry point for heroin and ATS entering China for transit to international markets and for domestic consumption. While the volume of police seizures of ATS has grown exponentially over recent years, the volume of heroin seizures has increased at a less rapid pace. Police seized 5.7 and 7.0 metric tons of heroin in 2006 and 2011, respectively. The amount of methamphetamines seized in these years was 5.9 and 14.3 metric tons respectively. Despite significant declines in poppy production in Burma due largely to successful crop replacement programs,[28, 29] large quantities of heroin continue to pour across the border. This is evident in continually huge annual heroin seizures most of which are located in Yunnan province on the Burmese border. The same can be said for methamphetamine seizures in Yunnan.[30] In all, 13.5 metric tons of narcotics were seized in Yunnan in 2011, a 46.8 percent increase from the previous year.

No single organized crime group monopolizes the drug trade in China, and trafficking groups are made up of tenuous and loose networks.[31] Most trafficking groups are relatively small and employ mules from one particular geographic area who share similar socioeconomic and ethnic backgrounds. Since manufacturing, trafficking, transporting, and smuggling stages are highly differentiated, most mules and traffickers are not aware of the identities of other group members or of the makeup of the organized crime group.[32, 33, 34] Heroin traffickers are nowadays using non-traditional transport routes and heroin is packaged into smaller lots with a greater number of mules carrying lighter loads to better conceal the narcotics.[35] The greater number of seizures over recent years can be attributed partly to improvements in transnational police operations between Chinese police and their counterparts in Burma, Thailand, Laos, and the Philippines. [36, 37, 38]

5. Combating Serious Drug Crime

The fifth and most police-intensive task, "combating serious drug crime," encourages interagency cooperation in investigating, prosecuting, and punishing serious drug crime. As noted earlier, policing and judicial personnel are highly responsive to the prevailing political narratives that dominate the general national policy agenda. In decades past, the "strike hard" policy encouraged legislative authorities to amend the PRC's first Criminal Law (1979) to increase punishment levels for social order crimes including homicide, robbery and drug crimes to enable the smooth implementation of "severe and swift punishment." [39] In the mid-2000s, the new criminal justice policy of "balancing leniency and severity" overtook "strike hard" as the dominant policing and judicial response to crime. This new policy encourages "severe punishment" to be given to a small minority of the most serious criminals and less harsh punishment to the vast majority of offenders. Article 347 amended Criminal Law (1997) stipulates that offenders convicted of transporting or trafficking over 50 grams of heroin can be sentenced to five years imprisonment, life imprisonment, or the death penalty. Despite the threshold for the death penalty of 50 grams, provincial courts tend to set their own benchmarks. In provinces where these offences are rife, the provincial courts nowadays set the punishment bar extremely high for drug mules who are not directly involved in organized criminal groups. In China's drug capital Yunnan province, for instance, offenders who transport or traffic less than 500 grams of heroin are not executed [40] and even in cases where individual offenders (usually poor rural workers) are found guilty of transporting one kilogram of heroin or more are rarely executed but are instead given a "suspended" death sentence which usually translates into a life imprisonment after two years. [41, 42] This lighter punishment is partly due to the reformist nature of the Yunnan Higher Court and their willingness to commit to the new "balancing leniency and severity" policy, and partly due to the fact that the sheer number of offenders convicted of these crimes makes it difficult or impractical to execute offenders on such as scale. "Leniency" policy as applied in Yunnan is in response to a now well-acknowledged fact that most offenders found guilty of drug transporting or trafficking crimes are poor rural workers who take on the dangerous tasks of transporting heroin across the Burmese border out of economic necessity. In contrast, in provinces where drug offences are rare, courts tend to punish these crimes more severely. In other provinces where drug trafficking is rare, "severe punishment" is more often than not applied to those found guilty of trafficking or transporting amounts approximating the 50 gram threshold in the criminal law.

"Severe punishment" policy is still in force for the most serious drug offenders who are involved in organized crime groups. "Serious drug cases," which have been on the rise for years, are those in which the criminal penalties are between five years imprisonment and the death penalty. Over a twenty-three-year period from 1982 to the end of 2005, police in China solved 166,500 serious drug cases involving 220,000 people.[43] In contrast, in one year alone in 2006, police solved 46,300 serious drug cases involving 56,200 suspects. In 2011 the figure was significantly higher: 101,700 cases involving 112,400 suspects. This rise can be partly attributed to increased criminal activity particularly in ATS manufacturing and trafficking. Another aspect of this increase can be attributed to police success in capturing both small-scale drug offenders and major drug lords due to greater interagency cooperation and involvement. Complex and large-scale criminal investigations require cooperation among specialized, general, and international policing agencies. China's cooperation with Burma, Laos, Thailand, and the Philippines in transnational drug crime operations such as the ongoing "Nail Eradication" is a strong feature of the state's commitment to track down major Chinese drugs operating in Asia. Since 2006, transport police, uniformed street police, and transnational counter-narcotics investigators work in unison with specialist counter-narcotics and border control police.[44, 45, 46]

While the enormous growth in drug crime has been mitigated in recent years, organized crime cultures have matured and taken more sophisticated forms. Hence the speed of China's transition from state planned economy to market economy has outpaced the capacity of the counter-narcotics authorities to truly curb the exponential growth of drug crime, given the opportunities that marketization has presented for serious crime to flourish in China today.

CONCLUSION

In the post-Mao period, that is, the last three decades, drug crime has not simply evolved in parallel with the development of the market but has been inextricably linked with the process of marketization. Introducing the market to work in tandem with the state has enabled and now sustains these criminal activities. Encouraging the socioeconomic conditions of marketization has created both the capacity and the will for drug crime.[47] In response to this situation, drug policy over these decades has been constructed around a political discourse that has favored protecting the nation's social stability and order at any cost. This privileging of stability and order allegedly facilitates the smooth advance of economic modernization.

Criminal law theory in China conceives of "social order" as a state of order or stability characterized by a stable social environment. Stable social order is manifest in society's orderly and stable economic production and the stable social relations between members of a community.[48] Drug crime damages the social order in many ways, not least of which is the health and lives of drug users, their families, and their communities. But Chinese authorities have concentrated their efforts on protecting the socioeconomic fallout rather than health damage inflicted by drugs. Their greatest challenge, however, is the elusive nature of organized crime that operates in and through China today. Increasing numbers of loosely organized criminal networks—local and regional—are involved in smuggling and trafficking and adept at evading law enforcement.

In summary, China's strong Maoist legacy ensured that post-Mao state responses to crime or disorder continued in the form of "strike hard" campaigns. China's War on Drugs campaign beginning in 2005 was originally conceived as a standard anti-crime campaign replete with expressive policing and punishment tactics and strategies. But the People's War subsequently shed its "strike hard" shell and became more bureaucratic, focusing on an all-round approach and inter-agency and intra-agency cooperation, both national and international. This is the hallmark of China's current drug policy.

NOTES

1. UNODC (United Nations Office on Drugs and Crime), *Patterns and Trends of Amphetamine-Type Stimulants and Other Drugs of Abuse in East Asia and the Pacific* (Vienna: UNODC, 2006).

2. UNODC (United Nations Office on Drugs and Crime), *Patterns and Trends of Amphetamine-Type Stimulants and Other Drugs of Abuse in East Asia and the Pacific* (Vienna: UNODC, 2011).

3. Murray Scot Tanner, "China Confronts Afghan Drugs: Law Enforcement Views of the 'Golden Crescent,'" CNA China Studies Report, Virginia, 2011. www.cna.org/research/2011/china-confronts-afghan-drugs-law-enforcement-views .

4. Susan Trevaskes, *Policing Serious Crime in China: from "Strike Hard" to "Kill Fewer"* (London: Routledge, 2010), 126.

5. Trevaskes, *Policing Serious Crime in China*.

6. Susan Trevaskes, *The Death Penalty in Contemporary China* (New York: Palgrave/ Macmillan, 2012).

7. Susan Trevaskes, "Severe and Swift Justice in China," *British Journal of Criminology* 47, no. 1 (2007): 23–41.

8. Trevaskes, *Policing Serious Crime in China*.

9. Trevaskes, *The Death Penalty in Contemporary China*.

10. Frank Peike, "The Communist Party and Social Management in China," *China Information* 26 (2012): 149–65.

11. Trevaskes, *Policing Serious Crime in China*.

12. Peike, *The Communist Party*, 149–65.

13. NNCC (National Narcotics Control Commission), *2006 Nian Zhongguo Jindu Baogao* (*National Narcotics Control Commission Annual Counternarcotics Report 2006*). Beijing: Ministry of Public Security, 2006.www.mps.gov.cn.

14. *Xinhua News,* "Anti-drugs Campaign Launched in 10,000 Recreation Venues in China." October 17, 2006. Accessed 25 February 2013.http://vlex.cn/vid/anti-drugs-campaign-launched-venues-197353559.

15. *Xinhua News,* "Beijing Ups Fight against Drug Abuse at Entertainment Venues," June 23, 2006. Accessed 25 February 2013.http://english.peopledaily.com.cn/200606/24/eng20060624_276749.html.

16. NNCC (National Narcotics Control Commission), *2012 Nian Zhongguo Jindu Baogao* (National Narcotics Control Commission Annual Counternarcotics Report, 2012). Beijing: Ministry of Public Security.www.jhak.com/jdzy/zgjdzy/20120710/7327.html.

17. Sarah Biddulph and Chuanyu Xie, "Regulating Drug Dependency in China: the 2008 PRC Drug Prohibition Law," *British Journal of Criminology* 51 (2011): 987–96.

18. Biddulph and Xie, *Regulating Drug Dependency,* 979, 987–96.

19. NNCC, *2012 Nian Zhongguo Jindu Baogao.*

20. Ko-lin Chin, *The Golden Triangle: Inside Southeast Asia's Drug Trade* (Ithaca: Cornell University Press, 2009).

21. Ko-lin Chin and Sheldon Zhang, "The Chinese Connection: Cross-border Drug Trafficking between Myanmar and China," Report published by the US Department of Justice, Office of Justice Programs, 2007.

22. Tanner, *China Confronts Afghan Drugs.*

23. Minwoo Yun and Euyoung Kim, "Evolution of North Korean Drug Trafficking: State Control to Private Participation," *North Korean Review* 6, no. 2 (2010): 55–64.

24. Beidi Chen, *Zhongguo Xidu Diaocha* (An Investigation into Drug Use in China) (Beijing: Xinhua Chubanshe, 2006).

25. Tanner, *China Confronts Afghan Drugs.*

26. Tanner, *China Confronts Afghan Drugs.*

27. Niklas Swanstrom, "Narcotics and China: An Old Security Threat from New Sources," *China and Eurasia Forum Quarterly* 4, no. 1 (2006): 113–31.

28. Chin, *The Golden Triangle.*

29. Chin and Zhang, *The Chinese Connection.*

30. APAIC (Asia and Pacific Amphetamine-Type Stimulants Information Centre). 2012. "China: Emerging Trends and Concerns." Accessed October 22, 2012.www.apaic.org/index.php?option=com_content&view=article&id=57&Itemid=70.

31. Chin and Zhang, *The Chinese Connection.*

32. Chin and Zhang, *The Chinese Connection.*

33. Chen, *Zhongguo Xidu Diaocha.*

34. Jinyun Liang, "Yunnan Jindu Douzheng Xingshi Pinggu. (Assessment of the Situation Regarding the People's War on Drugs in Yunnan province)." *Yunnan jingguan xueyuanbao* (*Yunnan Police Academy Journal*) 2 (2006): 1–7.

35. Liang, *Yunnan Jindu Douzheng Xingshi Pinggu,* 1–7.

36. US Department of State, *International Narcotics Strategy Report, Volume 1.* Accessed October 22, 2012./www.state.gov/j/inl/rls/nrcrpt/2012/index.htm.

37. NNCC (National Narcotics Control Commission), *2011 Nian Zhongguo Jindu Baogao* (*National Narcotics Control Commission Annual Counternarcotics Report 2011*). Beijing: Ministry of Public Security.www.mps.gov.cn.

38. NNCC, *2012 Nian Zhongguo Jindu Baogao*

39. Trevaskes, *Severe and Swift Justice,* 23–41.

40. Chumming Fan, "Shilun Sixing Anjian De Sifa Kongzhi." (Debates on Judicial Constraints in Death Penalty Cases)," in *Sixing Sifa Kongzhilun Jiqi Cuoshe* (The Death Penalty: Judicial Control and Alternative Punishments), ed. Jieluomei Ke'en and Zhao Bingzhi, pp. 149–55; 154 (Beijing: Falu Chubanshe).

41. Most higher courts these days have their own standardized sentencing guidelines on drug volumes in capital cases. Some, for example, set death penalty considerations at 150 or 300 grams, 400 grams or even over 500 grams. Judges can be guided by these amounts but also take other factors into consideration when sentencing. Note that one judge interviewed by the author put the Yunnan benchmark at 350 grams not 500 grams who noted that some drug mules

are given a suspended death sentence (then commuted to life imprisonment) for transporting drugs well in excess of 1000 grams.
42. Trevaskes, *The Death Penalty.*
43. Liang, *Yunnan Jindu Douzheng Xingshi Pinggu*, 1–7.
44. NNCC (National Narcotics Control Commission), *2007 Nian Zhongguo Jindu Baogao* (*National Narcotics Control Commission Annual Counternarcotics Report 2007*) (Beijing: Ministry of Public Security, 2007).www.mps.gov.cn.
45. NNCC, *2011 Nian Zhongguo Jindu Baogao.*
46. NNCC, *2012 Nian Zhongguo Jindu Baogao.*
47. Trevaskes, *Policing Serious Crime in China.*
48. Trevaskes, *Policing Serious Crime in China.*

BIBLIOGRAPHY

APAIC (Asia and Pacific Amphetamine-Type Stimulants Information Centre*)*. "China: Emerging Trends and Concerns." Accessed October 22, 2012. www.apaic.org/index.php?option=com_content&view=article&id=57&Itemid=70.
Biddulph, Sarah and Chuanyu Xie. "Regulating Drug Dependency in China: the 2008 PRC Drug Prohibition Law." *British Journal of Criminology* 51 (2011): 987–96.
Chen, Beidi. *Zhongguo Xidu Diaocha* (An Investigation into Drug Use in China). Beijing: Xinhua Chubanshe, 2006.
Chin, Ko-lin. *The Golden Triangle: Inside Southeast Asia's Drug Trad*e. Ithaca: Cornell University Press, 2009.
Chin, Ko-lin and Sheldon Zhang. "The Chinese Connection: Cross-border Drug Trafficking between Myanmar and China." Report published by the U.S Department of Justice, Office of Justice Programs, 2007.
Fan, Chunming. "Shilun Sixing Anjian De Sifa Kongzhi." (Debates on Judicial Constraints in Death Penalty Cases)." In *Sixing Sifa Kongzhilun Jiqi Cuoshe* (The Death Penalty: Judicial Control and Alternative Punishments), edited by Jieluomei Ke'en and Zhao Bingzhi, 149–155. Beijing: Falu Chubanshe.
Liang, Jinyun. "Yunnan Jindu Douzheng Xingshi Pinggu. (Assessment of the Situation Regarding the People's War on Drugs in Yunnan province)." *Yunnan jingguan xueyuanbao* (*Yunnan Police Academy Journal*) 2 (2006): 1–7.
NNCC (National Narcotics Control Commission). *2006 Nian Zhongguo Jindu Baogao* (*National Narcotics Control Commission Annual Counternarcotics Report 2006*). Beijing: Ministry of Public Security, 2006. www.mps.gov.cn.
NNCC (National Narcotics Control Commission). *2007 Nian Zhongguo Jindu Baogao* (*National Narcotics Control Commission Annual Counternarcotics Report 2007*). Beijing: Ministry of Public Security, 2007. www.mps.gov.cn.
NNCC (National Narcotics Control Commission). *2011 Nian Zhongguo Jindu Baogao* (*National Narcotics Control Commission Annual Counternarcotics Report 2011*). Beijing: Ministry of Public Security, 2011. www.mps.gov.cn.
NNCC (National Narcotics Control Commission). *2012 Nian Zhongguo Jindu Baogao* (*National Narcotics Control Commission Annual Counternarcotics Report* 2012) Beijing: Ministry of Public Security, 2012. www.jhak.com/jdzy/zgjdzy/20120710/7327.html.
Peike, Frank. "The Communist Party and Social Management in China." *China Information* 26 (2012): 149–65.
Swanstrom, Niklas. "Narcotics and China: An Old Security Threat from New Sources." *China and Eurasia Forum Quarterly* 4, no. 1 (2006): 113–31.
Tanner, Murray Scot. "China Confronts Afghan Drugs: Law Enforcement Views of the 'Golden Crescent'." CNA China Studies Report, Virginia, USA, 2011. www.cna.org/research/2011/china-confronts-afghan-drugs-law-enforcement-views.
Trevaskes, Susan. *Policing Serious Crime in China: from "Strike Hard" to "Kill Fewer."* London: Routledge, 2010; 126.

Trevaskes, Susan. "Severe and Swift Justice in China." *British Journal of Criminology* 47, no. 1 (2007): 23–41.

Trevaskes, Susan. *The Death Penalty in Contemporary China.* New York: Palgrave/Macmillan, 2012.

UNODC. (United Nations Office on Drugs and Crime). *Patterns and Trends of Amphetamine-Type Stimulants and Other Drugs of Abuse in East Asia and the Pacific.* Vienna: UNODC, 2006.

UNODC (United Nations Office on Drugs and Crime). *Patterns and Trends of Amphetamine-Type Stimulants and Other Drugs of Abuse in East Asia and the Pacific.* Vienna: UNODC, 2011.

US Department of State. *International Narcotics Strategy Report, Volume 1.* Accessed October 22, 2012. www.state.gov/j/inl/rls/nrcrpt/2012/index.htm.

Xinhua News. "Anti-Drugs Campaign Launched in 10,000 Recreation venues in China." October 17, 2006. Accessed 25 February 2013. http://vlex.cn/vid/anti-drugs-campaign-launched-venues-197353559.

Xinhua News. "Beijing ups Fight against Drug Abuse at Entertainment Venues" June 23, 2006. Accessed 25 February 2013.

Yun, Minwoo and Euyoung Kim. "Evolution of North Korean Drug Trafficking: State Control to Private Participation," *North Korean Review* 6, no. 2 (2010): 55–64.

Chapter Sixteen

Compulsory Drug Rehabilitation in China

Sarah Biddulph

China is not alone in relying heavily on compulsory measures for combating drug use and dependency. China's compulsory drug rehabilitation regime is also not alone in being subject to criticism on the grounds that it offends against basic human rights norms, is arbitrary and punitive,[1] and that it is ineffective.[2] Despite repeated international calls to close compulsory drug treatment facilities on the grounds that they are both unethical and inefficient[3] (see Baldwin et al. in this book), recent regulatory reforms have done nothing to diminish the scope of compulsory treatment orders.

The most recent significant reform to the regulation of compulsory drug treatment was passage of the PRC Drug Prohibition Law, (the "Law") which came into effect on 1 June 2008. The Drug Prohibition Regulations ("Regulations") were passed in June 2011 to provide more detailed implementing rules for aspects of the Law. The Law codifies China's drugs policy and articulates the administrative structure for combating the cultivation, manufacture, trafficking and use of illicit drugs. The Law asserts the need to adopt a humane approach to addressing problems of drug use and dependency.

The Chinese approach to dealing with drug use and dependency must be understood in the context of China's particular historical experience, where the struggle to eradicate opium addiction was heavily politicized both as a struggle against foreign incursions into Chinese sovereignty and as overcoming a source of national weakness. The success of the Communist Party of China ("CPC") in overcoming, or at least limiting, opium cultivation and addiction has been reified as not just a signifier of superior governance capacity but also as a sign of ethical superiority. Increasing incidence of use and dependency in China from the 1980s was thus not merely understood as a practical problem but also as a broader problem of governance.

To date, elimination or control of drug use and dependency has been regulated primarily as a problem of crime and social order. The central role played by the police in identifying and registering drug users, determining to impose compulsory treatment orders, in some cases carrying out the order, and, finally, supervising drug users after the end of these orders attests to the continuing primacy of social order considerations in the regulation of drug use and dependency. Against that background, the claims that the Law reflects the influence of both "Western" values and the Harmonious Society policy in characterizing drug dependent people as "sick" and "victims," suggests a considerable departure from earlier policy approaches.[4] This chapter evaluates these reforms. This chapter concludes that the Law has still not unequivocally embraced a human rights and health-oriented approach to treatment of drug-dependent people. It finds that many of mechanisms articulated in the Law reveal a "social management" orientation to dealing with drug dependency which continues to concentrate an interlocking set of administrative powers in the hands of the police.

POLICY ON DEALING WITH DRUG DEPENDENCY FROM THE 1980S TO 2007

Since the beginning of the reform period in the late 1970s, problems of drug cultivation, manufacture, trafficking, and use have worsened significantly. Law and policy have had to evolve quickly in response. Drug policy targets both supply and the demand. Important components of the strategy to attack the demand side of China's narcotic drugs problem have been anti-drugs education and propaganda, registration of drug users, compulsory drug rehabilitation, and social help and rescue in the community (*bang jiao* 帮教) for drug users and those released from compulsory treatment centers.[5] In addition to ongoing measures for demand reduction and the treatment of drug dependency, the state has waged periodic campaigns of suppression against drug manufacture and trafficking in an attempt to reduce supply, which is examined in more detail in the chapter by Trevaskes in this book. The most recent campaign was the nationwide People's War on Drugs which commenced in 2005 and remains ongoing. It aimed to control drug supply, curb the influence of drug-related crime, and halt the increase in drug addiction.[6,7] (See also Trevaskes's chapter in this book.)

In China, drug use itself is not a criminal offence. It is, however, still subject to punishment. Drug users and drug-dependent people comprise one of the groups targeted under policies introduced to strengthen management of groups considered to pose a threat to social order, as the problem of drug use is seen as closely connected to crime and one that seriously affects social order and stability.[8] Characterized as unlawful conduct, drug use and dependency are liable to be sanctioned by administrative measures imposed directly by the police.[9]

Drug users may be subject to administrative punishment and placed on the national register of drug users. If determined by the police to be drug-dependent, a person may be subject to a period of compulsory drug rehabilitation. The numbers of people sent to compulsory drug rehabilitation expanded significantly from the mid-1980s. The administrative detention of people determined as being drug dependent evolved from this time as a practical response to perceived crises in social order and management. At first, drug-dependent people were detained in police-run coercive drug rehabilitation centers for a period of between three and six months. Later, people who relapsed after release from detention were sent to another form of administrative detention, re-education through labor (RETL). These camps are operated by the justice department with drug-dependent people comprising only a portion of those incarcerated. The period of detention in this situation was between one and three years.[10] According to one estimate, in 2009 there were around five hundred thousand people detained in compulsory drug rehabilitation facilities at any one time.[11] However, detention has had little success in rehabilitating drug-dependent people, with the rate of relapse acknowledged to be extremely high, at least 85 percent.[12]

Despite efforts first to eliminate, then to control drug use and dependency, the rate of drug use and dependency in China has continued to climb. Not only has the number of drug users increased over time, the types of drugs used have changed, making the problem of rehabilitating drug users more complex. Heroin has been and remains the primary drug of addiction in China, but an increasing number of people are becoming addicted to "new" drugs such as ecstasy and ketamine hydrochloride, up from 2.5 percent percent of the total in 2001 to 9.5 percent in 2004.[13, 14]

The failure of strategies to cure drug dependency so far has forced some rethinking of strategies to reduce demand. In recent years, China has adopted a comprehensive HIV/AIDS strategy to confront the growth of HIV infections in the country. It is acknowledged that injecting drug use is one of the main vectors for HIV infection.[15] With that has been a growing acceptance of the need to strengthen harm reduction programs, to increase the availability of opportunities for voluntary rehabilitation, and to coordinate drug control policies better with harm reduction strategies.

As this brief background indicates, the Law was passed in an increasingly complex ideological and regulatory environment. The Law needed to go beyond a social management or punitive approach to coordinate better with harm reduction strategies and policies. It also needed to address problems with arbitrariness in the exercise of administrative powers to detain drug-dependent people. On the one hand there have been increasingly strident calls for urgent legal reform of police administrative and criminal coercive powers to improve fairness and accountability and to strengthen procedural protections. On the other hand, there is an ongoing demand for the law to embody principles of flexibility to enable the state's coercive apparatus to respond to conduct and groups perceived to undermine social order and stability. The Law enacted a range of interlocking measures which are discussed in the section below.

THE LEGAL REGIME FOR DRUG REHABILITATION

Harm Reduction and Voluntary Rehabilitation

The Law and Regulations seek to encourage people to undergo voluntary drug rehabilitation and promise that such people will not be punished if they undertake voluntary rehabilitation (Regulations article 9). The Law also gives some formal acknowledgment to the harm reduction strategies now being implemented in various parts of the country such as medical assisted treatment ("MAT") of opioid addiction and needle exchange programs, as well as programs to test and provide treatment for HIV/AIDS sufferers.[16] A person may also voluntarily place him- or herself on the register of drug users maintained by the local police. Those entering voluntary drug rehabilitation or harm reduction programs such as methadone or needle exchange programs must also be placed on the register (Law article 36). The Law requires that persons voluntarily placing themselves on the police register not be subject to any punishment (Article 62). However, as discussed below, being on the register renders a person liable to periodic and random drug testing by the police.

The Law permits local government to authorize establishment of not-for-profit treatment centers which are subject to supervision by the health department (Article 36). Despite the requirement that these centers are run on a not-for-profit basis, charges for both MAT and treatment in clinics remain high. Very few drug users have adequate personal funds, and so many rely on family to pay for treatment in clinics. Even among those families willing to support treatment in a private clinic, only the well-off have adequate resources to do so.[17]

Some provisions of the Regulations articulate a view that the privacy of people undergoing drug rehabilitation be protected by providing that government officials who release personal information will be subject to administrative, or, where serious, criminal sanctions (Article 43). The statement of this principle responds to the requirement that the right to health set out in Article 12 of the ICESCR includes a right to have personal information kept confidential. However, these regulations do not require that personal information be kept confidential from all but the treatment professionals responsible for the care of the person. Most important, this information is not kept confidential from the police. While in rehabilitation, patients are subject to zero-tolerance treatment, as the treatment center is obliged to report any drug use during the treatment period to the police. The person may then be subject to a coercive treatment order (Law article 37). Continuing police surveillance after undergoing participation in voluntary treatment and rehabilitation programs, discussed below, coupled with the high cost of treatment acts as a strong disincentive to further expansion of the scope of voluntary rehabilitation, even though the health department continues to seek to expand community based rehabilitation and MAT programs.

Registration of Drug Users

A person determined by the police, justice departments, or health department to be a drug user is to be put on a national register, the National Drug Prohibition Information System (Law Article 32, MPS Measures on Registration of Drug Users 20 July 2009, Article 3). Currently the register is maintained centrally within the Narcotics Control Bureau of the Ministry of Public Security ("MPS") (Article 7).

The register plays a critical role in the identification and management of drug users by the local police (MPS Measures on Registration of Drug Users 20 July 2009, Article 10). Management of registered drug users takes the form of "dynamic control" under which a person may be required by the police to take both periodic and random drug tests. Periodic testing is conducted monthly in the first year, bi-monthly in the second year, and quarterly in the third year.[18] Police may also conduct random drug tests, usually in the form of urine testing, in particular when the person uses their identity card for example to check into a hotel. A person may be subject to compulsory testing if they refuse to comply with a police directive to submit to testing (Law Article 32; MPS Regulations on Drug Testing Procedures Article 7).

One persistent complaint has been that random urine testing is often conducted in a way that undermines protections of both privacy and dignity.[19] A 2009 report compiled by the Open Society Institute suggests that the police have been requiring known drug users to undergo testing at random times and in ways that are intrusive, publicly humiliating, and disruptive of daily life and relationships.[20] There is thus a strong disincentive to being placed on the register, which inhibits those who are not already on the register from accessing voluntary treatment programs.

NON-CUSTODIAL TREATMENT ORDERS

One innovation in the Law is creation of non-custodial treatment orders. These are of two types. The first is an order by the police to undergo a three-year period of rehabilitation in the community ("Community Rehabilitation") for people determined to be drug dependent (Article 33).[21] The second is an order, again by the police, to undergo a period of between one and three years of Giving Up Drugs and Recovering Health ("Recovering Health") after release from a compulsory treatment center. This period may be served in the community (in which case it is carried out in the same way as a Community Rehabilitation order) or in a camp.

Local street committees in urban areas and village committees in rural areas have been made responsible for supervision of this type of order, which is carried out with police oversight. The efficacy of these orders thus depends very much on the capacity of street committees and local governments to allocate specialist resources to support drug-dependent people placed on this type of order. In some municipalities such as Shanghai and Beijing, social workers have been employed to carry out liaison and support work. Other areas of China, however, lack the resources required to fund such support personnel. The *Regulations* set out a number of restrictive requirements for compliance with a rehabilitation order. If a person fails to report to the street committee within the designated fifteen-day period, breaches the terms of the rehabilitation agreement by leaving the area without permission more than three times or on one occasion for more than thirty days, returns a positive drug test, or refuses or avoids a drug test more than three times he or she will be considered to be in serious breach of his or her rehabilitation agreement and may be subject to a compulsory treatment order.

Migrant workers who are living away from their place of household registration and who do not have a temporary residence registration in the place where they are living and working are placed at a disadvantage under this scheme. If ordered to undergo community-based rehabilitation, they will be required to return to the place of their household registration to report (Law Article 33). If they do not, they may be subject to a compulsory treatment order. This effectively excludes migrant workers living away from their permanent place of household registration from such programs as they will be obliged to leave the place where they are living and working if they do not have an urban registration.

CUSTODIAL TREATMENT ORDERS

The Law mandates a new detention power, Coercive Quarantine for Drug Rehabilitation ("CQDR"), for an initial period of two years to replace the pre-existing detention powers of coercive drug rehabilitation and drug deten-tion through RETL discussed above.[22, 23] The Law Article 47 provides that a person undergo evaluation at the end of the first year of detention to deter-mine how well he or she has reformed. If he or she determined to have reformed well, a recommendation may be made to the original decision maker to reduce his or her term of detention to one year. If, at the end of two years, the person is determined not to have rehabilitated well, a recommenda-tion may be made that the period of detention be extended for a further year, with the maximum period of detention being three years. Evaluation criteria are currently being implemented on a piecemeal basis in different detention centers and localities. Some make it relatively easy to obtain early release, others do not (see discussion in Biddulph and Xie, 2011, 9-11).[24]

Since implementation of the Law and Regulations there has been an ongoing process of determining which agency will be responsible for manag-ing the new CQDR centers. Arrangements differ from province to province. In Yunnan, for example, initially the police took over responsibility for man-agement of CQDR centers, but later this responsibility was transferred to the justice department. The Law required a major institutional reorganization of RETL camps. Some, which were already specialist drug detention centers, were rebadged as CQDR centers. In others, where drug-dependent people comprised only a portion of detainees, transfers took place either to remove drug-dependent people to CQDR centers or to remove other detainees so that the RETL camp could be converted into a CQDR center. This process has resulted in reallocation of both personnel and facilities both within the justice department and between the public security and justice departments.

There remains some ambiguity in the law about the physical arrange-ments for detention of drug dependent people as the Regulations (article 27) provide that the first three to six months will be served in police-run CQDR center and the person should then be transferred to a justice-department run CQDR center. In those localities where there are insufficient justice-operated facilities, the period in police-run CQDR may be extended to one year. CQDR thus cannot be seen as an improvement over the previous forms of detention. It actually *lengthens* the minimum amount of time a person must spend in compulsory rehabilitation.

The Law contains a commitment to rehabilitation and treatment of drug-dependent people by requiring appointment of medical staff and provision of medical and other forms of treatment to deal with addiction as well as to treat other diseases or illness of individual detainees (Articles 43, 44, 45). In reality many detention centers do not provide rehabilitation, and international NGOs report that many detention centers provide little, if any, medical treat-ment to detainees.[25, 26] A number of problems appear to be endemic in the system. These include: problems with infrastructure and management sys-tems, understaffing and inadequate training of guards, and chronic underfunding of detention facilities, resulting in poor or non-existent medical treatment and detainees being forced to work with little or no pay. Without adequate funding, long-term detention of between one and three years in these detention centers only punishes drug-dependent people without providing a sustainable basis for rehabilitation. For international organizations and NGOs, problems in the administration of CQDR centers sharpen the dilemma discussed by Baldwin and Thomson in this book—that is, whether to engage in programs with detention facilities to improve conditions and treatment programs or, if there is such engagement, whether that engagement compromises the basic demand that compulsory drug treatment centers be closed.

POST-RELEASE TREATMENT: RECOVERING HEALTH

After release from CQDR, a person may be subject to a further order by the original decision maker (the police at county level or above) to undergo a period of between one and three years of Recovering Health to consolidate their drug-free status. The people's government at county level and above is authorized to establish "giving up drugs, return to health centers" or to permit other groups to establish these centers in the public interest ("Recovering Health Centers") (Article 43) where people released from CQDR may go to live and work after release. To date, the RETL Bureau of the Ministry of Justice has been particularly active in the establishment of Recovering Health Centers.[27] In some cases, former RETL camps have been remodeled to provide vocational education, organize work, and provide other forms of assistance to people after they are released from CQDR.[28] In other areas, for example in Yunnan, Recovering Health Centers were established by the police on a trial basis even before passage of the Law. People living in rehabilitation centers can be required to work, but the regulations require that they be paid with reference to state wage policies (Regulations Article 42). While residence in these centers is officially voluntary, residents on entry agree to remain for a period of time and may not leave without permission during that period. There is a very real threat that a person under a recovering health order may be sent back to CQDR if they breach the terms of the rehabilitation agreement by reusing drugs.

CONCLUSION

Despite the rhetoric that the Law marks a more humane approach to the treatment of drug use and dependency, in critical respects it has failed to incorporate either a health-oriented or rights-based approach. An analysis of the powers set out in the Law reveals the continuing preponderance of social management and social order objectives in dealing with drug use and dependency. The 2011 Annual Report on Drug Control in China reported that in 2010, a majority of people placed on compulsory treatment orders were placed in detention, with 175,000 people sent to CQDR and a total of 96,000 placed in community treatment programs. The Law has also failed to incorporate strong procedural safeguards into police decision-making and so it remains difficult for a person to challenge the imposition of a compulsory treatment order to be served in the community or in a CQDR center.

NOTES

1. HRW (Human Rights Watch), "Where Darkness Knows No Limits: Incarceration, Ill-Treatment and Forced Labour as Drug Rehabilitation in China" (New York: HRW, 2010) www.hrw.org/reports/2010/01/07/where-darkness-knows-no-limits-0.

2. WHO-WPRO (World Health Organization-Western Pacific Regional Office), *Assessment of Compulsory Treatment of People who use Drugs in Cambodia, China, Malaysia and Viet Nam: An Application of Selected Human Rights Principles* (Manila: WHO-WPRO, 2009).

3. ILO/OHCHR/UNDP/UNESCO/UNPF/UNHCR/UNICEF/UNODC/UNWOMEN/WFP/WHP/ UNAIDS (International Labour Organisation, Office of the High Commissioner for Human Rights, United Nations Development Programme, United Nations Educational Scientific and Cultural Organisation, United Nations population Fund, United Nations High Commissioner for Refugees, United Nations Childrens Fund, United Nations Office on Drugs and Crime, United Nations Entity for Gender Equality and Empowerment of Women, World Food Programme, World Health Organisation and Joint United Nations Programme on HIV/AIDS). 2012. "Joint Statement: Compulsory Drug Detention and Rehabilitation Centers." Accessed October 17, 2012. www.ilo.org/aids/Whatsnew/WCMS_175377/lang--en/index.htm.

4. Dan Qi, "Zhi'an Zhixu Guanli Zhuanlun (Special Discussion of the Management of Public Order Administration)" (Zhongguo Renmin Gongan Daxue Chubanshe, Beijing, 2008).

5. Zhansheng Song, Zhimin Wang, Wannian Song, Wenqing Zhang, Yongzhi Song, and Yilin Liu (eds.), *Zhongguo Gong'an Dabaike Quanshu (Encyclopedia of China's Public Security) Vol.1* (Changchun: Jilin Renmin Chubanshe: Jilin People's Press, 2000), 161–62.

6. Xiaoyang Jiao, "People's War on Drugs sees Gains." *China Daily Online,* March 18, 2008. Accessed October 17, 2012. www.chinadaily.com.cn/china/2008npc/2008-03/18/content_6544494.htm.

7. Susan Trevaskes, *Policing Serious Crime in China* (London: Routledge, 2010), 127

8. Laojiao Ju Jiangsu, "The Hazards of Drug Abuse," *Jiangsu Drug Rehabilitation Web*, 20 June 2008. Accessed October 17, 2012. http://jsjiedu.com/jdkt/2008/0620/72.htm.

9. Sarah Biddulph, *Legal Reform and Administrative Detention Powers in China* (Cambridge: Cambridge University Press, 2007), 115–16.

10. Biddulph, *Legal Reform*, 115–16.

11. HRW, *Where Darkness Knows No Limits*, 11.

12. Jinpeng Liu, "Considering China's Drug Rehabilitation System from the Perspective of the High Relapse Rate," *Crime and Reform Research* 7 (2005) www.cqvip.com/qk/85511x/200507/16023004.html.

13. Su, 1998, twenty-six asserts that heroin accounts for over 87 percent of drug addicts in RETL.

14. Xi Shi, 石希. "The Proportion of Current Drug Addicts Nationwide who Abuse New Style Drugs Stands at 9.5 percent (滥用新型毒品的人数已占全国现有吸毒人员的 9.5 percent)." *People's Daily Online*, September 20, 2005, Accessed October 19, 2012.   http://society.people.com.cn/GB/1062/3711180.html.

15. The State Council's White Paper on Narcotics Control asserted that in 1999, 72.4 percent of people infected with HIV acquired their infection from injecting drug use at: www.

china.org.cn/e-white/1/1.V.htm , (accessed 24 August 2011). Others estimate that in the late 2000s injecting drug use accounted for 44 percent of HIV infection in China: Anderson et al., 2009: 6.

16. According to one Xinhua report, 307 methadone clinics in two-thirds of China's provinces had been opened by 2007; Xinhua 18 September 2007.

17. Li and Huang, 2008, estimate that between seven- and fifteen-day treatment costs between RMB 3,000 and 5,000.

18. Qiang Gao, "Guowuyuan Jiedu Tiaoli Sui Dabu Chuangxin Dan Xiaoqu Dongtai Guankong Reng Yaoyao Wu (Despite the Big Innovation in the State Council's Drug Prohibition Regulations, Abolition of Dynamic Control is Still Remote) 国务院戒毒条例虽大步创新 但消除动态管控仍遥遥无)." 21 July 2011. Accessed October 17, 2012. http://chinaaidsgroup. blogspot.com/2011/07/china-aids6671.html.

19. HRW, *Where Darkness Knows No Limits*.

20. OSI (Open Society Institute), 2009, *At What Cost?: HIV and Human Rights Consequences of the "Global War on Drugs."* New York: OSI, 54–55. www.opensocietyfoundations. org/reports/what-cost-hiv-and-human-rights-consequences-global-war-drugs.

21. For a discussion of the rules specifying standards for determining drug addiction see Sarah Biddulph and Chuanyu Xie, "Regulating Drug Dependency in China: the 2008 Drug Rehabilitation Law." *British Journal of Criminology* (2011): 1–19.

22. Taiyun Huang (ed.), *Zhonghua Renmin Gongheguo Jindu Fa Jiedu* (*Explanatory Reader on the PRC Illicit Drugs Prohibition Law*) (Beijing: China Legal System Publishing House, 2008).

23. Hong Yang and Chun Zhang, "Qiangzhi Geli Jiedu Qudai Laodong Jiaoyang Jiedu de Biyao yu Kexing (The Necessity and Feasibility for Forced Detoxificatin Replacing Detoxification via Re-education through Labour)," *Journal of Guangxi Administrative Cadre Institute of Politics and Law* 23 (2008): 82–86.

24. Biddulph and Xie, *Regulating Drug Dependency in China*, 978–96.

25. HRW (Human Rights Watch), *An Unbreakable Cycle: Drug Dependency Treatment, Mandatory Confinement and HIV/AIDS in China's Guangxi Province* (New York: HRW, 2008), 23–24.

26. HRW (Human Rights Watch), "Where Darkness Knows No Limits: Incarceration, Ill-Treatment and Forced Labour as Drug Rehabilitation in China" (New York: HRW, 2010), 31–33. www.hrw.org/reports/2010/01/07/where-darkness-knows-no-limits-0.

27. Re-education through Labour Bureau, Ministry of Justice, "Research Report on Perfecting Drug Treatment and Rehabilitation Work." *Renmin sifa (People's Judicature)* 1 (2009): 51–54.

28. Lan Li and Wu Huang, "Dangqian Woguo Jizhong Jiedu Moshi zhi Bijiao (A Comparison between Current Different Models for Giving up Drugs in China)" *Henan Sifa Jingguan Zhiye Xueyuan Xuebao* 6 (2008): 81–83.

BIBLIOGRAPHY

Biddulph, Sarah. *Legal Reform and Administrative Detention Powers in China*. Cambridge: Cambridge University Press, 2007, 115–16.

Biddulph, Sarah and Chuanyu Xie. "Regulating Drug Dependency in China: the 2008 PRC Drug Prohibition Law." *The British Journal of Criminology* 51, no. 6 (2011): 978–96.

Gao, Qiang. "Guowuyuan Jiedu Tiaoli Sui Dabu Chuangxin Dan Xiaoqu Dongtai Guankong Reng Yaoyao Wu (Despite the Big Innovation in the State Council's Drug Prohibition Regulations, Abolition of Dynamic Control is Still Remote) 国务院戒毒条例虽大步创新 但消除动态管控仍遥遥无)." 21 July 2011. Accessed October 17, 2012. http:// chinaaidsgroup.blogspot.com/2011/07/china-aids6671.html.

HRW (Human Rights Watch). *An Unbreakable Cycle: Drug Dependency Treatment, Mandatory Confinement and HIV/AIDS in China's Guangxi Province*. New York: HRW, 2008, 23–24.

HRW (Human Rights Watch). "Where Darkness Knows No Limits: Incarceration, Ill-Treatment and Forced Labour as Drug Rehabilitation in China." New York: HRW, 2010. www. hrw.org/reports/2010/01/07/where-darkness-knows-no-limits-0.

Huang, Taiyun (ed.). *Zhonghua Renmin Gongheguo Jindu Fa Jiedu (Explanatory Reader on the PRC Illicit Drugs Prohibition Law).* Beijing: China Legal System Publishing House, 2008.

ILO/OHCHR/UNDP/UNESCO/UNPF/UNHCR/UNICEF/UNODC/UNWOMEN/WFP/WHP/ UNAIDS (International Labour Organisation, Office of the High Commissioner for Human Rights, United Nations Development Programme, United Nations Educational Scientific and Cultural Organisation, United Nations population Fund, United Nations High Commissioner for Refugees, United Nations Childrens Fund, United Nations Office on Drugs and Crime, United Nations Entity for Gender Equality and Empowerment of Women, World Food Programme, World Health Organisation and Joint United Nations Programme on HIV/ AIDS). 2012. "Joint Statement: Compulsory Drug Detention and Rehabilitation Centers." Accessed October 17, 2012. www.ilo.org/aids/Whatsnew/WCMS_175377/lang--en/index. htm.

Jiangsu, Laojiao Ju. "The Hazards of Drug Abuse." *Jiangsu Drug Rehabilitation Web*, 20 June 2008. Accessed October 17, 2012. http://jsjiedu.com/jdkt/2008/0620/72.htm.

Jiao, Xiaoyang. "People's War on Drugs sees Gains." *China Daily Online,* March 18, 2008. Accessed October 17, 2012. www.chinadaily.com.cn/china/2008npc/2008-03/18/content_ 6544494.htm.

Li, Lan and Wu Huang. "Dangqian Woguo Jizhong Jiedu Moshi zhi Bijiao (A Comparison between Current Different Models for Giving up Drugs in China)" *Henan Sifa Jingguan Zhiye Xueyuan Xuebao* 6 (2008): 81–83.

Liu, Jinpeng. "Considering China's Drug Rehabilitation System from the Perspective of the High Relapse Rate." *Crime and Reform Research* 7 (2005) www.cqvip.com/qk/85511x/ 200507/16023004.html.

OSI (Open Society Institute). *At What Cost?: HIV and Human Rights Consequences of the "Global War on Drugs."* New York: OSI, 2009, 54–55. www.opensocietyfoundations.org/ reports/what-cost-hiv-and-human-rights-consequences-global-war-drugs.

Qi, Dan. "Zhi'an Zhixu Guanli Zhuanlun (Special Discussion of the Management of Public Order Administration)." Zhongguo Renmin Gongan Daxue Chubanshe, Beijing, 2008.

Re-education through Labour Bureau, Ministry of Justice. "Research Report on Perfecting Drug Treatment and Rehabilitation Work." *Renmin sifa (People's Judicature)* 1 (2009): 51–54.

Shi, Xi. 石希. "The Proportion of Current Drug Addicts Nationwide who Abuse New Style Drugs Stands at 9.5 percent (滥用新型毒品的人数已占全国现有吸毒人员的 9.5 percent)." *People's Daily Online*, September 20, 2005, Accessed October 19, 2012. http:// society.people.com.cn/GB/1062/3711180.html.

Song, Zhansheng, Zhimin Wang, Wannian Song, Wenqing Zhang, Yongzhi Song, and Yilin Liu (eds.). *Zhongguo Gong'an Dabaike Quanshu (Encyclopedia of China's Public Security) Vol.1* Changchun: Jilin Renmin Chubanshe (Jilin People's Press), 2000, 161–62.

Trevaskes, Susan. *Policing Serious Crime in China.* London: Routledge, 2010, 127

WHO-WPRO (World Health Organization-Western Pacific Regional Office). *Assessment of Compulsory Treatment of People who use Drugs in Cambodia, China, Malaysia and Viet Nam: An Application of Selected Human Rights Principles.* Manila: WHO-WPRO, 2009.

Yang, Hong and Chun Zhang. "Qiangzhi Geli Jiedu Qudai Laodong Jiaoyang Jiedu de Biyao yu Kexing (The Necessity and Feasibility for Forced Detoxificatin Replacing Detoxification via Re-education through Labour)." *Journal of Guangxi Administrative Cadre Institute of Politics and Law* 23 (2008): 82–86.

Chapter Seventeen

Alternatives to Criminal Justice

Drug Courts, Drug Diversion, and Decriminalization

Fifa Rahman

Criminal punishment of drug users has resulted in an undeniable social and public health cost. In recent times, however, there has been increased governmental and lawmaker understanding that a unilateral law-and-order approach to drug use simply does not make economic, social, and medical sense, and instead has resulted in increased crime, the spread of HIV, hepatitis C, and other blood-borne diseases, systemic human rights abuses, preventable overdose deaths, and numerous other social and economic costs to entire nations.

Keefer and Loayza state:

> In some places, social and cultural norms are so strong and social opprobrium regarding drug use so great that the tangible social and private costs of drug production may be irrelevant in the evaluation of drug policies. Instead, policy debate is driven by the disutility that nonusers feel from having certain drug users in their midst. [1]

In nations such as Switzerland and Portugal, among others, it seems that policy driven by "disutility" and stigma as illustrated above have been pushed aside in favor of approaches that deal with health and social symptoms associated with drug dependence. What has been demonstrated is that alternative approaches can result in reductions of crime, zero overdose deaths, a reduction of homelessness, and a reduction of adverse health outcomes, which include the spread of HIV.

This chapter describes alternatives to criminal punishment for drug use and drug dependence, including "problem-solving" drug courts which retain a judicial element, drug diversion practiced by police, "four pillar" systems, and decriminalization laws in tandem with evidence-based treatments, and discusses whether elements of these policies are transferable to Asia.

DRUG COURTS

Drug courts have been described as being a form of collaboration between criminal justice and public health and are a drug-diversion strategy. Drug diversion is intended to steer the offender away from incarceration and toward treatment and reintegration, and is based on the principle of "therapeutic jurisprudence," that is, the role of law as a therapeutic agent.[2] They are often referred to as "collaborative courts."[3]

American judge Leonard Edwards describes collaborative courts in his 2010 article:

> Collaborative courts are distinguished by a problem-solving focus, a team approach to decision making, integration of social and treatment services, judicial supervision and monitoring of the treatment process, community outreach, direct interaction between the client and the judge, accountability for adherence to the treatment plan, and a proactive role for the judge inside and outside the courtroom.[4]

Basically, individuals have the "option" to either attend drug court programs or be incarcerated. It is this characteristic which leads to the categorization of drug courts as "quasi-compulsory."[5] Individuals who elect to attend drug courts are diverted away from the criminal justice system and instead undergo an assessment process where a multidisciplinary team consisting of psychiatrists, social workers, and lawyers design a treatment and reintegration plan. This plan is monitored via regular drug court appearances, during which a judge supervises progress based on a "reward and sanction" system. Key features show, however, that treatment is not always evidence-based. Drug courts often require random urine testing, a minimum period of abstinence, curfews, and requirements to stay away from certain areas.[6]

Drug courts are different from regular criminal courts in several ways, in that they are multidisciplinary as opposed to consisting of solely legally trained individuals, less adversarial, and involve a change in the role of the judge.

However, their "quasi-compulsory" nature means that they retain the coercive element of criminal sanctions and continue to embrace prohibition ideology. The question is: Can coercion result in successful therapeutic outcomes?

Stevens et al. state that although entering treatment via criminal justice channels does not necessarily reduce motivation to adhere to treatment programs, success of the particular treatment program depends on actors in the quasi-compulsory treatment process being able to "deal with the essential contradictions that the care/control dichotomy presents."[7]

Urbanoski, however, contends that mandates from legal authorities result in lower autonomous motivation for treatment and lower cognitive engagement in treatment, meaning that although quasi-compulsory treatment guarantees physical presence, it "does not guarantee meaningful participation."[8] Furthermore, for coerced treatment to be in any way successful, some studies have found that "initial internal motivation" was necessary, and where this was not present, the tendency to drop out of these programs were higher.[9]

The Drug Policy Alliance in their 2011 report noted several key problems with American drug courts—that they did not improve public safety, that they inadequately assessed people's needs, and that they may not reduce costs.[10] The report recommended that existing drug courts incorporate health measures, and not necessarily abstinence, into drug court programs, and also that drug courts should prohibit incarceration as a sanction for failure in the drug court program.[11]

Arguably, whether coercion can result in successful therapeutic outcomes is dependent on many factors, such as ensuring that minor drug users are not brought within this system, choosing only internally motivated individuals, removing frequent urinalysis from programs, and ensuring that cost-benefit analyses prove that drug courts are necessarily more successful than voluntary treatment and widespread general health services. At present, the evidence base remains weak for drug courts.

The positive points remain that drug courts keep people out of jail and that many drug courts are less punitive than jails. Within the short term, drug court systems seem to be the most easily transferable to Asian government systems, seeing that their operation retains coercive elements, meaning that current structures could remain in place with only some modification. Embracing drug courts on a weak evidence base, however, may exacerbate negative outcomes.

POLICE DRUG DIVERSION

Drug diversion has been described as a "graduated series of interventions" to prevent a PWID from entering the criminal justice system as a result of his drug use.[12] For the purposes of this chapter, however, I will talk about police diversion in terms of any action taken by police pre-arrest or post-arrest to divert an individual away from the court system, incarceration, and in the case of countries like Malaysia, judicial corporal punishment.

In New South Wales, Australia, pre-arrest diversion means that the police can approach a potential arrestee and "caution" him, while at the same time providing referral information to harm reduction or treatment programs.[13] In some jurisdictions, the individual signs an agreement with police to attend particular programs. Agreements may contain terms and conditions as to how the program is carried out, including time periods for the completion of the program.[14] In the United Kingdom, social workers are situated in police stations to enable diversion to occur smoothly.[15]

Drug diversion exists in several jurisdictions to do several things, such as ensure an individual attends treatment, to improve chances of reintegration by ensuring the individual does not have a criminal record, and, predominantly, to break the drug-crime cycle. It is important to note here that while illicit drug use does not directly cause or initiate criminal behavior, studies have shown that drug dependence or heavy drug use is "related to the maintenance and frequency of offending,"[16] and the frequency of property offences.[17]

Across Asia, there are few places where individuals with criminal records can obtain jobs. These include work in rubber and palm oil plantation fields or self-employment selling food or items. Where employment is scant and reintegration remains difficult, "fundraising crimes" are the only source of income. Police drug diversion is intended to reduce criminal behavior by enabling reintegration. The question is: does it work?

Although there are many examples of diversion in practice, there is a dearth of evidence of its efficacy in academic literature.[18] Defenders of drug diversion state that it saves police resources to deal with more serious issues and that it reduces harms caused by incarceration. Critics state that it is quasi-compulsory treatment, therefore reducing motivation to attend treatment and that diversion opens the doors for arbitrary amounts of discretion on the part of the police.

The latter is especially important in many countries in Asia, where police brutality, urine sample contamination, and corruption continue to be a predominant feature in drug policing. Accountability mechanisms simply do not exist, and governments continue to ignore international recommendations of establishing Police Complaints Commissions.[19]

In such an environment, placing huge amounts of discretion to divert in the hands of police may exacerbate harms caused to persons who use drugs.

Arguably, the form of diversion contained in Portugal's drug policy system is the only existing form of diversion with evidence of efficacy, although not yet on crime statistics. Although not explicitly termed "police drug diversion," Portuguese policy of individuals being diverted post-arrest to a multidisciplinary body called the Dissuasion Commission (described in further detail below), is a form of diversion and has resulted in reduced HIV infections, fewer drug overdose deaths, and better overall health. The Dissuasion Commission, consisting of social workers, psychologists, and lawyers, helps refer individuals to health programs and social services but does not bind them to agreements. This model would remove a large amount of discretion from police hands and instead leave treatment aspects to health and social workers. As such, this model may be the most viable in countries where police accountability remains a problem and trained social workers are abundant. It is important to pinpoint, however, that decisions about diversion systems remain multi-faceted; issues of cultural suitability, availability of sustainable funding, geographic limitations, human rights protection, human resources, and general efficiency must be carefully considered in transferring models across borders.

DECRIMINALIZATION/DE FACTO DECRIMINALIZATION

Portugal decriminalized personal consumption of drugs in 2001 amid a devastating epidemic of harms associated with injecting drug use. By the end of the twentieth century, Portugal had the highest prevalence of problematic drug use (mainly from heroin) in Europe. Drug users had "high visibility," and there were widespread acquisitive crimes. Dr João Goulão, the Portuguese drug czar, stated that the situation got to a point where everyone knew someone with a heroin problem and understood that these persons weren't "bad" but instead were persons who needed treatment. Hence, there was public acceptance of drug use as a health issue and similarly public acknowledgement that incarceration policies were not only counterproductive, but also a waste of public funds.[20]

It is important to note that Portugal "decriminalized" and not "legalized" drugs. Greenwald explains: ". . . drug possession for personal use and drug usage itself are still legally prohibited, but violations of those prohibitions are deemed to be exclusively administrative violations and are removed completely from the criminal realm."[21]

In practice, the individual is taken to the police station, where drugs on his or her person are weighed. If the quantity of drugs is below the statutory threshold of ten days' consumption under Portuguese law, the individual is transferred to a Dissuasion Commission, a body consisting of social workers, sociologists, and/or psychologists who play a planning and monitoring role in the individual's life. At time of writing, the statutory threshold for ten days' consumption was 1 g for heroin and 25 g for cannabis.[22]

The Dissuasion Commission works creatively to design a program for the individual during a determined time. The interventions may include harm reduction services, psychosocial interventions, and/or referrals to employment and housing services.[23] The Dissuasion Commission has wide discretion, but each of its decisions is appealable.

The results were overwhelmingly positive; overdose deaths reduced, HIV infection reduced, and the policy proved that decriminalization did not increase drug tourism or drug use.[24]

The removal of criminal sanctions put people who use drugs in a position where they could access health services more readily without fear of prosecution, therefore increasing their ability to reintegrate into society.

Numerous reports recommend that other governments learn from Portuguese pragmatism in dealing with problematic drug use.[25, 26] Asian governments must keep in mind that Portuguese success is derived not only from a single decriminalization law but rather from the decriminalization law interacting with accessible, widespread, and qualified health and social work personnel throughout Portugal, as well as cooperation from the police.

Alternatively, governments could choose to derive elements from a four-pillar system akin to Switzerland and some parts of Germany. Switzerland's four pillars are: harm reduction, treatment, prevention, and law enforcement. Switzerland does not decriminalize possession of drugs but does not incarcerate for drug possession or consumption. Individuals found in possession of drugs are fined, and fines can range from CHF 150–300 (US $165–$330) up to a maximum of CHF 50,000 (US $54,981), depending on the quantity of the drugs.[27] Police do not have the power to arrest.

There are widespread voluntary health services throughout Switzerland. The ARUD Centre at Aussersihl, Zurich, for example, has methadone maintenance therapy, treatment with morphine in its slow-release formulation, physicians for internal medicine, psychotherapy, maternal health examinations, and social workers under one roof. The ARUD Centre at Stampfenbach has heroin-assisted therapy, physicians for internal medicine, social workers, and injection rooms, where nurses can ensure that individuals do not share needles and do not overdose.[28]

Swiss policy has also seen positive results. These results include reduction in HIV infection, reduction of overdose deaths, an increase in overall health of individuals, a reduction in street crimes, and reduced heroin use and initiation into heroin use. Heroin use has decreased to one-fifth of use prior to the implementation of the four-pillar policy.[29] This is attributed to the fact that medicalization of heroin use has resulted in heroin use becoming less attractive to younger users.[30] In regard to crime in Switzerland, Professor Martin Killias, member of the Swiss Federal Commission on Drugs, commented: "The drop in crime was immediate, important, and lasting."[31]

WHAT NOW, ASIA?

Drug policy advocates, concerned parliamentarians, physicians, health lawyers, and the community at large must take careful steps in adopting an entire new drug policy. Although it is clear that punitive policy is ineffective and costly, the implanting of entire models of drug policy into a different country without taking into account finances, human resources, and level of public knowledge about drug use can result in devastating failures.

Governments seeking to derive elements of the Portuguese Dissuasion Commission, for example, should ensure that there are sufficient qualified staff members, that those employees know how to assess an individual's needs, ensure that referrals to health services are quickly made, and that those individuals are monitored, among other things.

Enthusiastic governments must be aware that models presented here work in environments with long-established and well-oiled universal healthcare, unemployment benefits, and welfare systems, many of which does not exist in many Asian countries.

What can be foreseen is that some governments may reject better policies outright on the basis that they are "Western ways" and that they are contrary to religion, in spite of a plethora of evidence proving that they are effective. Political conservatism, although a major stumbling block, can be overcome by consistent and evidence-based campaigns for better drug policy. Csete noted:

> Switzerland's adoption of the policies and programs that it has placed under the four-pillars umbrella shows that pragmatic drug policy can be built even in an environment of political conservatism. It may need to be couched in some level of rhetoric about eventual abstinence and it may need to include explicitly strong support of policing, but with some level of respect for objective scientific evidence, harm reduction can be a strong part of drug policy among people of varying political persuasions.[32]

Resources aside, Asian governments would be wise to acknowledge successes found in more pragmatic and humane policy, including the reduction of street crime (which governments struggle so hard to reduce), and begin introducing the building blocks that can, in the near future, lead to effective and intelligent official drug policy.

NOTES

1. Phillip Keefer and Norman Loayza, *Innocent Bystanders: Developing Countries and the War on Drugs* (Washington, DC: The World Bank, 2010).

2. Glenn Took, "Therapeutic Jurisprudence and the Drug Courts: Hybrid Justice and its Implications for Modern Penalty," *Internet Journal of Criminology* (2005).

3. Leonard Edwards, "Sanctions in Family Drug Treatment Courts," *Juvenile and Family Court Journal* 61, no. 1 (2010): 55–62.

4. Edwards, *Sanctions*, 55–62.

5. Canadian HIV/AIDS Legal Network, "Impaired Judgment: Assessing the Appropriateness of Drug Treatment Courts as a Response to Drug Use in Canada," 2012. www.aidslaw.ca/publications/interfaces/downloadFile.php?ref=2034.

6. Canadian HIV/AIDS Legal Network, *Impaired Judgment*.

7. Alex Stevens, Daniele Berto, Ulrich Frick, Neil Hunt, Viktoria Kerschl, Tim McSweeney, Kerrie Oeuvray, Irene Puppo, Alberto Santa Maria, Susanne Schaaf, Barbara Trinkl, Ambros Uchtenhagen, and Wolfgang Werdenich, "Perceived Pressure and Motivation in Treatment for Drug Dependence: Results from a European Study of Quasi-Compulsory Treatment," *European Addiction Research* 12 (2006): 197–209.

8. Karen A. Urbanoski, "Coerced Addiction Treatment: Client Perspectives and the Implications of their Neglect," *Harm Reduction Journal* 7 (2010): 13–22.

9. Astrid Birgden, "A Compulsory Drug Treatment Program in Australia: Therapeutic Jurisprudence Implications," *Thomas Jefferson Law Review* 30 (2008): 367–90.

10. DPA (Drug Policy Alliance), *Drug Courts are not the Answer: Toward a Health-Centered Approach to Drug Use* (United States of America: DPA, 2011).

11. DPA, *Drug Courts are not the Answer.*

12. Catherine Spooner, Wayne Hall, and Richard Mattick, "A Strategic Overview of the Diversion of Drug-Related Offenders in NSW." NDARC Technical Report No. 96, A report commissioned by the NSW Intersectoral Taskforce on Recidivism of Drug & Alcohol Offenders, New South Wales, 2000. http://ndarc.med.unsw.edu.au/sites/ndarc.cms.med.unsw.edu.au/files/ndarc/resources/TR.096.pdf.

13. Jennifer Ogilvie and Kate Willis, "Police Drug Diversion in Australia." Criminal Justice Bulletin Series 3—March 2009, National Cannabis Prevention and Information Centre (Australian Government: Australian Institute of Criminology, Canberra, 2009). http://ncpic.org.au/ncpic/publications/aic-bulletins/pdf/police-drug-diversion-in-australia.

14. New Zealand Police, "Adult Diversion Scheme Policy." Accessed 18 September 2012. www.police.govt.nz/sites/default/files/diversion_policy_2011.pdf.

15. Mike Trace (chairman, International Drug Policy Consortium/Former UK Deputy Drug Czar), in discussion with the author, November 2011.

16. Spooner, Hall, and Mattick, *A Strategic Overview.*

17. Deborah Bradford and Jason Payne, "Illicit Drug Use and Property Offending among Police Detainees." Crime and Justice Bulletin No. 157, NSW Bureau of Crime Statistics and Research, Australian Government, 2012.

18. Ogilvie and Willis, *Police Drug Diversion.*

19. UN General Assembly, Human Rights Council, "Universal Periodic Review: Report of the Working Group on the Universal Periodic Review." June 3, 2009. http://daccess-dds-ny.un.org/doc/UNDOC/GEN/G09/137/38/PDF/G0913738.pdf?OpenElement.

20. Fifa Rahman, "Portuguese Drug Policy." Malaysian AIDS Council, Kuala Lumpur, 2012a. www.mac.org.my/v3/?page_id=367.

21. Glenn Greenwald, "Drug Decriminalization in Portugal: Lessons for Creating Fair and Successful Drug Policies" (Washington, DC: CATO Institute, 2009). www.cato.org/pubs/wtpapers/greenwald_whitepaper.pdf.

22. Artur Domosławski, "Drug Policy in Portugal: the Benefits of Decriminalising Drug Use" (Warsaw, Poland: Global Drug Policy Program, Open Society Foundations, 2011). www.soros.org/sites/default/files/drug-policy-in-portugal-english-20120814.pdf.

23. Rahman, *Portuguese Drug Policy.*

24. Domosławski, *Drug Policy in Portugal.*

25. Greenwald, *Drug Decriminalization in Portugal.*

26. Domosławski, *Drug Policy in Portugal.*

27. Fifa Rahman, "Swiss Drug Policy." Malaysian AIDS Council, Kuala Lumpur, 2012b. www.mac.org.my/v3/wp-content/uploads/2011/09/Swiss_Drug_Policy_Report.pdf.

28. Rahman, *Swiss Drug Policy.*

29. Carlos Nordt and Rudolf Stohler, "Incidence of Heroin Use in Zurich, Switzerland: A Treatment Case Register Analysis," *Lancet* 367, no. 9525 (2006): 1830–34.

30. Rahman, *Swiss Drug Policy.*

31. Rahman, *Swiss Drug Policy.*

32. Joanne Csete, "From the Mountaintops: What the World Can Learn from Drug Policy Change in Switzerland." Lessons for Drug Policy Series (New York: Open Society Foundations, 2010).

BIBLIOGRAPHY

Birgden, Astrid. "A Compulsory Drug Treatment Program in Australia: Therapeutic Jurisprudence Implications." *Thomas Jefferson Law Review* 30 (2008): 367–90.

Bradford, Deborah and Jason Payne. "Illicit Drug Use and Property Offending among Police Detainees." Crime and Justice Bulletin No. 157, NSW Bureau of Crime Statistics and Research, Australian Government, 2012.

Canadian HIV/AIDS Legal Network. "Impaired Judgment: Assessing the Appropriateness of Drug Treatment Courts as a Response to Drug Use in Canada." 2012. www.aidslaw.ca/publications/interfaces/downloadFile.php?ref=2034.

Csete, Joanne. "From the Mountaintops: What the World Can Learn from Drug Policy Change in Switzerland." Lessons for Drug Policy Series, New York: Open Society Foundations, 2010.

Domosławski, Artur. "Drug Policy in Portugal: the Benefits of Decriminalising Drug Use." Global Drug Policy Program, Open Society Foundations, Warsaw, Poland, 2011. www.soros.org/sites/default/files/drug-policy-in-portugal-english-20120814.pdf.

DPA (Drug Policy Alliance). *Drug Courts are not the Answer: Toward a Health-Centered Approach to Drug Use.* United States of America: DPA, 2011.

Edwards, Leonard. "Sanctions in Family Drug Treatment Courts." *Juvenile and Family Court Journal* 61, no. 1 (2010): 55–62.

Greenwald, Glenn. "Drug Decriminalization in Portugal: Lessons for Creating Fair and Successful Drug Policies." CATO Institute, Washington DC, 2009. www.cato.org/pubs/wtpapers/greenwald_whitepaper.pdf.

Keefer, Philip and Norman Loayza. *Innocent Bystanders: Developing Countries and the War on Drugs.* Washington, DC: The World Bank, 2010.

New Zealand Police. "Adult Diversion Scheme Policy." Accessed 18 September 2012. www.police.govt.nz/sites/default/files/diversion_policy_2011.pdf.

Nordt, Carlos and Rudolf Stohler. "Incidence of Heroin Use in Zurich, Switzerland: A Treatment Case Register Analysis." *Lancet* 367, no. 9525 (2006): 1830–34.

Ogilvie, Jennifer and Kate Willis. "Police Drug Diversion in Australia." Criminal Justice Bulletin Series 3—March 2009, National Cannabis Prevention and Information Centre, Australian Government: Australian Institute of Criminology, Canberra, 2009. http://ncpic.org.au/ncpic/publications/aic-bulletins/pdf/police-drug-diversion-in-australia.

Rahman, Fifa. "Portuguese Drug Policy." Malaysian AIDS Council, Kuala Lumpur, 2012a. www.mac.org.my/v3/?page_id=367.

Rahman, Fifa. "Swiss Drug Policy." Malaysian AIDS Council, Kuala Lumpur, 2012. www.mac.org.my/v3/wp-content/uploads/2011/09/Swiss_Drug_Policy_Report.pdf.

Spooner, Catherine, Wayne Hall, and Richard Mattick. "A Strategic Overview of the Diversion of Drug-Related Offenders in NSW." NDARC Technical Report No. 96, A report commissioned by the NSW Intersectoral Taskforce on Recidivism of Drug & Alcohol Offenders, New South Wales, 2000. http://ndarc.med.unsw.edu.au/sites/ndarc.cms.med.unsw.edu.au/files/ndarc/resources/TR.096.pdf.

Stevens, Alex, Daniele Berto, Ulrich Frick, Neil Hunt, Viktoria Kerschl, Tim McSweeney, Kerrie Oeuvray, Irene Puppo, Alberto Santa Maria, Susanne Schaaf, Barbara Trinkl, Ambros Uchtenhagen, and Wolfgang Werdenich. "Perceived Pressure and Motivation in Treatment for Drug Dependence: Results from a European Study of Quasi-Compulsory Treatment." *European Addiction Research* 12 (2006): 197–209.

Took, Glenn. "Therapeutic Jurisprudence and the Drug Courts: Hybrid Justice and its Implications for Modern Penalty." *Internet Journal of Criminology* (2005).

Trace, Mike (chairman, International Drug Policy Consortium/Former UK Deputy Drug Czar), in discussion with the author, November 2011.

UN General Assembly, Human Rights Council. "Universal Periodic Review: Report of the Working Group on the Universal Periodic Review." June 3, 2009. http://daccess-dds-ny.un.org/doc/UNDOC/GEN/G09/137/38/PDF/G0913738.pdf?OpenElement.

Urbanoski, Karen A. "Coerced Addiction Treatment: Client Perspectives and the Implications of their Neglect." *Harm Reduction Journal* 7 (2010): 13–22.

Chapter Eighteen

Capital Punishment for Drug Offenses

Fifa Rahman

Asia is the next important frontier for policy debate and legal change with respect to capital punishment.

—Johnson and Zimring, 2009 [1]

Despite overwhelming evidence that the death penalty does not reduce drug supply or demand, it continues to be prescribed in thirty-two countries and territories across the globe, although only six of these countries make it an operational part of their criminal justice systems. [2] Table 18.1 illustrates the situation in East and Southeast Asia.

In relation to capital punishment for drug offenses these nations face an undeniable truth: that most persons executed for drug offenses are low-level drug carriers recruited by syndicates to carry drugs across borders. Those who transport drugs across borders are often female and are given packages or suitcases to transport; those caught for trafficking are also overwhelmingly uneducated and are of modest financial backgrounds. Some people on death row for drug offenses are females who were arrested with a male companion: it is not entirely implausible in such situations that the drug manufacturer or dealer is the male and that the female was snared into a death sentence by default.

In countries where there is a mandatory death penalty based on a statutory threshold quantity, judges are given no discretion to take into account factors which ordinarily could and should have a determining influence on whether the individual lives or dies. These include financial circumstance, motives behind the transport or traffic of drugs, knowledge of the contents of the package or luggage, age of offender, and whether it was a first offense. The fact that there is no opportunity for mitigation, and no discretion on the part

Country	Status: Death Penalty for Drugs
Brunei	Abolitionist in practice, mandatory death penalty for drugs.[i]
Cambodia	Abolished in constitution in 1993.
East Timor	Abolished since independence by constitution in 2002.
Indonesia	Prescribed in narcotics law, discretionary death penalty.
Japan	No death penalty for drugs. Only murder or treason.
Laos	Abolitionist in practice, mandatory death penalty for drugs.
Malaysia	Prescribed in Dangerous Drugs Act 1952, actively sentences, mandatory death penalty for drugs.
Myanmar	Abolitionist in practice.
North Korea	Prescribed in law since 2008.[ii]
Philippines	Abolished in constitution in 1987.
Singapore	Prescribed in Misuse of Drugs Act 1973, mandatory death penalty.
South Korea	Abolitionist in practice.[iii]
Taiwan	Prescribed in Drug Control Act, discretionary death penalty.[iv]
Thailand	Prescribed in Narcotics Act 1979,[v] discretionary death penalty.
Vietnam	Prescribed in Penal Code[vi], death sentences are official state secrets.

Table 18.1. i. Ibid.
ii. Ibid.
iii. Ibid.
iv. Ibid.
v. Ibid.
vi. Ibid.

of the judge, means that sentences handed out are often arbitrary, heart-rending, and destructive.

It is this emotive factor, however, reinforced by pressure from international organizations, that may be a key factor behind recent discussions by governments on the possibility of moratoria, restoring discretion to judges, and/or complete abolition. In this chapter, I will provide a background of the situation in East and Southeast Asia, discuss the potential for reform, public and judicial opinion of the death penalty, and whether these do or even should influence policy decisions on the death penalty.

WHY RETAIN CAPITAL PUNISHMENT?

Retentionist governments often argue that the death penalty for drug offenses is justified because it reduces drug use and drug supply. In 2010, K. Shanmugam, Singapore's law minister, stated that the laws are needed to prevent an "unstoppable stream of such people" from dealing drugs.[3]

This oft-used excuse, of deterrence, is one that has not been conclusively proved. Griffith Edwards et al. comment that the death penalty "cannot rationally be expected to be an effective instrument of deterrence."[4] And further, "Not only is there a dearth of tangible evidence as to efficacy, but a large body of research on the general issue of deterrents suggests strongly that likelihood of detection is a more important deterrent than intensity of punishment."[5]

This is evident from the fact that despite actively handing down death sentences for drug offenses, such countries continue to have drug use and drug dependence little different from their non-death penalty neighbors. Such rates of use may be reflected in budgets: in Malaysia, the Ministry of Home Affairs estimated that based on the 2012 allocated National Anti-Drug Agency budget, a total of RM 62 million (US $19.65 million) will be spent on treatment and "rehabilitation" of persons who use drugs.[6]

Meanwhile, in 2008, China had the highest number of methamphetamine seizures in the world.[7] In East and Southeast Asia in 2011 there were an estimated 2,870,000 people using amphetamine-type substances and 4,990,000 persons using opiates.[8] Of injecting drug users worldwide, the largest proportion is in China.[9]

Despite these and many other statistics that indicate that neither drug seizures nor drug use is influenced by the active imposition of death sentences, countries continue to claim that the death penalty is an effective deterrent.

In addition, a 2010 study showed that public support for the death penalty does not directly correlate to deterrence as an individual sentencing philosophy.[10] In the survey conducted in Singapore—which practices the mandatory death penalty for drug trafficking—60 percent of respondents supported the death penalty, yet only 13 percent endorsed deterrence as a sentencing philosophy.[11] Taiwan recently reinstated the death penalty, but only 28 percent of respondents embraced deterrence as the main consideration in sentencing, compared to the 83 percent who support the death penalty—the highest in the world.[12]

Persons in favor of the death penalty ("retentionists") may argue that individual perception of what the death sentence should do cannot be compared with the actual effects of the death penalty. The fact remains, however, that there is no conclusive evidence at all that the death penalty affects entry and use of drugs. The above study draws yet another conclusion about the ideas surrounding the death penalty and deterrence—that they do not necessarily correlate. The question is: If the death penalty clearly does not deter, and the people who support the death penalty do not necessarily think that it deters, how else can we justify its application to drug offenses?

Politicians argue that abolition of the death penalty is not possible because public support for the death penalty is high, and therefore legislating for abolition would be akin to political suicide. In October 2011, Malaysian de facto law minister Dato' Seri Nazri Aziz spoke about the possibility of abolition and stated: "we follow the majority."[13]

Ben Brown et al. argue that it is "possible for the public to support capital punishment in nations where the practice has long been abandoned."[14] England, which is abolitionist and has not carried out any executions since 1964, has a 50 percent public support for the death penalty.[15] In 2004, England acceded to the 13th Protocol of European Convention of Human Rights which prohibits the death penalty outright—despite 55 percent of Britons in 2004 supporting the death penalty.

Estonia is abolitionist and has 64 percent support for the death penalty. The Russian Federation has the ninth-highest percentage of support for the death penalty in the world, at 67 percent, and is categorized as "abolitionist in practice,"[16] which means that although they retain the death penalty in their laws, they have not carried out executions within the past ten years and have an established practice of not carrying out executions.[17]

According to Eric Neumayer, "the global trend towards abolition is mainly politically determined rather than by cultural, social and economic factors."[18] This means that although politicians argue that abolition of the death penalty is dependent on public support, it is entirely more likely that abolition is dependent less on public support and more on political will.

MALAYSIA: MANDATORY DEATH PENALTY AND PRESUMPTION OF TRAFFICKING

Under the purview of the Dangerous Drugs Act,[19] Malaysia metes out a mandatory death penalty to persons found to be trafficking in drugs.[20] The operation of this section is subject to several other provisions of the Act, notably Sections 2 and 37. Section 2 of the Act defines the act of trafficking as:

> [D]oing of any of the following acts, that is to say, *manufacturing*, importing, exporting, keeping, concealing, buying, selling, giving, receiving, storing, administering, *transporting*, carrying, sending, delivering, procuring, supplying or distributing any dangerous drug.[21] [Emphasis added.]

The scope of this section is large—meaning that persons hired to maintain equipment in a methamphetamine laboratory, for example, could possibly fall within its ambit. Section 37 contains a presumption that anyone found in possession of a statutory threshold of drugs or more is presumed to be a trafficker unless the contrary is proven.[22] In addition, statutory quantities for the presumption of trafficking in Malaysian law are relatively low compared to thresholds across Asia; in Malaysia, 15 grams of heroin,[23] 200 grams of cannabis,[24] and 50 grams of amphetamines.[25] The only nation that has lower threshold quantities is Indonesia: Indonesian law prescribes the death penalty for the production, import, export, or distribution of 5 grams[26] of Class 1 narcotics in a non-tree/plant form which includes heroin, cannabis, cocaine, and ecstasy.[27] Indonesia prescribes a similar penalty for "selling, buying, becoming a middle person in narcotics buying or selling, exchanging, handing over, or receiving Class 1 narcotics."[28]

It is important to note, however, that Indonesian judges have the discretion to mete out jail sentences instead of the death penalty, which is not the case in Malaysia. It is often argued by advocates that restoring discretion to judges may be a strategic first step toward abolition. Others argue that it is possible to immediately call for a formal moratorium on capital punishment for drug offenses.

Either way, the mandatory death penalty means that judges cannot take into account family circumstances, such as if the individual has a young child and is a single mother, or that the individual transported drugs to pay for legal fees or loans, financial backgrounds, knowledge of contents of packages given to them or the fact, terminal illnesses or psychiatric illnesses that the individual might have, or that the individual was raised in a drug-manufacturing family and had been coerced into the business. The mandatory death penalty, in itself, prescribes for arbitrariness by eliminating the possibility for mitigation. The following cases may illustrate this.

Realization of this arbitrariness was recognized in the Indian case that was successful in striking down the mandatory death penalty; the case held that the use of discretion was "indispensable" to cases where the death penalty was an option, and that to mete out the death penalty without this discretion would be to act unfairly.[29]

Noor Atiqah	Jacqueline Quiamno	Mariko Takeuchi
Noor Atiqah is a Singaporean single mother who was arrested at the age of 25, carrying a suitcase containing 370 grams of heroin. She had been given the suitcase by a Ghanaian friend, and was not aware of its contents. Nevertheless, she was sentenced to death. Recently, however, the Court of Appeal overturned this sentence on the basis that it was the Ghanaian who was the actual trafficker, amended the charge, and gave her a 12-year sentence instead.	Jacqueline Quiamno was arrested at the age of 19 with 3.9 grams of cocaine at the entrance of Kuala Lumpur International Airport on 28 June 2005. Despite only being a pub singer in the Philippines, the judge rejected her defense that she was a mere carrier, and sentenced her to death.	Mariko Takeuchi was arrested in possession of 3.5 kilograms of methamphetamines in her suitcase. Despite her stating that she had no knowledge of the contents of the bag and that an Iranian colleague had given her the suitcase in Dubai, High Court Judge Siti Mariah stated that it Takeuchi had suspicious motives in spite of her claims, and sentenced her to death. She was 35 years old at the time of arrest, and was working as a nurse in Tokyo.
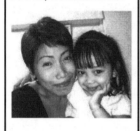		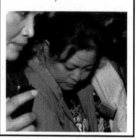

Figure 18.1

Malaysia may have also realized the arbitrary nature of the mandatory death penalty, or even the death penalty as a whole. In the 2009 United Nations Universal Periodic Review, in response to recommendations of an outcome report, Malaysia stated that it was considering proposed amendments to anti-drug trafficking legislation to reduce the penalty to life imprisonment.[30] Interestingly, Malaysia also stated that it prescribes the death penalty only for "serious crimes,"[31] despite several reports implying that drug offenses are not serious crimes.[32, 33]

Beginning in 2010, the Malaysian death penalty abolition agenda seemed to pick up speed. In August 2010, Law Minister Dato' Seri Nazri Aziz expressed the view that government should not take life.[34] In the same report, however, he pointed out that there was no political will to abolish. On October 13, 2011, a public forum was held in Kuala Lumpur discussing the possibility of abolition of capital punishment. Three hundred and sixty people attended, and debate was heated. On the same day, a newspaper article was released stating that abolition would only be considered if public support for abolition was high.[35] Also on October 13, 2011, the Malaysian Bar Council president called for an immediate moratorium.[36] A year later, in October 2012, the de facto law minister announced that the application for a moratorium was to be discussed with the prime minister.[37]

There may be several factors behind the recent increased governmental interest toward considering capital punishment reform. These may include pressure from abolitionist nations and international organizations, possible judicial reservations on meting out the death penalty, and empathy emanating out of the case of a young Malaysian sentenced to death in Singapore for trafficking. Brief details of the latter are contained in figure 18.2.

Out of efforts by Malaysians to save Vui Kong, several questions arose: How can countries successfully save their citizens overseas if they themselves actively hand out death sentences? Can countries expect clemency from others where they have not shown the same courtesy?

Malaysia's de facto Law Minister argued in October 2012 along the same lines: "So if we want to save the Malaysian 'drug mules' (overseas), a large number of whom were not aware they were being used, how can we appeal to those countries while we ourselves hang such offenders. It doesn't make sense."

INDONESIA: TRANSNATIONAL POLICE COOPERATION AND DEATH PENALTY ACTIVISM

Discussions on the death penalty in Indonesia have been focused on trafficking by foreigners, the high number of Indonesians in prisons or on death row in neighboring countries for drug offenses, and the high support for the death penalty at home.

Indonesia has become notorious for the trials of high-profile trafficking cases, in particular of Australian citizens such as Schapelle Corby and the Bali Nine. There is no doubt that arrests, convictions, and executions of

---

Yong Vui Kong

Yong Vui Kong was arrested at the age of 18 ½ years at the Malaysia-Singapore border carrying 47.27 grams of heroin, and was sentenced to death in 2007. The son of a dishwasher from Sabah, in East Malaysia, Vui Kong moved to Malaysia's capital, Kuala Lumpur in 2002, and found it difficult to make ends meet. He was working as a runner for a drug dealer at the time

of his arrest.

Figure 18.2

citizens of abolitionist nations result in tensions between nations. Eric Neumayer commented: "The execution of foreigners who are citizens of abolitionist countries commonly creates political tensions between governments."[38] Australia has utilized diplomatic means in the past to negotiate for the lives of its citizens.[39] In addition to that, where arrests are made as a result of surveillance or information provided by abolitionist nations, there seems to be the necessity for a "balancing exercise" between cooperation in regard to transnational crime, and the need to protect citizens. Finlay comments: "While it can be argued that such cooperation is simply a practical necessity given the retention of the death penalty by key regional neighbours such as Indonesia, Singapore and Vietnam, it has also been suggested that it risks undermining Australia's stated commitment to the abolition of the death penalty and the protection of human rights."[40] These conflicts are evident in the Bali Nine case.

The Indonesian Bali Nine case involved nine Australian citizens who were arrested in Bali for an attempt to traffic heroin from Indonesia to Australia on April 17, 2005. The arrests occurred pursuant to information received from the Australian Federal Police on their suspicions that a group of Australians were "importing a narcotic substance from Bali to Australia."[41] This information was conveyed to the Indonesian National Police via a letter from Paul Hunniford, who was the Senior Liaison Officer for the Australian Federal Police in Bali at the time.[42] The youngest member, Michael Czugaj, was only eighteen years old at the time of arrest, and was found with 1.75 kilograms of heroin strapped to his legs and chest and was sentenced to life imprisonment. Scott Rush, who was arrested with 1.3 kilograms of heroin at Bali's Ngurai Rai International Airport, was initially sentenced to life imprisonment at the District Court but was sentenced to the death penalty instead on appeal at the Bali High Court in September of 2006, and on appeal at the Indonesian Supreme Court, this was reduced again to life imprisonment.[43]

Myuran Sukumaran and Andrew Chan, the two members of the Bali Nine who were deemed to be the "ringleaders" and planners of the operation, were sentenced to death in October 2005 and have exhausted all their appeals with no change to the sentences.[44] They now await the firing squad or a decision of clemency by the president of Indonesia. During these trials in particular, Kevin Rudd, the then opposition foreign affairs spokesperson stated, "When it comes to the death penalty applied to Australian citizens, we then seek, with the Government, to intervene on a bipartisan basis to obtain clemency."[45] Alexander Downer, foreign minister at the time, similarly stated that it was also Australia's policy to appeal for clemency.[46]

Meanwhile, in Australia the role of the federal police was roundly criticized by the Australian public;[47] however it was held by Justice Finn in the case of *Rush v. Commissioner of Police*[48] that the Australian police had acted lawfully. In balancing Australia's legal obligation to combat transnational crime and their commitment to abolition of the death penalty, Justice Finn referred [49] to the American case of *Rodriguez v. United States*[50] and quoted: "Deciding what competing values will or will not be sacrificed to the achievement of a particular objective is the very essence of legislative choice."[51]

This in turn has been criticized as Australia prioritizing international and mutual criminal assistance over commitment to abolition.[52] Sifris in 2007 argues: "there is no reason why these two commitments cannot be reconciled and valued equally."[53] At the time of this writing, Sukumaran and Chan still face the death penalty in Indonesia, and arguments such as these will continue to arise.

Arrests of foreigners accused of transporting drugs are a key focus of anti-death penalty activists in Indonesia. Death penalty activism in Indonesia is carried out by local NGOs such as Imparsial and Lebuh Masyarakat, the European Union delegations to Indonesia, and lawyers working on individual cases. Reprieve, a UK-based organization, assists in constitutional challenges to the death penalty in retentionist countries and assists with trials of British citizens under threat of the death penalty for drugs.

Indonesia is beginning to see increased advocacy on the death penalty in recent times. On October 10, 2011, an anti-death penalty forum supported by the EU Delegation to Indonesia and Imparsial took place in Jakarta, and was attended by ambassadors, lawyers, as well as members of the public.[54]

In addition, the president of Indonesia, Bambang Yudhyono, has expressed that no executions would occur during his term as president. His aversion to the death penalty can also be seen in his 2011 official decision to "carry out advocacy and legal assistance for Indonesian citizens and Indonesian laborers overseas that are undergoing legal process, in particular those that are facing or threatened by the death penalty."[55]

CHINA: SECRET EXECUTIONS AND RECENT REFORMS

Statistics on the death penalty in China are state secrets,[56] but it is widely believed to have the largest death row in the world. Amnesty International states that figures are in the thousands per year.[57] Dui Hua Foundation, an organization that focuses on human rights in China, stated that approximately four thousand people were executed in China in 2011.[58, 59] In addition to that, China has fifty-five death penalty offenses in the criminal law.[60]

These high figures, however, are a reduction from previous years. This is as a result of recent substantive reforms to reduce the number of capital offenses in the criminal law and the procedural reforms to institutionalize more rigorous reviews in death penalty cases. The wide use of the death penalty with a two-year delay (or a two-year "reprieve") before execution has also helped in limiting the application of death penalty because for virtually all the offenders, the death penalty is converted to life imprisonment after the two year reprieve. In fact, in 2006, the former chief justice, Xiao Yang, of the Supreme People's Court (SPC) "instructed judges to avoid handing down death sentences with immediate execution, for all but the most heinous criminals."[61] Susan Trevaskes discusses reforms in her 2008 article, discussing that punishment ideology is currently a balance between two dicta: "Kill Fewer, Kill Cautiously," and *Yan da* which means "Strike Hard."[62] Although recent reforms in China are indicative of a slow embrace of the latter after Wang Shengjun became the chief justice in 2007 replacing Xiao Yang, it can be said that current practice in China involves "balancing leniency and severity," with the SPC and provincial high courts making serious efforts to reduce the number of death penalty in China.[63]

While overall death penalty cases may have declined in China in recent years, the death penalty for drug trafficking and manufacturing may have been on the increase. Indeed, drug trafficking may have overtaken murder as the offense that attracts the highest number of death penalties in some provinces and is certainly one of the few offenses (murder, robbery, and assault causing death) for which the death penalty is regularly imposed. China has adopted a dual penalty policy for drug offenses. On the one hand, legislative efforts have been made to institutionalize community correction, drug treatment and rehabilitation. On the other, the harshest penalty is routinely used on the more serious cases of drug manufacturing and trafficking.

In 2010, the police investigated about 13,000 drug offenses, arrested about 16,000 individuals suspected of drug offenses, and confiscated 5.5 tons of various drugs, an increase of 35.7 percent, 37.1 percent, and 36.8 percent over the previous year.[64] In 2010, courts in China tried 59,234 drug cases and sentenced 66,298 offenders. The number of so-called serious drug offenses, offenses attracting the penalties from five years' imprisonment to death penalty, is 18,961.[65]

There is no mandatory death penalty for drug offenses, and judges exercise discretion in sentencing after considering the nature of the case, including quality and quantity of drug involved, and the record of the offenders, including previous criminal record and cooperation with the investigation. But the quantity of the drug involved has become the most significant determinant in determining death penalty and the amount that may trigger death penalty varies from one province to another. The more serious the drug problem is, the higher the trigger amount is. While, under the criminal law, the trigger amounts of trafficking in heroin and other hard drugs is 50 grams, provincial courts set different trigger amount ranging from 100 grams in Gansu province to 500 grams in Yunnan province.[66]

In spite of the positive step toward reduction of death sentences in China, laws remain harsh and the use of death penalty for drug trafficking is particularly frequent. By way of illustration: in December of 2011, five individuals were sentenced to death and another two were sentenced to death with a two-year reprieve for trafficking a total of 6 kilograms of mostly heroin.[67] Also in December, a thirty-five-year-old Filipino man was executed in China for trafficking 1.5 kilograms of heroin from Malaysia, despite appeals from Philippines' President Benigno Aquino III for China to spare his life.[68]

China is still a long way from any talk of abolition, or in particular, abolition in regard to drug offenses given the the perceived seriousness of drug problem in China and the political sensitivity of the matter. Kandis Scott comments: "The new SPC rules will diminish the number of executions, satisfy a public that is presently committed to capital punishment, and postpone radical change. However, the fact that Chinese authorities rely on current conditions to explain preserving the death sentence may signal openness to significant changes in the future."[69]

CONCLUSION

As shown from the above arguments and examples, debates on the death penalty in East and Southeast Asia are lively and range around issues of human rights, transnational criminal obligations, support for the death penalty, purported deterrent effect, and political will. Although there is increasing potential and support toward abolition, persistent advocacy and political will is lacking.

Death penalty abolitionists in China continue to face significant obstacles toward abolition of the death penalty for drug offenses; however, recent reforms are encouraging and only open up the door to increased anti-death penalty efforts.

NOTES

1. David T. Johnson and Franlin E. Zimring, *The Next Frontier: National Development, Political Change, and the Death Penalty in Asia* (New York: Oxford University Press, 2009).

2. HRI (Harm Reduction International), *The Death Penalty for Drug Offences: Global Overview 2011* (London: HRI, 2011).

3. The minister's comments were published in a May 10, 2010 edition of the *Today* newspaper, which is no longer available online, but was quoted in a summary of Civil Appeal No 144 of 2010, *Yong Vui Kong v Attorney-General* (April 4, 2011) per Chan Sek Keong CJ at Para 5. Accessed December 22, 2011. http://app.supremecourt.gov.sg/data/doc/ManagePage/3721/Yong%20Vui%20Kong%20v%20Attorney-General%20CA%20144%202010%20-%20Summary%20Judgement%20by%20Chief%20Justice%20Chan%20Sek%20Keong.pdf.

4. Griffith Edwards, Tom Babor, Shane Darke, Wayne Hall, John Marsden, Peter Miller, and Robert West, "Drug Trafficking: Time to Abolish the Death Penalty." *Addiction* 104, no. 8 (2009): 1267.

5. Edwards et al., *Drug Trafficking*, 1267.

6. Ministry of Home Affairs. "Statistics given by the Ministry of Home Affairs in response to a question by Member of Parliament Haji Ahmad Lai Bujang in the Malaysian *Dewan*

Rakyat (House of Representatives)." November 10, 2011. Accessed December 27, 2011. https:/
/docs.google.com/document/d/1y2YTC05k9DM-AdkSu9GAlar1iat8BnJahhhpTJYg8gc/edit.

7. UNODC (United Nations Office on Drugs and Crime), *2008 World Drug Report* (Geneva: UNODC, 2009).

8. UNODC (United Nations Office on Drugs and Crime), *2010 World Drug Report* (Geneva: UNODC, 2011), 24.

9. UNODC, *2010 World Drug Report*, 30.

10. James Unnever, "Global Support for the Death Penalty." *Punishment & Society* 12, no. 4 (2010): 463, 468.

11. Unnever, *Global Support*, 468.

12. Unnever, *Global Support*, 468.

13. Bernama, "Nazri: Abolition of Death Penalty Would Depend on Public Opinion." *The Star Online*, October 13, 2011. Accessed December 28, 2011. http://thestar.com.my/news/story.asp?file=/2011/10/13/nation/20111013225050&sec=nation.

14. Ben Brown, Wm. Reed Benedict, and Kevin Buckler, "Support for the Death Penalty in Developing Democracies: A Binational Comparative Case Study." *International Criminal Justice Review* 20, no. 4 (2010): 398, 407.

15. Unnever, *Global Support*, 473.

16. AI (Amnesty International), "Death Sentences and Executions 2010" (London: Amnesty International, 2011), 44.

17. Amnesty International, *Death Sentences and Executions 2010*, 45.

18. Eric Neumayer, "Death Penalty: The Political Foundations of the Global Trend towards Abolition," *Human Rights Review* 9 (2008): 241–42.

19. *Dangerous Drugs Act 1952*, Act 234 (Laws of Malaysia).

20. Id., s39B.

21. Id., s2.

22. Id., s37(da).

23. Id., s37(da)(i).

24. Id., s37(da)(vi).

25. Id., s37(da)(xii).

26. Undang-Undang Republik Indonesia, Nomor 35 Tahun 2009 Tentang Narkotika, Article 113(2) [Laws of the Republic of Indonesia, Number 35 of Year 2009 on Narcotics, Article 113(2)]

27. Id., Schedule 1.

28. Id., Article 114(2).

29. *Indian Harm Reduction Network v. The Union of India* (2010) High Court of Judicature, Bombay, criminal writ petition no. 1784 of 2010, June 2010 quoted in Harm Reduction International, *The Death Penalty for Drug Offences: Global Overview 2011* at 14.

30. UNHRC (United Nations Human Rights Council), *Universal Periodic Review: Report of the Working Group on the Universal Periodic Review, Addendum, Malaysia.* Agenda Item No. 6, A/HRC/11/30/Add.1., para 10, 2009. Accessed January 14, 2012. http://daccess-dds-ny.un.org/doc/UNDOC/GEN/G09/137/38/PDF/G0913738.pdf?OpenElement.

31. UNHRC, *Universal Periodic Review*, para 10.

32. UNHRC (UN Human Rights Committee), *UN Human Rights Committee: Concluding Observations: Kuwait* , July 27, 2000, CCPR/CO/69/KWT. Accessed October 24, 2012; para 13. www.unhcr.org/refworld/docid/3df36be44.html.

33. Rick Lines, "A 'Most Serious Crime'? The Death Penalty for Drug Offences and International Human Rights Law," *Amicus Journal* 21 (2010): 21.

34. Rashvinjeet S. Bedi, "Abolish Death Penalty, It's Wrong to Take Someone's Life, Says Nazri," *The Star Online*, August 29, 2010. Accessed January 12, 2012. http://thestar.com.my/news/story.asp?file=/2010/8/29/nation/6893246&sec=nation.

35. Bernama, "Nazri: Abolition of Death Penalty Would Depend on Public Opinion." *The Star Online*, October 13, 2011. Accessed December 28, 2011. http://thestar.com.my/news/story.asp?file=/2011/10/13/nation/20111013225050&sec=nation.

36. *The Malaysian Bar*, "Press Release: Abolish the Death Penalty Now." (October 13, 2011) Accessed January 14, 2012. www.malaysianbar.org.my/press_statements/press_release_abolish_the_death_penalty_now.html.

37. *New Straits Times*, "Possible Moratorium on Death Sentence Pending Govt's Final Decision," *New Straits Times*, October 20, 2012. Accessed October 24, 2012. www.nst.com.my/latest/possible-moratorium-on-death-sentence-pending-govt-s-final-decision-1.159690#.

38. Neumayer, *Death Penalty: The Political Foundations*, 242.

39. Colman Lynch, "Indonesia's Use of Capital Punishment for Drug Trafficking Crimes: Legal Obligations, Extralegal Factors, and the Bali Nine Case," *Columbia Human Rights Law Review* 40 (2009): 523.

40. Lorraine Finlay, "Exporting the Death Penalty? Reconciling International Police Cooperation and the Abolition of the Death Penalty in Australia," *Sydney Law Review* 33 (2011): 95.

41. *Rush v. Commissioner of Police* [2006] FCA 12.

42. *Rush*, para 22.

43. Finlay, *Exporting the Death Penalty?* 99.

44. Finlay, *Exporting the Death Penalty?* 99.

45. Lynn Bell, "Bali Nine Death Penalties Confirmed." *ABC News*, September 6, 2006. Accessed February 8, 2012. www.abc.net.au/pm/content/2006/s1734717.htm.

46. Hamish Fitzsimmons, "Govt to Seek Clemency over Bali Nine Death Sentences," *ABC News*, September 6, 2009. Accessed February 8, 2012. www.abc.net.au/7.30/content/2006/s1734780.htm.

47. Finlay, *Exporting the Death Penalty?* 99.

48. *Rush*.

49. *Rush*, para 70

50. *Rodriguez v. United States* 480 US 522 (1987) at 526.

51. *Rodriguez*, 526.

52. Ronli Sifris, "Balancing Abolitionism and Cooperation on the World's Scale: The Case of the Bali Nine," *Federal Law Review* 35, no. 1 (2007): 81.

53. Sifris, *Balancing Abolitionism*, 81.

54. Imparsial, "Inggris Anti Hukuman Mati (The English are Anti-Death Penalty)." Accessed February 8, 2012. www.imparsial.org/id/latest-news/inggris-anti-hukuman-mati.html.

55. Presiden Republik Indonesia (The President of the Republic of Indonesia), "Keputusan Presiden Republik Indonesia Nomor 17 Tahun 2011 Tentang Satuan Tugas Penanganan Kasus Warga Negara Indonesia/Tenaga Kerja Indonesia di Luar Negeri yang Terancam Hukuman Mati (Decision of the President of the Republic of Indonesia Number 17 Year 2011 about a Workforce on Cases of Indonesian Citizens and Labourers Overseas Threatened by the Death Penalty." Accessed February 3, 2012. www.presidenri.go.id/DokumenUU.php/725.pdf.

56. Kandis Scott, "Why Did China Reform Its Death Penalty?" *Pacific Rim Law and Policy Journal* 19, no. 1 (2010): 63–64.

57. Amnesty International, *Death Sentences and Executions 2010*, 5.

58. Dui Hua Foundation, "Criminal Justice." Accessed January 18, 2012. http://duihua.org/wp/?page_id=136.

59. Johnson and Zimring, *The Next Frontier*.

60. Lu Hong and Terance D. Miethe, *China's Death Penalty: History, Law, and Contemporary Practices*. New York: Routledge, 2007; 54–55. There were sixty-eight capital offenses in the 1997 Criminal Law. In 2011, the National People's Congress Standing Committee amended the Criminal Law and abolished death penalty for thirteen economic offenses.

61. Susan Trevaskes, "The Death Penalty in China Today: Kill Fewer, Kill Cautiously," *Asian Survey* 48, no. 3 (2008): 393.

62. Trevaskes, "The Death Penalty in China," 393.

63. Trevaskes, "The Death Penalty in China," 393.

64. Xin Zhomg Du, "2011 年中国禁毒报告 (2011 Anti-Drug Report)." 北京禁毒在线 *Beijing Anti-Drug Online*. State Drug Prohibition Commission, Drug Prohibition Report 2011. Accessed October 24, 2012. www.jhak.com/topic/2011-05/29/content_5773.html.

65. Jun Gong Sun, "最高法院：2010年以来毒品犯罪案件审理情况 (Supreme Court: Drug-Related Criminal Cases since 2010)." Eastern Eye on Law, SPC News Release, June 21, 2011. Accessed October 24, 2012. www.dffy.com/fazhixinwen/sifa/201106/23813.html.

66. Xu Anzh, "Death Penalty on Drug Offences and Judicial Experiences" *Faxue Pinglun (Law Review)* 162, no. 4 (2010): 38.

67. Xinhua, "7 Drug Traffickers Sentenced to Death." *China Daily*, December 23, 2011. Accessed January 25, 2012. www.chinadaily.com.cn/china/2011-12/23/content_14317625.htm.

68. Alexa Oleson, "China: Filipino Drug Trafficker Executed." *Huffington Post*, December 8, 2011. Accessed January 25, 2012. www.huffingtonpost.com/2011/12/08/china-filipino-drug-trafficker-executed_n_1136046.html.

69. Scott, *Why Did China Reform*, 68.

BIBLIOGRAPHY

Anzh, Xu. "Death Penalty on Drug Offences and Judicial Experiences" *Faxue Pinglun (Law Review)* 162, no. 4 (2010): 38.
Bedi., Rashvinjeet S. "Abolish Death Penalty, It's Wrong to Take Someone's Life, Says Nazri." *The Star Online*, August 29, 2010. Accessed January 12, 2012. http://thestar.com.my/news/story.asp?file=/2010/8/29/nation/6893246&sec=nation.
Bell, Lynn. "Bali Nine Death Penalties Confirmed." *ABC News*, September 6, 2006. Accessed February 8, 2012. www.abc.net.au/pm/content/2006/s1734717.htm.
Bernama. "Nazri: Abolition of Death Penalty Would Depend on Public Opinion." *The Star Online*, October 13, 2011. Accessed December 28, 2011. http://thestar.com.my/news/story.asp?file=/2011/10/13/nation/20111013225050&sec=nation.
Brown, Ben, Wm. Reed Benedict, and Kevin Buckler. "Support for the Death Penalty in Developing Democracies: A Binational Comparative Case Study." *International Criminal Justice Review* 20, no. 4 (2010): 398; 407.
Dangerous Drugs Act 1952, Act 234 (Laws of Malaysia)
Du, Xin Zhong. "2011 年中国禁毒报告 (2011 Anti-Drug Report)." 北京禁毒在线 *Beijing Anti-Drug Online*. State Drug Prohibition Commission, Drug Prohibition Report 2011. Accessed October 24, 2012. www.jhak.com/topic/2011-05/29/content_5773.html.
Dui Hua Foundation. "Criminal Justice." Accessed January 18, 2012. http://duihua.org/wp/?page_id=136.
Edwards, Griffith, Tom Babor, Shane Darke, Wayne Hall, John Marsden, Peter Miller, and Robert West. "Drug Trafficking: Time to Abolish the Death Penalty." *Addiction* 104, no. 8 (2009): 1267
Fitzsimmons, Hamish. "Govt to Seek Clemency over Bali Nine Death Sentences." *ABC News*, September 6, 2009. Accessed February 8, 2012. www.abc.net.au/7.30/content/2006/s1734780.htm.
Hong, Lu and Terance D. Miethe. *China's Death Penalty: History, Law, and Contemporary Practices*. New York: Routledge, 2007; 54–55.
HRI (Harm Reduction International). *The Death Penalty for Drug Offences: Global Overview 2011*. London: HRI, 2011.
Imparsial, "Inggris Anti Hukuman Mati (The English are Anti-Death Penalty)." Accessed February 8, 2012. www.imparsial.org/id/latest-news/inggris-anti-hukuman-mati.html.
Indian Harm Reduction Network v. The Union of India (2010) High Court of Judicature, Bombay, criminal writ petition no. 1784 of 2010, June 2010 quoted in Harm Reduction International, *The Death Penalty for Drug Offences: Global Overview 2011* at 14.
Johnson, David T. and Franlin E. Zimring. *The Next Frontier: National Development, Political Change, and the Death Penalty in Asia*. New York: Oxford University Press, 2009.
Lines, Rick. "A 'Most Serious Crime'? The Death Penalty for Drug Offences and International Human Rights Law." *Amicus Journal* 21 (2010): 21.

Lynch, Colman. "Indonesia's Use of Capital Punishment for Drug Trafficking Crimes: Legal Obligations, Extralegal Factors, and the Bali Nine Case." *Columbia Human Rights Law Review* 40 (2009): 523.

Ministry of Home Affairs. "Statistics given by the Ministry of Home Affairs in response to a question by Member of Parliament Haji Ahmad Lai Bujang in the Malaysian *Dewan Rakyat* (House of Representatives)." November 10, 2011. Accessed December 27, 2011. https://docs.google.com/document/d/1y2YTC05k9DM-AdkSu9GAlar1iat8BnJahhhpTJYg8gc/edit.

Neumayer, Eric. "Death Penalty: The Political Foundations of the Global Trend towards Abolition." *Human Rights Review* 9 (2008): 241–42.

New Straits Times. "Possible Moratorium on Death Sentence Pending Govt's Final Decision." *New Straits Times*, October 20, 2012. Accessed October 24, 2012. www.nst.com.my/latest/possible-moratorium-on-death-sentence-pending-govt-s-final-decision-1.159690#.

Oleson, Alexa. "China: Filipino Drug Trafficker Executed." *Huffington Post*, December 8, 2011. Accessed January 25, 2012. www.huffingtonpost.com/2011/12/08/china-filipino-drug-trafficker-executed_n_1136046.html.

Presiden Republik Indonesia (The President of the Republic of Indonesia), "Keputusan Presiden Republik Indonesia Nomor 17 Tahun 2011 Tentang Satuan Tugas Penanganan Kasus Warga Negara Indonesia/Tenaga Kerja Indonesia di Luar Negeri yang Terancam Hukuman Mati (Decision of the President of the Republic of Indonesia Number 17 Year 2011 about a Workforce on Cases of Indonesian Citizens and Labourers Overseas Threatened by the Death Penalty." Accessed February 3, 2012. www.presidenri.go.id/DokumenUU.php/725.pdf.

Rodriguez v. United States 480 US 522 (1987).

Scott, Kandis. "Why Did China Reform Its Death Penalty?" *Pacific Rim Law and Policy Journal* 19, no. 1 (2010): 63–64.

Sifris, Ronli. "Balancing Abolitionism and Cooperation on the World's Scale: The Case of the Bali Nine." *Federal Law Review* 35, no. 1 (2007): 81.

Sun, Jun Gong. "最高法院：2010年以来毒品犯罪案件审理情况 (Supreme Court: Drug-Related Criminal Cases since 2010)." Eastern Eye on Law, SPC News Release, June 21, 2011. Accessed October 24, 2012. www.dffy.com/fazhixinwen/sifa/201106/23813.html.

The Malaysian Bar. "Press Release: Abolish the Death Penalty Now." (October 13, 2011) Accessed January 14, 2012. www.malaysianbar.org.my/press_statements/press_release_abolish_the_death_penalty_now.html.

Trevaskes, Susan. "The Death Penalty in China Today: Kill Fewer, Kill Cautiously." *Asian Survey* 48, no. 3 (2008): 393.

Undang-Undang Republik Indonesia, Nomor 35 Tahun 2009 Tentang Narkotika, Article 113(2) [Laws of the Republic of Indonesia, Number 35 of Year 2009 on Narcotics, Article 113(2)].

UNHRC (UN Human Rights Committee). *UN Human Rights Committee: Concluding Observations: Kuwait*, 27 July 2000, CCPR/CO/69/KWT. Accessed October 24, 2012; para 13. www.unhcr.org/refworld/docid/3df36be44.html.

UNHRC (United Nations Human Rights Council). *Universal Periodic Review: Report of the Working Group on the Universal Periodic Review, Addendum, Malaysia.* Agenda Item No. 6, A/HRC/11/30/Add.1.; para 10, 2009. Accessed January 14, 2012. http://daccess-dds-ny.un.org/doc/UNDOC/GEN/G09/137/38/PDF/G0913738.pdf?OpenElement.

Unnever, James. "Global Support for the Death Penalty." *Punishment & Society* 12, no. 4 (2010): 463; 468.

UNODC (United Nations Office on Drugs and Crime). *2008 World Drug Report.* Geneva: UNODC, 2009.

UNODC (United Nations Office on Drugs and Crime). *2010 World Drug Report.* Geneva: UNODC, 2011; 24.

Xinhua. "7 Drug Traffickers Sentenced to Death." *China Daily*, December 23, 2011. Accessed January 25, 2012. www.chinadaily.com.cn/china/2011-12/23/content_14317625.htm.

Yong Vui Kong v. Attorney-General (4 April 2011), Civil Appeal No 144 of 2010.

Chapter Nineteen

Treatment for Drug Dependence in Asia

Marek Chawarski, Richard Schottenfeld,[1] and B. Vicknasingam[2]

This chapter provides an overview of the societal responses to drug dependence in the Asian region, focusing in particular on the transition from approaches based predominantly on criminal justice system and/or punitive measures to the introduction of medical treatments and public health approaches. Despite stringent law enforcement efforts and, in some settings, harsh punishment for drug users or drug dealers, the prevalence of illicit drug use and addiction and associated medical and social consequences (including HIV/AIDS) continued to increase substantially in the Asian region. The growing epidemic of illicit drug use and concerns that injection drug use was fueling the HIV/AIDS epidemic in the region prompted calls for acceptance of science- or evidence-based guidelines regarding public health responses to addiction and HIV prevention and led to the introduction of public health and medical approaches in several countries in Asia beginning in the mid- to late-1990s.

After providing a brief description of the medical model of addiction treatment and the components of medical treatments, the chapter discusses some of the challenges faced and problems encountered in the Asian region in making the transition to the medical approach, reviews some of the research conducted in the region regarding the efficacy and effectiveness of various treatments and treatment components, and concludes with a discussion of some of the current challenges faced in scaling up effective treatments and addressing emerging problems with new drugs and the opportunities for reducing drug addiction and associated problems in Asia.

TRANSITION FROM CRIMINAL JUSTICE SYSTEM AND PUNITIVE APPROACHES TO PUBLIC HEALTH AND MEDICAL TREATMENTS

Until recently, in most countries in Asia the primary responsibility to provide prevention, rehabilitation, and intervention services for illicit drug use and associated problems was given to specialized anti-narcotic branches of the government, public security, and the police. The long-standing reliance on deterrence and punishment resulted from broad societal and religious factors, which viewed illicit drug use and dependence as a moral problem or a vice, rather than as a public health or social problem. Deterrence focused primarily on efforts to punish drug users and drug dealers, often with very harsh criminal penalties. Many of the rehabilitation efforts were delivered on an involuntary basis, often for prolonged periods (one to two years or longer) in specially designated rehabilitation centers. Most of such residential rehabilitation centers are based on a penitentiary model, which confines the rehabilitants into a highly regulated and restrictive environment where illicit drugs are not easily available; these centers may also provide some educational and rehabilitation services in addition to work and limited recreational activities. For most rehabilitants, however, the transition from drug abstinence in a prison-like environment to prolonged recovery following release is difficult, and relapse rates following release have generally been very high. Often poorly equipped psychologically or emotionally to make the transition, without adequate social or family supports or employment opportunities, and facing the added stress of the stigma associated with incarceration or detention, very few individuals released from the residential centers are able to avoid relapse in settings where drugs continue to be readily available.[3, 4]

In addition to the problems with the conditions of confinement, negative labeling and stigmatization of drug rehabilitants, lack of specific and efficacious treatment interventions, and high relapse rates following discharge from involuntary, residential treatment, the focus on deterrence and punishment failed to stem the growing epidemic of drug problems. Misuse of illicit substances and the incidence of HIV infections among individuals misusing illicit drugs as well as in general populations continued to rise during the 1990s and 2000s,[5, 6] and drug use emerged throughout Asia as the major driver of the HIV/AIDS epidemic in the region during this period.[7] These failures of the primary public security measures prompted many governments in the region to reevaluate their overall approaches and policies toward tackling these important social problems. As a result, some governments, including Malaysia, Indonesia, China, Taiwan, Thailand, Myanmar, Vietnam, and Cambodia, allowed introduction and dissemination of health-care based or medical approaches, including medication-assisted treatments with buprenorphine or methadone. Because of important social, cultural, legal, or religious concerns, in all of these countries (described in previous chapters), the newly introduced health care or medical approaches did not replace but were allowed to coexist simultaneously with the traditional public security measures.

MEDICAL MODEL AND TREATMENTS OF DRUG DEPENDENCE

The principles of good medical practice for medically oriented treatments for drug dependence are rooted in a conceptualization of substance use disorders as closely resembling other chronic, medical disorders (e.g., diabetes, hypertension, or asthma) with regard to disease etiology, progression or natural history, treatment approach, and response to treatment.[8] This conceptualization is based on accumulated scientific evidence indicating that repeated and prolonged intake of many commonly misused illicit substances (opioids, ATS, other stimulants, benzodiazepines) results in dysregulation of normal brain functioning, which contributes to preoccupation with the drug and drug use, craving, impulsivity, and loss of control over drug use or compulsive use, despite adverse consequences of drug use, in addition to tolerance and physical dependence. The initial decision to use a drug reflects a complex interplay of individual and social factors (and also genetic factors, which may influence risk-taking behaviors and impulsivity). The transition from occasional use to dependence or addiction is also influenced by genetic, social, psychological, and neurobiological factors and vulnerabilities: the transition brings into play powerful neurobiological changes in addition to the powerful psychological, emotional, and social dynamics implicated in addiction. Behaviors that initially might have been relatively easy to discontinue become increasingly more resistant to change following this transition. The progression is similar to what occurs in the development of adult-onset diabetes (Type II diabetes) or hypertension, medical disorders that, like addictions, are persistent and associated with substantial increased morbidity and mortality risk. Prior to the onset of diabetes or hypertension for many patients, poor dietary habits and a lack of sufficient physical exercise contribute to the development of obesity, insulin-intolerance, or elevated blood pressure, especially in individuals at higher familial or genetic risk. Initially, changes in diet and exercise may be sufficient to reverse these processes, but once the individual develops diabetes or sustained hypertension, life-style changes alone may not be sufficient to reverse the biological changes or disease progression. Following the onset of diabetes or hypertension, effective treatment involves a combination of medication treatments, to address the biological factors implicated in the disease process, in addition to behavioral or lifestyle changes (e.g., regular exercise, dietary changes, and weight loss).

Components of Medical Treatments of Addictive Disorders

Medications

Medical treatments for addictive disorders may include both medications and psychosocial interventions to assist patients in their efforts to reduce or cease drug use, reduce the harmful consequences of their addiction, and improve their health and overall functional status and well-being. Medications used to treat addictive disorders may have one or more targets, including elimination, reduction, or prevention of drug-withdrawal symptoms; prevention or amelioration of drug craving or urges; reduction, attenuation, or blockade of the rewarding effects of drugs; alleviation of emotional or mental distress, which may contribute to craving and relapse; or improvement of emotional, cognitive, or decision-making functioning of the patient or reduction of impulsivity. For example, opioid antagonist medications, such as naltrexone, block or reduce the rewarding effects of opioids (and possibly also alcohol) and may also reduce craving through brain pathways involved in regulating craving. Opioid agonist medications (e.g., methadone or buprenorphine) used either for gradual short-term detoxification treatment or as long-term maintenance medications can greatly help to reduce opioid withdrawal symptoms, reduce drug cravings, reduce/attenuate/block the rewarding effects of illicit opiates, and possibly also stabilize mood and reduce impulsivity. Consequently, opioid antagonist medications and opioid agonist maintenance can play an important role in treatment of opioid dependence, as discussed in this section.

As reviewed in this section, there is substantial and compelling evidence supporting the efficacy and effectiveness of opioid agonist maintenance treatment for opioid dependence and strong evidence supporting the efficacy for selected patients of opioid antagonist maintenance treatment for opioid dependence and for alcohol dependence. Currently, however, there are no medications that have established efficacy for treating amphetamine-type stimulant dependence or dependence on other drugs. Consequently, this section on medication treatments focuses on medications used to treat opioid dependence.

Medications play an important role in medically supervised withdrawal from opioids ("detoxification"). A variety of medication regimens are efficacious in preventing or alleviating withdrawal symptoms and facilitating achievement of abstinence. Several reviews of the many regimens are available.[9, 10, 11, 12] In the absence of longer-term medical treatments to prevent relapse, however, detoxification alone is rarely effective in promoting recovery and may instead leave the patient at substantially increased risk for overdose death. Consequently, this chapter focuses on longer-term, medication maintenance treatments for opioid dependence.

Medication treatment with opioid antagonists (e.g., oral naltrexone or extended-release injection naltrexone) is an appealing option for some patients and many policymakers, because opioid antagonists have no abuse liability or rewarding or other noticeable mood- or mind-altering effects. Additionally, patients can discontinue taking opioid antagonists without experiencing any withdrawal. Antagonist maintenance treatment may also reduce overdose risk, but patients may overdose if they attempt to override the blockade by taking greater quantities of opioid drugs. Patients are also at a greatly increased risk of overdose after they discontinue the opioid antagonist, since they have lost tolerance to opioids and may even be supersensitive to opioid effects and overdose risk. In order to prevent the patient from experiencing severe opioid withdrawal precipitated by initiating of opioid antagonist treatment, patients first need to complete a medical withdrawal or detoxification, often in an inpatient or residential setting, before starting antagonist maintenance treatment.

Opioid antagonist maintenance treatment with naltrexone has demonstrated some efficacy in some settings and populations, but problems with low patient acceptability and poor medication adherence or retention in treatment have greatly limited the observed effectiveness of opioid antagonist treatments, especially with oral administration of naltrexone. With oral naltrexone, patients must take the pill daily (or higher doses three times per week); patients who forget to take the medication or stop taking it quickly lose any protective effects of the naltrexone within a few days and are then at high risk of relapse and overdose. Combining antagonist maintenance treatment with behavioral or psychosocial treatments may also improve the efficacy of antagonist maintenance treatment for some patients. Long-acting injectable formulations of naltrexone may also improve the overall effectiveness of antagonist maintenance treatment by improving medication adherence. To date, however, there are no countries or settings where opioid antagonist maintenance treatment has been effectively disseminated or scaled up to provide treatment to more than a very small proportion of opioid-dependent individuals. While individual patients and selected patient groups may benefit from opioid antagonist maintenance treatment—and antagonist maintenance treatment represents an important and useful treatment option for these patients—because of its limited reach and patient acceptability, from a public health perspective, opioid antagonist maintenance treatment has not had a major public health impact for the treatment of opioid dependence and prevention of problems associated with opioid dependence.

Opioid agonist maintenance treatments with methadone (MMT) or the partial agonist buprenorphine (BMT) address many of the potential targets for medical treatments of opioid dependence. Long-acting opioid agonists can be administered orally (e.g., methadone) or sublingually (e.g., buprenorphine) on a daily basis to prevent withdrawal or craving, which serve as some of the major drivers of illicit opioid use among opioid-dependent individuals. Oral or sublingual administration substitutes a considerably safer form of administration for injection drug use, which puts patients at high risk of infectious disease (e.g., hepatitis C or HIV). Oral or sublingual administration of the maintenance dose to a patient who has been consistently maintained at the daily dose does not cause euphoria or impair cognitive functioning. Unlike the use of heroin or other illicit opioid use, which destabilize mood and functioning by leading to a cycle throughout the day of initial production of euphoric effects followed by anxiety and withdrawal symptoms, once daily administration of opioid agonist maintenance medications helps stabilize mood within a "normal" range throughout a twenty-four-hour period. Additionally, once a patient has been slowly brought to and remains consistently at a sufficient dose, craving is absent or greatly reduced, and the patient has developed high tolerance to illicit opioids, so that heroin or other illicit drug use produces little or no rewarding effects.

From both an individual and a societal perspective, opioid agonist maintenance treatment has substantial public health and societal benefits. Opioid agonist maintenance treatment is generally very well tolerated by patients, and its high patient acceptability has facilitated rapid uptake of this treatment by patients and high retention in treatment. MMT and BMT produce substantial reductions in illicit opioid dependence, substantial reductions in mortality and morbidity risk associated with addiction, substantial protective benefits against HIV transmission, and substantial reductions in criminal activity and improvements in family, vocational, and social functioning. Because they are so effective as treatment for opioid dependence, can be scaled up rapidly, and are appealing as a treatment to a high proportion of opioid-addicted individuals (especially after some of the myths about problems caused by the treatment have been dispelled), MMT and BMT are considered essential medical treatments for opioid dependence. As reviewed in the following paragraphs, the effectiveness of MMT and BMT are substantially improved when medication maintenance is combined with psychosocial interventions, counseling or behavioral treatment.

Psychosocial Interventions, Counseling, and Behavioral Therapies

Psychosocial interventions employed in medical treatments of addictive disorders typically aim to improve patients' treatment engagement, medication adherence, and ongoing recovery efforts. Psychosocial interventions may include education about harmful effects of drugs and drug-use lifestyle; training in new and effective recovery skills and strategies and improved decision-making skills; guidance and encouragement in the patients' efforts to develop a lifestyle supportive of prolonged recovery from addictive disorders; behavioral monitoring of illicit drug use and goal attainment to identify when treatment is working effectively or when treatment may need to be adjusted to work more effectively; and implementation of graduated behavioral contingencies designed to encourage treatment adherence, abstinence from illicit drug use, and attainment of other treatment goals. Psychosocial interventions that are most commonly used in treatment of addictive disorders are based on broad cognitive-behavioral, motivational, and educational principles and approaches and are most effective when offered for a prolonged time in outpatient settings by trained specialty personnel (e.g., therapists, drug counselors, social workers, nurses).

Psychosocial interventions for addictive disorders are efficacious on their own,[13, 14, 15] and, at present, constitute the only medical interventions with proven efficacy for addiction to some drugs. (e.g., methamphetamine or other stimulants) for which currently there are no proven effective medication treatments. Psychosocial interventions are also an important component of effective medication maintenance treatments for addiction.[16] In medication-assisted or medically oriented treatments, education and counseling promote a recovery process. The detailed diagnosis of the disorder by the doctor or the medical team and education about the disease process and the recovery process provides the patient an understanding of the disease and recovery process and helps encourage adherence to the medications and full treatment regimen. Monitoring of the patient for progress in achieving psychosocial or behavioral goals or for signs of continued illicit drug use or relapse are critical components of treatment. Behavioral monitoring includes observation of the patient, self-report by the patient, and urine toxicology testing. Patients and medical practitioners need to appreciate that cycles of remission, followed by relapse, followed by remission may be common, especially early in the course of recovery. Monitoring of treatment progression is essential to ensure early detection of illicit drug use or relapse and appropriate modifications of treatment, including medication dose adjustments, changes in the frequency or focus of counseling, or implementation of interventions to retain patients in treatment or improve medication adherence or adherence to other components of treatment.

Conceptualization of substance dependence as a chronic and often persistent or relapsing medical disorder opens an opportunity to apply more general principles of best medical practices during the treatment of individuals seeking treatment for illicit substance use disorders and to adapt well-established evidence-based medical practice protocols pertaining to treatments of other chronic diseases. Consequently, treatment of illicit substance misuse disorders becomes less stigmatizing, more acceptable to the patients and societies, and can be made more available though dissemination of such treatments across the existing and typically well established networks of general health care services that already exist in many countries in the region.

Treatment setting: An increasing body of clinical research and accumulating clinical experience supports the feasibility and effectiveness of providing medical treatments for addictive disorders, including opioid agonist or antagonist maintenance treatment, in a variety of general medical practice or clinic settings.[17, 18] When offered and provided in primary medical care clinics or physician offices by trained medical personnel, medical treatments for addictive disorders have been found, in studies conducted by our research group and others, to be appealing and acceptable to patients and effective in reducing illicit drug use and adverse consequences of illicit drug use and improving functioning.[19, 20] Patient and provider satisfaction with opioid agonist maintenance treatment in primary care settings or physician office-based practices has been quite high.[21, 22, 23, 24, 25, 26, 27] The results of these studies indicate that significant recovery from opiate dependence can be achieved by many patients through medication-assisted or medically oriented treatments offered in general practice or primary care settings. The results of several small studies also support the feasibility of providing behavioral counseling along with opioid agonist maintenance treatment in primary medical care of physician office-based settings as well as the impact of behavioral counseling on improving drug-dependence treatment outcomes.[28, 29, 30, 31] Several other large-scale randomized clinical trials are also currently underway evaluating the effectiveness of these treatments in Asia and evaluating the impact of providing behavioral counseling in addition to opioid agonist maintenance treatment; when completed, these studies will build the evidence to better evaluate the efficacy of treating drug-dependent individuals in medical settings and the essential components of effective treatment.

CHALLENGES IN MAKING THE TRANSITION TO PUBLIC HEALTH AND MEDICAL APPROACHES AND PROBLEMS ENCOUNTERED

1. Problems with Medication Diversion and Abuse

Introduction of buprenorphine maintenance treatment, using buprenorphine mono-tablets (Subutex®) containing buprenorphine only (BUP), in Malaysia and Singapore in 2002[32, 33] was followed by a rapid uptake. In Malaysia, importation of BUP increased from 2 kg in 2002 to 12 kg in 2005 and 14 kg in 2006, and the number of general practitioners (GPs) prescribing BUP increased from less than 50 in 2002 to more than 500 in 2006.[34] Initially, any practicing, licensed general practitioner was allowed to prescribe Subutex for treatment of opiate dependence and to dispense the medication in their private offices; no detailed guidelines, training, or oversight of prescription and/ or dispensation procedures were offered or required. This largely unregulated approach may have facilitated the availability, accessibility, and rapid dissemination of buprenorphine treatment. Unfortunately, however, the rapid treatment implementation and dissemination model utilized in Malaysia, Singapore, and Indonesia resulted in frequent prescribing and dispensing of weekly or monthly take-home supplies of Suboxone for patients from the beginning of treatment and to widespread problems with diversion of buprenorphine for non-medically prescribed use or dependence, including injection drug use.[35, 36, 37] In response to the problems of diversion and misuse of BUP, Singapore reversed its drug treatment policy, significantly limiting availability or entirely discontinuing agonist maintenance treatments in 2006, while Malaysia adopted a multi-pronged strategy addressing some of the factors that may have contributed to the diversion problems.

In 2006, as part of their effort to reduce problems associated with buprenorphine diversion and abuse, the Malaysian government agencies started to offer a mandatory, brief (eight-hour workshop) training about agonist maintenance treatment for prescribing physicians. Starting in 2007, Buprenorphine mono-tablet (BUP) were replaced with a tablet combining buprenorphine and naloxone, an opioid antagonist. The buprenorphine/naloxone (BNX) combination tablet (Suboxone®) was designed to reduce the abuse liability of buprenorphine. Taken sublingually, as prescribed, the opioid antagonist, naloxone, in the BNX is minimally absorbed and does not precipitate withdrawal in opioid-dependent individuals or interfere with the efficacy of buprenorphine. When BNX is injected by an opioid-dependent individual, however, the naloxone in the BNX can precipitate severe withdrawal, and consequently the combination tablet may reduce the likelihood of BNX IDU.[38] In addition, Malaysia implemented a nationwide registry of patients receiving BNX. All prescribing physicians or treatment centers in Malaysia are required to record identities and basic demographic characteristics of patients receiving Suboxone treatment, including amounts of medications dispensed.

These changes in policy reduced but did not entirely eliminate the problems, as documented by our own research[39] and research by others.[40] Further efforts aimed at developing specific and detailed medical protocols, as well as improved training, and ongoing monitoring of prescribing, dispensing, and overall medical management of addiction treatment regimens, are necessary to further limit the diversion, misuse, or dependence on maintenance medications and to improve the overall addiction treatment efficacy.

2. Lack of Sufficient Numbers of Trained Medical Personnel

The current availability of medication-assisted treatments for substance misuse disorders is limited across the Asian region in part because of the relatively small number of general medical practitioners or other physicians trained to provide such treatment. Many physicians or other health professionals are also initially reluctant to treat individuals with addictions, because of a lack of training or experience and because of concerns that treatment will not be effective or that addicted patients will pose management problems that they are unable to handle in their practice setting. Physicians or other health care providers may be particularly reluctant to treat patients who are dependent on substances for which currently there are no efficacious medications (e.g., amphetamine type stimulants, benzodiazepines, ketamine, club drugs, or marijuana), especially given their lack of training or experience providing counseling or behavioral treatments.

Additionally, even when medical treatments for addictive disorders are being scaled up, such as is occurring currently with regard to opioid agonist maintenance treatment in many countries in the region, the lack of highly trained, experienced medical personnel leads to problems in treatment implementation and less than optimal service delivery. Examples of deficiencies that we observed often in many newly implemented treatment programs include insufficient or incomplete diagnostic evaluation when initiating the treatment (e.g., leading, for example, to administration of opioid agonist maintenance treatment to individuals who were not dependent on opioids or to the failure to diagnose co-occurring benzodiazepine use or dependence, which could compromise the safety of patients prescribed opioid agonist maintenance treatment) and both too rapid or too slow medication induction phases of opioid agonist maintenance treatment, resulting in sometimes dangerously high medication doses in the first days of treatment, or in very low, suboptimal maintenance doses throughout the entire treatment. Additionally, the combination of a very strong reliance on the medication components of treatment with frequent requests or demands by patients to receive additional medications to alleviate anxiety symptoms or sleep difficulties, which might best be managed by behavioral or psychosocial counseling, frequently results in overprescribing of benzodiazepine medications. These medications can become problem drugs for the recovering patient and can increase the risk of adverse consequences, including overdose, when abused or combined with illicit drug use. Consequently, in general, the use of benzodiazepines in treatment of addictions should be limited. In many treatment implementation efforts we also observed a lack of monitoring of treatment progression. Many programs or providers rarely or never conduct urine toxicology testing to objectively assess ongoing illicit drug use and many fail to assess regularly through self-report ongoing illicit drug use, medication compliance, changes in risk behaviors, or improvements in medical or functional status. The accuracy of patients' self-report can be improved by interviewing the patient in a private setting, ensuring confidentiality of the information obtained, asking questions and responding to the patient in a non-judgmental and non-punitive fashion, and conducting urine toxicology testing to verify self-report and encourage accuracy in disclosure.

Some of these limitations can be overcome by introducing or extending addiction training curricula during the medical education programs or by providing additional addiction training and certification to physicians and other health care providers. Development of local centers of excellence for drug dependence treatment, clinical research, and training will facilitate scale-up of effective medical treatments throughout Asia and also play a critical role in the development and evaluation of improved medical treatment protocols for addictive disorders.

3. Program of Systemic Factors Impeding the Effectiveness of Dissemination Efforts

Treatment costs and other treatment program factors have also impeded effective scale-up and dissemination efforts. The high cost as well as the payment structure of many opioid agonist maintenance treatment services (e.g., requiring fixed, additional payments for each day of treatment) deters many opioid-dependent individuals from seeking treatment or from taking a sufficiently high dose of the opioid agonist maintenance medication on a regular daily basis to obtain full benefits of treatment. In some settings, patients come for their maintenance dose only when they have sufficient funds to cover the cost of treatment for that day. When patients need to pay on a daily basis for each dose of the maintenance medication, patients may also decide on a day-to-day basis whether they would prefer to pay for the maintenance medication dose or use the money to purchase heroin or other opioids illicitly. Providing opioid agonist maintenance medications for free or at a very low cost, having patients pay in advance for a week or a month of maintenance treatment, or charging a flat fee for the maintenance medication regardless of dose (so that taking an adequate dose does not cost the patient more than taking a subtherapeutic dose) may shift the contingencies to encourage regular, daily adherence with an optimal dose of the opioid agonist medication during maintenance treatment. Other burdens of drug dependence treatments (e.g., a requirement for daily attendance or inconvenient locations or operating hours of the clinics) may be barriers to treatment entry or regular attendance and treatment adherence. Moreover, drug counseling or other forms of psychosocial or ancillary services are only rarely provided (due to both the lack of trained personnel and the lack of understanding or appreciation of the role and importance of counseling). When they are provided, many patients perceive them as an unnecessary burden or sometimes punishment, resulting in low attendance rates in such services. In many settings, a combination of such implementation factors or limitations has resulted in a situation where patients most often engage in treatments for only very short periods of time or intermittently navigate between short periods of recovery and ongoing illicit drug use for extended periods of time. While such treatments offer some help, and may contribute somewhat to the reduction or curtailment of the illicit drug use and associated problems, the overall effectiveness of such treatment are significantly reduced.

In some settings, police have responded to the provision of medical treatments for addictive disorders by stepping up law enforcement activities immediately outside of the treatment program, targeting individuals who use the program for increased surveillance or detention, or entering the program premises to arrest patients. Needless to say, these misguided efforts can have a chilling effect of enrollment or continued participation in drug dependence treatment and undercut national efforts to expand medical treatments as one essential component of an effective public health policy.

4. Emergence of Other Drugs, in Addition to Heroin and Opiods

Historically opium and opiate-based drugs (e.g., heroin and morphine) were the dominant illicit and problem drugs in the Asian region. Recently, many countries in Asia experienced a dramatic, epidemic increase in use, misuse, or dependence on amphetamine-type stimulants,[41, 42, 43, 44, 45] and in some regions also ketamine, club drugs, or other synthetic or plant-based drugs.[46] While currently there are no medication-based treatments that are approved or highly efficacious for dependence of amphetamine-type stimulants, benzodiazepines, ketamine, club drugs, or marijuana, some patients presenting with such problems can achieve good progress when treated by medical providers using psychosocial approaches and possibly also some available medications that appear promising as potential treatments while research to discover new and more efficacious treatments is still ongoing.

5. Misconceptions about Opioid Agonist Maintenance Treatment

Medication-assisted treatments are often incorrectly put under the umbrella of drug replacement or drug-substitution therapies, especially opioid agonist maintenance treatment. The term "drug replacement or drug-substitution therapy" in itself is confusing and frequently leads to misinterpretation and misattribution of the roles that medications play in the recovery process. For most patients, medications cannot fully replace or substitute for the desirable effects of illicit drugs taken in intimate, private, or social settings; therefore, many continue to interchangeably use prescribed maintenance medications and illicit drugs. However, this severely undermines the effectiveness of opioid agonist maintenance treatment. In some settings, interchangeable use of illicit opioids and agonist medications has also been inadvertently promoted by policies or treatments that fail to provide adequate doses of maintenance medications or fail to ensure adequate medication adherence (as evidenced by frequent missed medications). Additionally, provision of opioid agonist maintenance medications without adequate supervision or efforts to deter diversion for non-medically prescribed use may also contribute to ineffective maintenance treatment or lead to problems with abuse of the maintenance medication. Opioid agonist medications have misuse/abuse potential and, when dispensed without regulations, oversight, or monitoring, can easily lead to significant diversion problems. When misused, these medications can cause health, social, and life's opportunity problems akin to those resulting from misuse of other illicit substances. Finally, in the context of very low purity/quality of street drugs in Southeast Asia, pharmaceutically produced medications can also become highly desirable illicit substances and can fuel the spread of illicit substance misuse problems in the region.[47, 48, 49, 50, 51]

When medication-assisted treatments are mislabeled as drug replacement or drug substitution therapies, the role that the medication plays in the recovery process is also often overemphasized. Medications falsely become viewed as the primary or the only agent of recovery. Very little additional services or recovery support is offered or provided besides the dispensation of the medications. Both treatment providers and the recovering individuals are readily inclined to treat any ancillary co-occurring symptoms with additional medications, often incompatible with the opioid agonist maintenance medication (e.g., prescription of benzodiazepines for sleep problems or anxiety in MMT or BMT). Recovering individuals themselves solidify their entrenched view that discomforts or problems can only be treated with medications or drugs and that they cannot otherwise learn to cope with these problems successfully without resorting to drug use. This self-defeating view contributes to the persistence of drug dependence during MMT or BMT.

The term drug substitution or drug-replacement therapy also continues to fuel social stigma of such treatments due to misinterpretation of these treatments as the replacement of one addiction with another. In some parts of Southeast Asia and/or in some portions of societies in the region, if recovery is achieved through drug substitution or drug-replacement therapy, it is perceived at best as partial and lesser than "a full recovery," associated with the achievement of prolonged substance- and medication-free abstinence.

Contrary to this misperception or misunderstanding about medical treatments for addiction (and specifically about opioid agonist maintenance treatment), in medication-assisted treatments, the medications are not the only or the primary agents of recovery. Opioid agonist maintenance medications, when taken regularly, as prescribed, and at a sufficient dose, can provide a stable base for the patient to engage in meaningful recovery activity. Similar to treatments for other chronic medical conditions (e.g., diabetes or high blood pressure), the potential facilitative effect of medications should be combined with monitoring of treatment progress or symptoms recurrence, adjustment or change of treatment regimens as necessary (e.g., in response to a lack of adequate progress) and changes in patients' daily behavioral patterns, activity levels, and lifestyle that support stable, long-term recovery and help prevent symptom reoccurrence or disease progression or complications.

OPPORTUNITIES AND NEEDS

Many of the challenges and needs faced in Asia with regard to effective dissemination of medically oriented treatments for substance-use disorders can be successfully addressed by expanding medical and social and behavioral science education curricula to include more extensive training and certification in addiction medicine and in psychosocial or behavioral interventions for substance dependence disorders. A model based on country- or region-wide centers of excellence for drug dependence treatment, research, and training could be particularly promising. Collaborative efforts between practitioners, researchers, and educators focused on developing local expertise, developing and adapting treatment guidelines targeting unique or specific patient characteristics, developing or adapting treatment protocols utilizing local resources or infrastructure, and adapted to the specific local cultural, social, and economic contexts can accelerate progress that has been made so far in transitioning from criminal justice approaches to medical and public health approaches. Several countries in Asia, including Malaysia, China, Taiwan, and Thailand among others, have accumulated extensive experience and technological know-how and have developed local expertise during their own implementation and dissemination efforts aimed at introducing and expanding medication-assisted treatments for substance-dependence disorders. Current achievements stemming from these initial efforts combined with best research and practice evidence collected in other parts of the world could be used as springboards to train drug dependence clinicians and clinical researchers in Asia. Centers of excellence could also help to hone research and clinical skills for professionals from outside the center, help to develop treatment monitoring and evaluation protocols, and conduct research and development on medical treatments for locally relevant or newly emerging substance dependence problems in Asia (e.g., ATS, ketamine, other plant-based or synthetic drugs).

NOTES

1. Yale University School of Medicine, New Haven, CT.
2. Centre for Drug Research, Universiti Sains Malaysia.
3. Jamila K. Stockman and Steffanie A. Strathdee, "HIV Among People Who Use Drugs: A Global Perspective of Populations at Risk," *Journal of Acquired Immune Deficiency Syndromes* 55 (2010): S17–S22.
4. Kanna Hayashi, M-J Milloy, Nadia Fairbairn, Karyn Kaplan, Paisan Suwannawong, Calvin Lai, Evan Wood, and Thomas Kerr, "Incarceration Experiences among a Community-

Recruited Sample of Injection Drug Users in Bangkok, Thailand," *BMC Public Health* 9 (2009): 492.

5. UNODC (United Nations Office on Drugs and Crime), *World Drug Report 2010* (Vienna: UNODC, 2011).

6. UNODC (United Nations Office on Drugs and Crime), *World Drug Report 2011* (Vienna: UNODC, 2012).

7. UNODC, *World Drug Report 2011*.

8. Thomas A. McLellan, A. Thomas, David C. Lewis, Charles P. O'Brien, and Herbert D. Kleber, "Drug Dependence, a Chronic Medical Illness. Implications for Treatment, Insurance, and Outcomes Evaluation," *JAMA*. 284, no. 13 (2000): 1689–95.

9. Richard P. Mattick, Courtney Breen, Jo Kimber, and Marina Davoli, "Methadone Maintenance Therapy versus No Opioid Replacement Therapy for Opioid Dependence," *Cochrane Database of Systematic Reviews* 3 (2009). CD002209. DOI: 10.1002/14651858.CD002209.pub2.

10. Richard P. Mattick, Jo Kimber, Courtney Breen, and Marina Davoli, "Buprenorphine Maintenance versus Placebo or Methadone Maintenance for Opioid Dependence," *Cochrane Database of Systematic Reviews* 2 (2008), CD002207. DOI: 10.1002/14651858.CD002207.pub3.

11. Jennifer C. Veilleux, Peter J. Colvin, Jennifer Anderson, Catherine York, and Adrienne J. Heinz, "A Review of Opioid Dependence Treatment: Pharmacological and Psychosocial Interventions to treat Opioid Addiction," *Clinical Psychology Review* 30 (2010): 155–66.

12. Silvia Minozzi, Laura Amato, Simona Vecchi, Marina Davoli, Ursula Kirchmayer, and Annette Verster, "Oral Naltrexone Maintenance Treatment for Opioid Dependence," *Cochrane Database of Systematic Reviews* 4 (2011), CD001333. DOI: 10.1002/14651858.CD001333.pub4.

13. Kathleen M. Carroll, "Integrating Psychotherapy and Pharmacotherapy to Improve Drug Abuse Outcomes," *Addictive Behaviors* 22 (1997): 233–45.

14. Lissa Dutra, Georgia Stathopoulou, Shawnee L. Basden, Teresa M. Leyro, Mark B. Powers, and Michael W. Otto, "A Meta-Analytic Review of Psychosocial Interventions for Substance Use Disorders," *American Journal of Psychiatry* 165 (2008): 179–87.

15. Veilleux et al., *A Review of Opioid Dependence*, 155–66.

16. Thomas A. McLellan, Isabelle O. Arndt, David S. Metzger, George E. Woody, and Charles P. O'Brien, "The Effects of Psychosocial Services in Substance Abuse Treatment," *Journal of Addictions Nursing* 5, no. 2 (1993): 38–47.

17. David A. Fiellin, Michael V. Pantalon, Marek C. Chawarski, Brent A. Moore, Lynn E. Sullivan, Patrick G. O'Connor, and Richard S. Schottenfeld, "Counseling plus Buprenorphine-Naloxone Maintenance Therapy for Opioid Dependence," *New England Journal of Medicine* 355, no. 4 (2006): 365–74.

18. David A. Fiellin, Patrick G. O'Connor, Juliana P. Pakes, Marek C. Chawarski, Michael V. Pantalon, and Richard S. Schottenfeld, "Methadone Maintenance in Primary Care: a Randomized Controlled Trial," *JAMA* 286 (2001): 1724–31.

19. Chawarski et al., *Lifetime ATS Use*, 177–80.

20. Richard S. Schottenfeld, Marek C. Chawarski, and Mahmud Mazlan, "Maintenance treatment with Buprenorphine and Naltrexone for Heroin Dependence in Malaysia: A Randomized Double-Blind Placebo-Controlled Trial," *Lancet* 371 (2008): 2192–200.

21. Declan T. Barry, Brent A. Moore, Michael V. Pantalon, Marek C. Chawarski, Lynn E. Sullivan, Patrick G. O'Connor, Richard S. Schottenfeld, and David A. Fiellin, "Patient Satisfaction with Primary Care Office-based Buprenorphine/Naloxone Treatment," *Journal of General Internal Medicine* 22 (2007): 242–45.

22. David A. Fiellin, Brent A. Moore, Lynn E. Sullivan, William C. Becker, Michael V. Pantalon, Marek C. Chawarski, Declan T. Barry, Patrick G. O'Connor, and Richard S. Schottenfeld, "Long-term Treatment with Buprenorphine/Naloxone in Primary Care: Results at 2–5 Years," *The American Journal on Addictions* 17 (2008): 116–20.

23. David A. Fiellin, Michael V. Pantalon, Julianna Pakes, Patrick G. O'Connor, Marek C. Chawarski, and Richard S. Schottenfeld, "Treatment of Heroin Dependence with Buprenor-

phine in Primary Care," *American Journal of Drug and Alcohol Abuse* 28, no. 2 (2002): 231–41.

24. Fiellin et al., *Methadone Maintenance*, 1724–31.

25. Brent A. Moore, David A. Fiellin, Declan T. Barry, Lynn E. Sullivan, Marek C. Chawarski, Patrick G. O'Connor, and Richard S. Schottenfeld, "Primary Care Office-Based Buprenorphine Treatment: Comparison of Heroin and Prescription Opioid Dependent Patients," *Journal of General Internal Medicine* 22 (2007): 527–30.

26. Lynn E. Sullivan, Brent A. Moore, Marek C. Chawarski, Michael V. Pantalon, Declan T. Barry, Patrick G. O'Connor, Richard S. Schottenfeld, and David A. Fiellin, "Buprenorphine/Naloxone Treatment in Primary Care is associated with Decreased HIV Risk Behaviors," *Journal of Substance Abuse Treatment* 35 (2008): 87–92.

27. Lynn E. Sullivan, Brent A. Moore, Marek C. Chawarski, Richard S. Schottenfeld, Patrick G. O'Connor, and David A. Fiellin, "Buprenorphine Reduces HIV Risk Behavior among Opioid Dependent Patients in Primary Care," *Journal of General Internal Medicine* 20 (Suppl.1) (2005): 172.

28. Marek C. Chawarski, Wang Zhou, and Richard S. Schottenfeld, "Behavioral Drug and HIV Risk Reduction counseling (BDRC) in MMT Programs in Wuhan, China: A Pilot Randomized Clinical Trial," *Drug and Alcohol Dependence* 115 (2011): 237–39.

29. Marek C. Chawarski, Mahmud Mazlan, and Richard S. Schottenfeld, "Behavioral Drug and HIV Risk Reduction Counseling (BDRC) with Abstinence-Contingent Take-Home Buprenorphine: A Pilot Randomized Clinical Trial," *Drug and Alcohol Dependence* 94 (2008): 281–84.

30. Fiellin et al., *Counseling plus Buprenorphine-Naloxone*, 365–74.

31. David A. Fiellin, Michael V. Pantalon, Marek C. Chawarski, Lynn E. Sullivan, Declan T. Barry, P. O'Connor, and R. S. Schottenfeld, "Counseling and Attendance Requirements for Buprenorphine Treatment in Primary Care," *Journal of General Internal Medicine* 20 (Suppl.1), (2005): 173–74.

32. C. E. Lee, "Tackling Subutex Abuse in Singapore," *Singapore Medical Journal.* 47 (2006): 919.

33. Schottenfeld et al., *Maintenance Treatment*, 2192–2200.

34. Balasingam Vicknasingam, Mahmud Mazlan, Marek C. Chawarski, and Richard S. Schottenfeld, "Injecting Buprenorphine in Malaysia: Demographic and Drug Use Characteristics of Buprenorphine Injectors." Paper presented at the College on Problems of Drug Dependence (CPDD) 69th Annual Scientific Meeting, Quebec City, Canada, June 16–21, 2007.

35. R. Douglas Bruce, Sumathi Govindasamy, S. Laurie Sylla, Marwan S. Haddad, Adeeba Kamarulzaman, and Frederick Altice, "Case Series of Buprenorphine Injectors in Kuala Lumpur, Malaysia," *American Journal of Drug Alcohol Abuse* 34 (2008): 511–17.

36. McLellan et al., *Drug Dependence, A Chronic Medical Illness*, 1689–95.

37. Balasingam Vicknasingam, Mahmud Mazlan, Richard S. Schottenfeld, and Marek C. Chawarski, "Injection of Buprenorphine and Buprenorphine/Naloxone Tablets in Malaysia," *Drug and Alcohol Dependence* 111 (2010): 44–49.

38. John Mendelson and Reese T. Jones, "Clinical and Pharmacological Evaluation of Buprenorphine and Naloxone Combinations: Why the 4:1 Ratio for Treatment?" *Drug Alcohol Dependence* 70 (2003): S29–37

39. Vicknasingam et al., *Injection of Buprenorphine*, 44–49.

40. R. Douglas Bruce, Sumathi Govindasamy, Laurie Sylla, Adeeba Kamarulzaman, and Frederick Altice, "Lack of Reduction in Buprenorphine Injection after Introduction of Co-formulated buprenorphine/naloxone to the Malaysian Market," *American Journal of Drug and Alcohol Abuse* 35 (2009): 68–72.

41. Chawarski et al., *Lifetime ATS Use*, 177–80.

42. Grant Colfax, Glenn-Milo Santos, Priscilla Chu, Eric Vittinghoff, Andreas Pluddemann, Suresh Kumar, and Carl Hart, "Amphetamine-group Substances and HIV," *Lancet* 376 (2010): 458–74.

43. Louisa Degenhardt, Bradley Mathers, Mauro Guarinieri, Samiran Panda, Benjamin Phillips, Steffanie A. Strathdee, Mark Tyndall, Lucas Wiessing, Alex Wodak, John Howard, and the Reference Group to the United Nations on HIV and Injecting Drug Use, "Meth/ampheta-

mine Use and Associated HIV: Implications for Global Policy and Public Health," *International Journal of Drug Policy* 21 (2010): 347–58.

44. Rebecca McKetin, Nicholas Kozel, Jeremy Douglas, Robert Ali, Balasingam Vicknasingam, Johannes Lund, and Jih-Heng Li, "The Rise of Methamphetamine in Southeast and East Asia," *Drug Alcohol Review* 2 (2008): 220–28.

45. UNODC (United Nations Office on Drugs and Crime), *Patterns and Trends of Amphetamine-Type Stimulants and Other Drugs: Asia and the Pacific.* A Report from the Global SMART Programme (Vienna: UNODC, 2011).

46. Jih-Heng Li, Balasingam Vicknasingam, Yuet-Wah Cheung, Wang Zhou, Adhi Wibowo Nurhidayat, Don C. Des Jarlais, and Richard S. Schottenfeld, "To Use or not to Use: an Update on Licit and Illicit Ketamine Use," *Substance Abuse and Rehabilitation.* 2 (2011): 11–20.

47. Shane Darke, Joanne Ross, Maree Teesson, and Michael Lynskey, "Health Service Utilization and Benzodiazepine use among Heroin Users: Findings from the Australian Treatment Outcome Study (ATOS)." *Addiction* 98, no. 8 (2003): 1129–35.

48. Balasingam Vicknasingam and V. Navaratnam, "The Use of Rapid Assessment Methodology to Compliment Existing National Assessment and Surveillance Data: A Study among Injecting Drug Users in, Penang, Malaysia," *International Journal of Drug Policy* 19 (2008): 90–93.

49. Bruce et al., *Case Series*, 511–17.

50. Bruce et al., *Lack of Reduction*, 68–72.

51. Vicknasingam et al., *Injection of Buprenorphine*, 44–49.

BIBLIOGRAPHY

Barry, Declan T., Brent A. Moore, Michael V. Pantalon, Marek C. Chawarski, Lynn E. Sullivan, Patrick G. O'Connor, Richard S. Schottenfeld, and David A. Fiellin. "Patient Satisfaction with Primary Care Office-based Buprenorphine/Naloxone Treatment." *Journal of General Internal Medicine* 22 (2007): 242–45.

Bruce, R. Douglas, Sumathi Govindasamy, S. Laurie Sylla, Marwan S. Haddad, Adeeba Kamarulzaman, and Frederick Altice, "Case Series of Buprenorphine Injectors in Kuala Lumpur, Malaysia," *American Journal of Drug Alcohol Abuse* 34 (2008): 511–17.

Bruce, R. Douglas, Sumathi Govindasamy, Laurie Sylla, Adeeba Kamarulzaman, and Frederick Altice. "Lack of Reduction in Buprenorphine Injection after Introduction of Co-formulated buprenorphine/naloxone to the Malaysian Market." *American Journal of Drug and Alcohol Abuse* 35 (2009): 68–72.

Carroll, Kathleen M. "Integrating Psychotherapy and Pharmacotherapy to Improve Drug Abuse Outcomes." *Addictive Behaviors* 22 (1997): 233–45.

Chawarski, Marek C., Vicknasingam Balasingam, M. Mazlan, and Richard S. Schottenfeld, "Lifetime ATS Use and Increase HIV Risk among Not-in-Treatment Opiate Injectors in Malaysia," *Drug and Alcohol Dependence* 124 (2012): 177–80.

Chawarski, Marek C., Mahmud Mazlan, and Richard S. Schottenfeld, "Behavioral Drug and HIV risk Reduction Counseling (BDRC) with Abstinence-contingent Take-home Buprenorphine: A Pilot Randomized Clinical Trial," *Drug and Alcohol Dependence* 94 (2008): 281–84.

Chawarski, Marek C., Wang Zhou, and Richard S. Schottenfeld, "Behavioral Drug and HIV Risk Reduction counseling (BDRC) in MMT Programs in Wuhan, China: A Pilot Randomized Clinical Trial," *Drug and Alcohol Dependence* 115 (2011): 237–39.

Colfax, Grant, Glenn-Milo Santos, Priscilla Chu, Eric Vittinghoff, Andreas Pluddemann, Suresh Kumar, and Carl Hart, "Amphetamine-group Substances and HIV," *Lancet* 376 (2010): 458–74.

Darke, Shane, Joanne Ross, Maree Teesson, and Michael Lynskey, "Health Service Utilization and Nenzodiazepine use among Heroin Users: Findings from the Australian Treatment Outcome Study (ATOS)." *Addiction* 98, no. 8 (2003): 1129–35.

Degenhardt, Louisa, Bradley Mathers, Mauro Guarinieri, Samiran Panda, Benjamin Phillips, Steffanie A. Strathdee, Mark Tyndall, Lucas Wiessing, and Alex Wodak, John Howard, and the Reference Group to the United Nations on HIV and Injecting Drug Use. "Meth/ampheta-mine use and associated HIV: Implications for Global Policy and Public Health." *International Journal of Drug Policy* 21 (2010): 347–58.

Dutra, Lissa, Georgia Stathopoulou, Shawnee L. Basden, Teresa M. Leyro, Mark B. Powers, and Michael W. Otto. "A Meta-Analytic Review of Psychosocial Interventions for Substance Use Disorders." *American Journal of Psychiatry* 165 (2008): 179–87.

Fiellin, David A., Brent A. Moore, Lynn E. Sullivan, William C. Becker, Michael V. Pantalon, Marek C. Chawarski, Declan T. Barry, Patrick G. O'Connor, and Richard S. Schottenfeld, "Long-term Treatment with Buprenorphine/Naloxone in Primary Care: Results at 2–5 Years." *American Journal on Addictions* 17 (2008): 116–20.

Fiellin, David A., Patrick G. O'Connor, Juliana P. Pakes, Marek C. Chawarski, Michael V. Pantalon, and Richard S. Schottenfeld. "Methadone Maintenance in Primary Care: a Randomized Controlled Trial." *JAMA* 286 (2001): 1724–31.

Fiellin, David A., Michael V. Pantalon, Marek C. Chawarski, Lynn E. Sullivan, Declan T. Barry, P. O'Connor, and R. S. Schottenfeld, "Counseling and Attendance Requirements for Buprenorphine Treatment in Primary Care," *Journal of General Internal Medicine* 20 (Suppl.1), (2005): 173–74.

Fiellin, David A., Michael V. Pantalon, Marek C. Chawarski, Brent A. Moore, Lynn E. Sullivan, Patrick G. O'Connor, and Richard S. Schottenfeld, "Counseling plus Buprenorphine-Naloxone Maintenance Therapy for Opioid Dependence" *New England Journal of Medicine* 355, no. 4 (2006): 365–74.

Fiellin, David A., Michael V. Pantalon, Julianna Pakes, Patrick G. O'Connor, Marek C. Chawarski, and Richard S. Schottenfeld, "Treatment of Heroin Dependence with Buprenorphine in Primary Care," *American Journal of Drug and Alcohol Abuse* 28, no. 2 (2002): 231–41.

Hayashi, Kanna, M-J. Milloy, Nadia Fairbairn, Karyn Kaplan, Paisan Suwannawong, Calvin Lai, Evan Wood, and Thomas Kerr, "Incarceration Experiences among a Community-Recruited Sample of Injection Drug Users in Bangkok, Thailand," *BMC Public Health* 9 (2009): 492.

Lee, C. E. "Tackling Subutex Abuse in Singapore." *Singapore Medical Journal* 47 (2006): 919.

Li, Jih-Heng, Balasingam Vicknasingam, Yuet-Wah Cheung, Wang Zhou, Adhi Wibowo Nurhidayat, Don C. Des Jarlais, and Richard S. Schottenfeld, "To Use or Not To Use: An Update on Licit and Illicit Ketamine Use," *Substance Abuse and Rehabilitation.* 2 (2011): 11–20.

Mattick, Richard P., Courtney Breen, Jo Kimber, and Marina Davoli. "Methadone maintenance therapy versus no opioid replacement therapy for opioid dependence." *Cochrane Database of Systematic Reviews* 3 (2009), CD002209. DOI: 10.1002/14651858.CD002209.pub2.

Mattick, Richard P., Jo Kimber, Courtney Breen, and Marina Davoli. "Buprenorphine Maintenance versus Placebo or Methadone Maintenance for Opioid Dependence." *Cochrane Database of Systematic Reviews* 2 (2008), CD002207. DOI: 10.1002/14651858.CD002207.pub3.

McKetin, Rebecca, Nicholas Kozel, Jeremy Douglas, Robert Ali, Balasingam Vicknasingam, Johannes Lund, and Jih-Heng Li. "The Rise of Methamphetamine in Southeast and East Asia." *Drug Alcohol Review* 2 (2008): 220–28.

McLellan, A. Thomas, Isabelle O. Arndt, David S. Metzger, George E. Woody, and Charles P. O'Brien, "The Effects of Psychosocial Services in Substance Abuse Treatment." *Journal of Addictions Nursing* 5, no. 2 (1993): 38–47.

McLellan, A. Thomas, David C. Lewis, Charles P. O'Brien, and Herbert D. Kleber, "Drug Dependence, a Chronic Medical Illness. Implications for Treatment, Insurance, and Outcomes Evaluation." *JAMA* 284, no. 13 (2000): 1689–95.

Mendelson, John and Reese T. Jones. "Clinical and Pharmacological Evaluation of Buprenorphine and Naloxone Combinations: Why the 4:1 Ratio for Treatment?" *Drug Alcohol Dependence* 70 (2003): S29–37.

Minozzi, Silvia, Laura Amato, Simona Vecchi, Marina Davoli, Ursula Kirchmayer, and Annette Verster. "Oral naltrexone maintenance treatment for opioid dependence." *Cochrane Database of Systematic Reviews* 4 (2011), CD001333. DOI: 10.1002/14651858.CD001333.pub4.

Moore, Brent A., David A. Fiellin, Declan T. Barry, Lynn E. Sullivan, Marek C. Chawarski, Patrick G. O'Connor, and Richard S. Schottenfeld. "Primary Care Office-based Buprenorphine Treatment: Comparison of Heroin and Prescription Opioid Dependent Patients." *Journal of General Internal Medicine* 22 (2007): 527–30.

Schottenfeld, Richard S., Marek C. Chawarski, and Mahmud Mazlan. "Maintenance treatment with Buprenorphine and Naltrexone for Heroin Dependence in Malaysia: a Randomized Double-Blind Placebo-controlled trial." *Lancet* 371 (2008): 2192–2200.

Stockman, Jamila K. and Steffanie A. Strathdee. "HIV Among People Who Use Drugs: A Global Perspective of Populations at Risk." *Journal of Acquired Immune Deficiency Syndromes* 55 (2010): S17–S22.

Sullivan, Lynn E., Brent A. Moore, Marek C. Chawarski, Michael V. Pantalon, Declan T. Barry, Patrick G. O'Connor, Richard S. Schottenfeld, and David A. Fiellin. "Buprenorphine/ naloxone Treatment in Primary Care is associated with Decreased HIV Risk Behaviors." *Journal of Substance Abuse Treatment* 35 (2008): 87–92.

Sullivan, Lynn E., Brent A. Moore, Marek C. Chawarski, Richard S. Schottenfeld, Patrick G. O'Connor, and David A. Fiellin. "Buprenorphine Reduces HIV Risk Behavior among Opioid Dependent Patients in Primary Care." *Journal of General Internal Medicine* 20 (Suppl.1) (2005): 172.

UNODC (United Nations Office on Drugs and Crime). *Patterns and Trends of Amphetamine-Type Stimulants and Other Drugs: Asia and the Pacific.* A Report from the Global SMART Programme. Vienna: UNODC, 2011.

UNODC (United Nations Office on Drugs and Crime). *World Drug Report 2010.* Vienna: UNODC, 2011.

UNODC (United Nations Office on Drugs and Crime). *World Drug Report 2011.* Vienna: UNODC, 2012.

Veilleux, Jennifer C., Peter J. Colvin, Jennifer Anderson, Catherine York, and Adrienne J. Heinz. "A Review of Opioid Dependence Treatment: Pharmacological and Psychosocial Interventions to treat Opioid Addiction." *Clinical Psychology Review* 30 (2010): 155–66.

Vicknasingam, Balasingam and Navaratnam, V. "The Use of Rapid Assessment Methodology to Compliment Existing National Assessment and Surveillance Data: A Study among Injecting Drug Users in, Penang, Malaysia." *International Journal of Drug Policy* 19 (2008): 90–93.

Vicknasingam, Balasingam, Mahmud Mazlan, Marek C. Chawarski, and Richard S. Schottenfeld. "Injecting Buprenorphine in Malaysia: Demographic and Drug Use Characteristics of Buprenorphine Injectors." Paper presented at the College on Problems of Drug Dependence (CPDD) 69th Annual Scientific Meeting, Quebec City, Canada, June 16–21, 2007.

Vicknasingam, Balasingam, Mahmud Mazlan, Richard S. Schottenfeld, and Marek C. Chawarski. "Injection of Buprenorphine and Buprenorphine/Naloxone Tablets in Malaysia." *Drug and Alcohol Dependence* 111 (2010): 44–49.

Chapter Twenty

The Future of Drug Law Reform in Asia

Alex Wodak

HIV SPREAD AMONG AND FROM PEOPLE WHO INJECT DRUGS IN ASIA

Asia, home to almost half the world's population, is now the center of global economic activity. In coming decades, increasing income and wealth are bound to have far-reaching social, political, and economic effects. Education standards are rising and will ensure increasing interest in and respect for human rights.

The recent decades of rapid economic growth in China and India coincided with a time when Asia was forced to confront the serious threat of epidemic spread of HIV. In most Asian countries, HIV spreading first among and then from people who inject drugs represented the greatest threat of an HIV epidemic spreading among the general population (see des Jarlais et al.'s chapter in this book). When the seriousness of the HIV epidemic among people who inject drugs was first raised in Asia in the early 1990s, authorities in every Asian country denied vehemently that HIV could ever take root in their country. Each country asserted that even if HIV was ever accepted as a serious threat, harm reduction would never be countenanced as an acceptable control framework.

One by one, each country ultimately accepted the reality that their population was at risk of serious health, social, and economic consequences from an HIV epidemic beginning among people who inject drugs. Authorities also accepted that the package of effective HIV prevention measures we now call "harm reduction" represented the only realistic way of averting this serious threat. The entrenched commitment to drug prohibition delayed the introduction of effective HIV prevention.[1] Eventually countries were forced to choose between maintaining their long-standing and often strident commitment to punitive drug policies, with the associated high risk of an HIV epidemic, and allowing some policy flexibility in order to avert disaster. Fortunately, almost all major countries in Asia chose to accept greater policy flexibility. That acceptance however took almost two decades to achieve. Harm reduction measures began to be adopted widely across Asia in the 1990s. Twenty years later the scale of implementation is still well short of that required to control the HIV epidemic and is still grossly underfunded. The scale of implementation in the early 2010s is now slowly increasing but at a rate that will ensure that HIV will still be a major problem in Asia for decades to come.

This remarkable change in attitudes to harm reduction, affecting the health and well-being of billions of people in Asia, was achieved with modest resources. The persistent efforts of perhaps a score of Asian people and another score of international harm reduction advocates achieved this change in just two decades. In those countries where harm reduction eventually prevailed, the impressive health, social, and economic benefits that followed from relatively minor expenses in sharp contrast with the abundant evidence of failure from expensive and often draconian drug law enforcement measures. The HIV era has been a turning point in attitudes to drug problems that had been defined for over half a century as essentially a criminal justice issue. The green shoots of drug law reform are now starting to sprout in Asia.

Although the dramatic impact of the HIV pandemic on deaths, disease, suffering, and economic costs are, quite appropriately, the effects that are most often emphasized, there have been some important benefits. It seems almost perverse to mention benefits flowing from the HIV pandemic. But there have been benefits and these include a greater respect for the powerful interaction between public health and human rights, improvement in universal hygiene in operating theaters and the acceptance of human-rights-based approaches to groups at high risk of HIV (such as men who have sex with men, sex workers, and people who inject drugs). Increased support for drug law reform is one of the benefits flowing from international responses to HIV. Indeed UN Secretary-General Ban Ki-Moon noted that "In addition to criminalizing HIV transmission, many countries impose criminal sanctions for same-sex sex, commercial sex and drug injection. Such laws constitute major barriers to reaching key populations with HIV services. Those behaviors should be decriminalized, and people addicted to drugs should receive health services for the treatment of their addiction."[2]

GLOBAL DRUG PROHIBITION: THE BEGINNINGS OF REFORM

In the second decade of the twenty-first century, global drug prohibition is slowly starting to unravel.[3] It has been a long time coming. The first country in the world to challenge the international drug policy straight jacket was the Netherlands in the 1970s, followed by Switzerland in the early 1990s, and then Portugal in 2001.[4] Modest reforms resulted in worthwhile health, social, and economic benefits including a reduction in drug overdose deaths, HIV infections, problematic drug use, and crime.[5] In each country, drug treatment was expanded and considerably improved, and far greater emphasis was given to health and social interventions. In the Netherlands, the cannabis market was partially regulated. Portugal removed criminal sanctions from people found to be in possession of quantities of street drugs below a threshold defined to be consistent with personal consumption. These people were referred for health and social assessment and possible drug treatment. The community in the Netherlands, Switzerland, and Portugal has strongly and consistently supported these reforms.

In recent years, the international impetus for drug law reform has shifted from Europe to Latin America. In 2007, the Latin America Commission on Drug Policy issued a report signed by former presidents of Brazil, Mexico, and Colombia which was very critical of conventional drug policy. This was taken further in 2011 when the Global Commission on Drug Policy concluded "the global war on drugs has failed, with devastating consequences for individuals and societies around the world."[6] Several Central American countries have been devastated by the "War on Drugs" in recent years and this is now fueling significant drug law reform in Latin America. On August 8, 2012, President José Mujica of Uruguay made international history when he referred a bill to his country's legislature that would allow the regulated sale of cannabis.[7]

Drug law reform has also been gathering pace in the in the United States in the last decade. This is particularly important as the United States has been the most important country in the establishment and maintenance of global drug prohibition. At present eighteen states plus the District of Colombia now permit medicinal use of cannabis and three states (Colorado, Washington, and Oregon) will vote on regulated cannabis on November 6, 2012. Support for the legalization of marijuana rose in annual Gallup polls of US citizens from 12 percent in 1969 to 50 percent in 2011 while opposition fell from 84 percent in 1969 to 46 percent in 2011.[8] Some candidates running for political office in 2012 who support drug law reform defeated opponents who have been strongly supporters of the "War on Drugs."

THE IMPACT OF INCREASING INEQUALITY ON ILLICIT DRUGS

Disparities in income and wealth have been increasing in many developed and developing countries in recent decades. There is increasing evidence that inequality exacerbates illicit drug problems. Canadian researchers found in the 1970s that rats accommodated in cages with "ghetto-like" conditions consumed nineteen times more sweetened morphine than rats kept in quiet cages with ample food, water, and toys and at temperatures these animals prefer.[9] Although these findings were published in a reputable journal and replicated by other researchers, they have been rarely referred to. The notion that "addiction is a brain disease," a biological reductionist approach to illicit drugs, has been more popular in the United States and vigorously exported to other countries.

A follow up study of US soldiers who had fought in the Vietnam War and become dependent on heroin or opium found that almost all had stopped their drug use after returning home to normal civilian life.[10] Those who continued to use heroin after returning to the United States had generally used heroin before leaving for military service in Vietnam. The findings of this study were interpreted as showing that catastrophic conditions can increase the likelihood of heroin use.

A study of inequality in developed countries found that many major public health problems including illicit drug use were more common in countries with greater inequality.[11] (Mannava et al. discuss this further in their chapter in this book). Countries with less inequality, such as Japan and the Scandinavian countries, generally had lower levels of these public health problems including illicit drug use. In many countries, authorities have relied on mass and school-based education to reduce the demand from drugs despite evidence of only modest and delayed benefit. There has been less interest in the possibility of reducing inequality to reduce the demand for drugs.

THE POLITICAL REALITIES OF DRUG LAW REFORM
AND CIVIL SOCIETY

Acceptance of the need for drug law reform is now growing slowly in many Asian countries. However change is slow because bad policy is still good politics. With the political system jammed on drug law reform, change can only happen through pressure from civil society. The political obstacles to reform affect countries with democratic systems of government but also impede the reform process in countries with other forms of government. Drug law reform is slow to progress in Asia partly because civil society is still very weak in most Asian countries.

In recent decades, global drug production and consumption have continued to increase while the price of street drugs has continued to fall.[12] Even staunch supporters of drug prohibition, such as the then executive director of the UNODC, have been forced to question whether the current global drug policy was "fit for purpose" while also acknowledging the seriousness of the unintended negative consequences.[13, 14] In recent years the trickle of countries questioning the international orthodoxy has begun to increase.

Efforts to reduce the harm from drugs are now being extended to attempts to reduce the harm from drug policy in recognition of the fact that the pernicious effects of drugs supplied by a black market can be difficult to separate from direct harm arising from the drugs themselves.[15] There is increasing consideration of regulating the supply of drugs while recognizing the substantial political difficulties of achieving this.[16] Young people are often adept at the new social media, and this is now changing political realities on many questions in many countries. It may well be that political reform, including drug policy reform in Asia, will in future be influenced increasingly by the use of social media by young people.

The economics of the drug trade ensures that as long as demand for drugs remains strong, drug prohibition will fail. In recent decades, the reality has been that any attempt to adopt a policy that respected the inexorable economic forces of the drug market would fail politically. The irresistible force of economics confronted the immovable mountain of politics. However, while the laws of economics are immutable, what is politically possible can change over time. A growing number of senior politicians now admit privately that their national drug policy does not work. Some now feel able to say this in public. Effective strategies for drug law reform will differ between countries and depend on how politics is organized in each country. But the one constant is the critical role of civil society in achieving change.

In many countries, it was the relentless efforts of civil society in the last three decades which forced effective HIV policies onto a reluctant political system. This example should be an encouraging precedent for global efforts now underway to reform drug policy. Civil society has many strengths. These including diversity of members, representation of groups at high risk, and representation of young people. Young people are most at risk from drugs, most at risk from a punitive drug policy, and will have to contend longer than the rest of the community with the consequences of a failed drug policy.

Few people in developed countries realize the magnitude of the collateral damage from drug prohibition in producer and transit countries. A quarter century ago, the world's major producer of illicit opium was Burma. Since the 1990s, Afghanistan has been the world's major producer of illicit opium. The huge opium and heroin trade in west Asia has continued to corrupt and destabilize Afghanistan and Pakistan. The production and trade in amphetamine-type substances (ATS) has now largely replaced the opium trade in Southeast Asia. Aerial and satellite surveillance has forced the lucrative production of illicit drugs beyond easy detection of law enforcement and thus contributed to this transition from opium to ATS (see McKetin et al. in this book). A few years before the HIV epidemic was first recognized, the world was warned of the inadvertent pro-heroin effects of anti-opium policies in Laos, Thailand, and Hong Kong. [17] These policies eradicated opium smoking, which had been largely confined to elderly men, only to see this relatively benign habit replaced by heroin injecting among young and sexually active men, thus preparing the conditions for potential epidemic spread of HIV in the most populous area of the world.

Most social reforms take many decades. Drug law reform in Asia may also require many decades, but the rate of recent change in the Americas suggests that change may start occurring faster than many people think. Civil society may be able to achieve change that is not possible from within the conventional political process.

WHAT DOES DRUG LAW REFORM ENTAIL?

The threshold step in drug law reform is redefining drugs as primarily a health and social issue. More than half a century of treating illicit drugs as a criminal justice problem has failed comprehensively. Funding for health and social measures will have to be increased toward levels enjoyed for decades by drug law enforcement. Change should be incremental and carefully evaluated. There are many options for drug law reform. It is better to think of drug law reform as a process rather than an event. To some extent that process has already started in countries that have already established needle syringe programs and opioid substitution treatment with methadone and buprenorphine. Research will play a critical role in drug law reform.

The most important step is to improve drug treatment. Specifically, capacity should be expanded to meet demand, quality raised to the level of other health services, and flexibility increased. Heroin-assisted treatment should be provided for the few percent of heroin users who are severely dependent and have not benefited from multiple previous treatments.

Ultimately cannabis should be controlled by taxation and regulation. Regulation would include hard-to-get but easy-to-lose licenses for cultivation and wholesale and retail sale; labels with health warnings, information for consumers seeking help, and product data; proof of age at purchase; and bans on advertising and donations from the cannabis industry to political parties. Hypothecation of cannabis taxes could generate funding for drug prevention and treatment. Cannabis laws would probably have to pass through stages first with reduction of criminal sanctions and then reduction of civil penalties before consideration of regulated sale. Medicinal cannabis should be treated as a separate issue.

Supervised injecting facilities are needed near major illicit drug markets when these spill over into neighboring streets, parks, and supermarkets.

If these reforms do not provide sufficient benefit, there may be a case for considering the commercial sale of small quantities of dilute and carefully selected psychoactive drugs. Edible opium was taxed and regulated and available for sale in Australia until 1906. In the United States, Coca Cola contained cocaine until 1903.

Prevention and treatment of drug problems in correctional facilities should be of at least the same standard as in the community.

CONCLUSION

Global drug prohibition began in Asia with a meeting convened by the United States in Shanghai, China, in 1909. It developed slowly and culminated in the negotiation of three international drug treaties between 1961 and 1988. Efforts to control the HIV epidemic were hampered because the entrenched commitment to drug prohibition obstructed and delayed the implementation of effective prevention strategies. A century after it began, serious review of global drug prohibition is underway because drug law enforcement is now recognized to be relatively ineffective, often accompanied by serious unintended negative consequences and expensive.

Drug law reform is now being seriously considered in many parts of the world including Asia. This will take different forms in different countries. Global drug prohibition required that all countries had to adopt similar policies regardless of their situation. Drug law reform will allow countries to adopt policies best suited to their own conditions.

Drug law reform will evolve in Asia as Asian countries undergo rapid change fueled by the dramatic economic, political, and social changes now underway. This will involve a process of learning to come to terms with the world we actually live in rather than a world that some might dream of.

NOTES

1. Global Commission on Drug Policy. "The War on Drugs and HIV/AIDS: How the Criminalization of Drugs fuels the Global Pandemic" (Rio de Janeiro: Global Commission on Drug Policy, 2012). http://globalcommissionondrugs.org/wp-content/themes/gcdp_v1/pdf/GCDP_HIV-AIDS_2012_REFERENCE.pdf .

2. UN General Assembly. Progress made in the Implementation of the Declaration of Commitment on HIV/AIDS and the Political Declaration on HIV/AIDS. *Report of the Secretary-General Ban Ki-Moon, Sixty-third Session, Agenda item 41, 7 May 2009.* (A/63/812)

3. Global Commission on Drug Policy. "War on Drugs." Report of the Global Commission on Drug Policy, Rio de Janeiro, 2011. www.globalcommissionondrugs.org/wp-content/themes/gcdp_v1/pdf/Global_Commission_Report_English.pdf.

4. Caitlin Hughes and Alex Stevens, "What Can We Learn From The Portuguese Decriminalization of Illicit Drugs?" *British Journal of Criminology* 50, no. 6 (2010): 999–1022.

5. Bob Douglas, Alex Wodak, and David McDonald, "Alternatives to Prohibition. Illicit Drugs: How can we Stop Killing and Criminalising Young Australians," Report of the Second Australia 21 Roundtable on Illicit Drugs held at The University of Melbourne, Australia, July 6, 2012, www.australia21.org.au/publications/press_releases/A21_Alternatives_to_Prohibition_SEP_12.pdf.

6. Global Commission, *War on Drugs*, 2011.

7. Damien Cave, "South America Sees Drug Path to Legalization," *New York Times*, July 29, 2012. Accessed October 17, 2012. www.nytimes.com/2012/07/30/world/americas/uruguay-considers-legalizing-marijuana-to-stop-traffickers.html?pagewanted=all.

8. Gallup Poll, "Record-High 50% of Americans Favor Legalizing Marijuana Use." Accessed October 17, 2012. www.gallup.com/poll/150149/record-high-americans-favor-legalizing-marijuana.aspx

9. Bruce K. Alexander, Barry L. Beyerstein, Patricia F. Hadaway, and Robert B. Coambs, "Effects of Early and Later Colony Housing on Oral Ingestion of Morphine in Rats," *Psychopharmacology Biochemistry and Behavior* 58 (1981): 175–79.

10. Lee N. Robins, Darlene H. Davis, and Donald W. Goodwin, "Drug Use by U.S Army Enlisted Men in Vietnam: A Follow Up on their Return Home." *American Journal of Epidemiology* 19, no. 4 (1974): 235–49.

11. Richard G. Wilkinson and Kate Pickett, *The Spirit Level: Why More Equal Societies Almost Always Do Better* (London: Allen Lane, 2009).

12. Global Commission, *War on Drugs*, 2011.

13. Commission on Narcotic Drugs. "Making Drug Control 'Fit for Purpose': Building on the UNGASS Decade." *Report by the Executive Director of the United Nations Office on Drugs and Crime as a contribution to the review of the twentieth special session of the General Assembly, Fifty-first Session, Item 3 of the Provisional Agenda, 10 – 14 May 2009.* (E/CN.7/2008/CRP.17).

14. UNODC (United Nations Office of Drugs and Crime), "The 51st Session of the Commission on Narcotic Drugs: UNODC Executive Director Antonio Maria Costa," March 10, 2008. www.unodc.org/unodc/en/about-unodc/speeches/2008-03-10.html.

15. David J. Nutt, Leslie A. King, Lawrence D. Phillips, for the Independent Scientific Committee on Drugs. "Drug Harms in the UK: a Multicriteria Decision Analysis," *Lancet* 376, no. 9752 (2010): 1558–65.

16. Stephen Rolles, "An Alternative to the War on Drugs," *British Medical Journal* 341 (2010): c3360. DOI: http://dx.doi.org/10.1136/bmj.c3360.

17. Joseph Westermeyer, "The Pro-Heroin Effects of Anti-Opium Laws in Asia." *Archives of General Psychiatry* 33, no. 9 (1976): 1135–39.

BIBLIOGRAPHY

Alexander, Bruce K., Barry L. Beyerstein, Patricia F. Hadaway, and Robert B. Coambs. "Effects of Early and Later Colony Housing on Oral Ingestion of Morphine in Rats." *Psychopharmacology Biochemistry and Behavior* 58 (1981): 175–79.

Cave, Damien. "South America Sees Drug Path to Legalization." *New York Times*, July 29, 2012. Accessed October 17, 2012. www.nytimes.com/2012/07/30/world/americas/uruguay-considers-legalizing-marijuana-to-stop-traffickers.html?pagewanted=all.

Commission on Narcotic Drugs. "Making Drug Control 'Fit for Purpose': Building on the UNGASS Decade." *Report by the Executive Director of the United Nations Office on Drugs and Crime as a contribution to the review of the twentieth special session of the General Assembly, Fifty-first Session, Item 3 of the Provisional Agenda, 10–14 May 2009.* (E/CN.7/2008/CRP.17).

Douglas, Bob, Alex Wodak, and David McDonald. "Alternatives to Prohibition. Illicit Drugs: How Can We Stop Killing and Criminalising Young Australians." Report of the Second Australia 21 Roundtable on Illicit Drugs held at The University of Melbourne, Australia, July 6, 2012. www.australia21.org.au/publications/press_releases/A21_Alternatives_to_ Prohibition_SEP_12.pdf.

Gallup Poll. "Record-High 50% of Americans Favor Legalizing Marijuana Use." Accessed October 17, 2012.www.gallup.com/poll/150149/record-high-americans-favor-legalizing-marijuana.aspx.

Global Commission on Drug Policy. "War on Drugs." Report of the Global Commission on Drug Policy, Rio de Janeiro, 2011.www.globalcommissionondrugs.org/wp-content/themes/ gcdp_v1/pdf/Global_Commission_Report_English.pdf.

Global Commission on Drug Policy. "The War on Drugs and HIV/AIDS: How the Criminalization of Drugs fuels the Global Pandemic." Rio de Janeiro: Global Commission on Drug Policy, 2012.http://globalcommissionondrugs.org/wp-content/themes/gcdp_v1/pdf/GCDP_ HIV-AIDS_2012_REFERENCE.pdf.

Nutt, David J., Leslie A. King, Lawrence D. Phillips, for the Independent Scientific Committee on Drugs. "Drug Harms in the UK: a Multicriteria Decision Analysis." *Lancet* 376, no. 9752 (2010): 1558–65.

Robins, Lee N., Darlene H. Davis, and Donald W. Goodwin. "Drug Use by U.S Army Enlisted men in Vietnam: A Follow up on their Return Home. *American Journal of Epidemiology* 19, no. 4 (1974): 235–49.

Rolles, Stephen. "An Alternative to the War on Drugs." *British Medical Journal* 341 (2010): c3360. DOI: http://dx.doi.org/10.1136/bmj.c3360.

UN General Assembly. Progress made in the Implementation of the Declaration of Commitment on HIV/AIDS and the Political Declaration on HIV/AIDS. *Report of the Secretary-General Ban Ki-Moon, Sixty-third Session, Agenda item 41, May 7, 2009.* (A/63/812)

UNODC (United Nations Office of Drugs and Crime). 2008. "The 51st Session of the Commission on Narcotic Drugs: UNODC Executive Director Antonio Maria Costa." March 10, 2008. www.unodc.org/unodc/en/about-unodc/speeches/2008-03-10.html.

Westermeyer, Joseph. "The Pro-Heroin Effects of Anti-Opium Laws in Asia." *Archives of General Psychiatry* 33, no. 9 (1976): 1135–39.

WilkinsonRichard G. and KatePickett. *The Spirit Level: Why More Equal Societies Almost Always Do Better.* London: Allen Lane, 2009.

Index

About the Contributors

Simon Baldwin has lived and worked in Asia for the past ten years. He has spent the past three years living in Vietnam where he was the global technical adviser from FHI on issues relating to HIV and illicit drug use. Simon's work has focused on the structural drivers of HIV among people who use drugs. He is especially interested in the role of drug policy reform in reducing harm. He also works tirelessly to address the ethical and human rights concerns associated with extrajudicial compulsory detention of drug users. Simon has published several articles on drug use in the Asia and Pacific region. He is currently working as a consultant based in Indonesia.

Sarah Biddulph is associate professor and reader in the law school at The University of Melbourne. She teaches and researches in the area of Chinese law. Her work focuses on contemporary Chinese administrative law, criminal procedure, labor, comparative law, and the law regulating social and economic rights. Her recent publications include: *Legal Reform and Administrative Detention Powers in China* (2007) and she was coeditor of *Examining Practice Interrogating Theory: Comparative Legal Studies in Asia* (2008). She has been working on a project with Associate Professor Sean Cooney and Professor Zhu Ying looking at the regulatory responses to wages arrears in China. She currently holds a research fellowship from the ARC to work on the recent reforms to the police administrative detention powers in China. This project includes an examination of reforms to compulsory detention for treatment of drug-dependent people.

Heidi Bramson has worked in the field of HIV prevention, with a particular focus on the drug-using community, for over a decade. She has experience in community-based outreach and organizing, as well as in public health research design and management. Heidi is currently a project director at The Baron Edmond de Rothschild Chemical Dependency Institute at Beth Israel Medical Center in New York City. Her interests are in public health law and policy, with an emphasis on racial and economic health disparities, and women's health. Heidi obtained a master's in public health from The Johns Hopkins Bloomberg School of Public Health, and attained her juris doctor from Rutgers School of Law-Newark.

Marek C. Chawarski, PhD, is associate professor of psychiatry in the Substance Abuse Division at Yale University School of Medicine. His research and teaching involves international collaborative efforts in Asia, the Middle East, and Europe that are focused on the development of improved interventions for treatment of substance abuse targeting high risk individuals (e.g., opiate-dependent, IDU, with long history of drug use, and multiple treatment failures) and training programs for researchers and clinicians in the area of substance use. His current research includes the development of a behavioral intervention to help patients seeking and participating in substance use treatment improve their treatment engagements, to increase their chances of succeeding in treatment, and to reduce their risk of HIV and other infectious diseases. His international collaborative research and training activities aim to develop and implement effective substance use treatment approaches to treat drug dependence and to reduce HIV and other infectious diseases risks in diverse cultural, ethnic, and religious populations, primarily in Asia but also in other parts of the world.

Nick Crofts is a professorial fellow in the School of Population Health at the University of Melbourne. He has worked in blood-borne virus epidemiology and in harm reduction in most countries in Asia for more than twenty years; his current major interest, arising from this work, is in the intersection of law enforcement and public health. He is a founding director of the Centre for Law Enforcement and Public Health.

Joanne Csete is senior program officer of the Global Drug Policy Program at the Open Society Foundations. She was previously an associate professor at the Columbia University Mailman School of Public Health, executive director of the Canadian HIV/AIDS Legal Network, founding director of the HIV Program at Human Rights Watch, and an assistant professor at the University of Wisconsin–Madison. She worked in Africa for over ten years, including as chief of program planning at the regional office of UNICEF in Nairobi. She holds a doctorate from Cornell University, a master's degree in public health from Columbia, and a bachelor's degree in economics from Princeton University.

Don C. Des Jarlais, PhD, is director of research for the Baron Edmond de Rothschild Chemical Dependency Institute at Beth Israel Medical Center, a Senior Research Fellow with the National Development and Research Institutes, Inc. and a guest investigator at Rockefeller University in New York. He began his research on AIDS in 1982. As a leader in the fields of AIDS and injecting drug use, Dr. Des Jarlais has published extensively on these topics including papers in the *New England Journal of Medicine*, the *Journal of the American Medical Association*, *Science*, and *Nature*. He has been particularly active in international research, having collaborated on studies in twenty-five different countries. He serves as a consultant to various institutions, including the Centers for Disease Control and Prevention, the National Institute on Drug Abuse, the National Academy of Sciences, and the World Health Organization. He is a former commissioner for the US National Commission on AIDS, and is currently a core group member of the UNAIDS Reference Group on HIV and Injecting Drug Use. In 2010 Dr. Des Jarlais was elected to the US President's Emergency Plan for AIDS Relief (PEPFAR) Scientific Advisory Board (SAB).

Kate Dolan is a professor and also the head of the Program of International Research and Training at the National Drug and Alcohol Research Centre, UNSW in Australia. She was involved in starting the first needle and syringe program in Australia in 1986 and has studied drug use and infectious diseases among prison populations since 1989. She conducted a randomized controlled trial of the NSW prison methadone program. She established a drug treatment clinic for women in Iran in 2007. Her most recent project was an examination of supply, demand, and harm reduction strategies for Australian prisoners.

Jimmy Dorabjee has been engaged in a range of harm reduction and development activities for over twenty years. From 2001 till 2010, Jimmy was the principal fellow harm reduction at the Burnet Institute for Medical Research and Public Health, Centre for Harm Reduction and Centre for International Health, Australia working on Burnet projects in Asia. Before this, Jimmy was program manager for Drug Treatment & Harm Reduction Projects at SHARAN, a pioneering community development NGO in New Delhi. While at SHARAN, he began Asia's first buprenorphine substitution program for injecting drug users in India in 1992. In 1998 and 2000, he conducted two rounds of multicenter rapid assessments on injecting drug use in India and expanded the SHARAN harm reduction program to five major Indian cities. In 1996, Jimmy was a founding member of the Asian Harm Reduction Network and was its chairman till 2002. Jimmy's extensive experience and commitment to harm reduction program development has gained him international recognition, and in 2001, he was awarded the National Rolleston

Award by the International Harm Reduction Association. Jimmy continues to consult in Asia with a special interest in building capacity of networks and communities affected by drug use. He is currently a member of the UN Regional Task Force on Injecting Drug Use and HIV/AIDS in Asia and the Pacific and the Interagency Reference Group, UNAIDS Technical Support Facility for South Asia, core member of the Reference Group to the United Nations on HIV and Injecting Drug Use, Board Member and Member of the Management Committee of the Coalition of Regional Networks on HIV/ AIDS in Asia and the Pacific (7 Sisters), founding member and Chairperson of the Asian Network of People who Use Drugs (ANPUD), and an Executive Member of Response Beyond Borders, the Asian Consortium on Drugs, HIV, AIDS and Poverty (ACDHAP).

Jonathan Feelemyer works as an epidemiologist in the Baron Edmond de Rothschild Chemical Dependency Institute of Beth Israel Medical Center. During his work at the institute, Jonathan has worked closely with national and international researchers to examine trends among persons who inject drugs and their mixing patterns with other high-risk populations including sex workers and men who have sex with men. His focus has been on HIV, HCV, and other blood-borne infections and harm reduction programs targeted at these high-risk groups. Previous to this, Jonathan worked on a National Drug Abuse Study under the direction of the Substance Abuse and Mental Services Administration (SAMHSA), examining trends in major drugs of abuse and adverse events in hospitals and emergency rooms across the country. This data was used to report on trends in drugs of abuse in the United States among the general population, allowing for harm reduction workers in different locations to tailor their harm reduction programs appropriately based on SAMHSA yearly reports.

Asmin Fransiska is a lecturer at the law faculty of Atmajaya University, Jakarta, since 2005, on several subjects such as Human Rights Law, Children and Women Protection Law, and European Law. She has a master's degree (LLM with honors) from the Northwestern University School of Law, Chicago. In 2004, she worked as a UN-Fulbright Fellow in the Rule of Law Division at the Office of High Commissioner for Human Rights (OHCHR), Geneva, Switzerland. She is also a coordinator of Indonesian Drug Policy Reform (ICDPR).

Holly Hagan, RN, MPH, PhD, is a professor at the NYU College of Nursing. Her program of research has focused on the infectious disease consequences of illicit drug use. She has led a number of NIH-funded studies, including several that have examined the etiology of blood-borne viral transmission associated with drug administration practices and to estimate prevalence and incidence of viral hepatitis, sexually transmitted infections, and HIV in people who use illicit drugs. Dr. Hagan has gained an international reputation from her studies of hepatitis C virus infection in people who inject drugs, and her work on the etiology, epidemiology, and prevention of HCV has informed harm reduction practices in the United States and abroad.

Faisal Ibrahim has master of public health and a master of primary health care management. He is currently a professor of Public Health at Universiti Putra Malaysia and was formerly the harm reduction program consultant in the Malaysian Ministry of Health. He is currently working together with UNICEF on a project on children and families affected by HIV/AIDS. He is also a committee member of the Islamic Religious Council of Perlis.

David Jacka, MBBS, MPH, FAChAM, has worked in the area of HIV since 1989, Injecting Drug Use, Drug Dependence Treatment and Harm Reduction since 1993, and until December 2006 he was deputy director of the Centre for Harm Reduction at the Burnet Institute in Melbourne and Drug Treatment Specialist in community and custodial settings in Australia. Since January 2007 he has worked within WHO as a drug treatment specialist and adviser on HIV prevention programming for IDU in Indonesia, Myanmar, Cambodia, and Vietnam. He is currently the medical officer for Comprehensive HIV Prevention at the World Health Organization Country Office, Vietnam and advisor to the large World Bank/DFID/Global Fund HIV Prevention Programmes there.

Karyn Kaplan is the cofounder and director of Policy and Development at the Thai AIDS Treatment Action Group (TTAG), a PLWHA-run HIV and human rights advocacy organization based in Bangkok. Karyn has worked on HIV/AIDS for marginalized populations in Thailand since 1988, and with her partner and TTAG co-founder, Paisan Suwannawong, was the 2009 recipient of the John M. Lloyd Foundation International HIV/AIDS Leadership Award. Karyn has authored and coauthored numerous human rights and public health publications, including *Human Rights Documentation and Advocacy: A Guide for Organizations of People Who Use Drugs* (2009).

Shui Shan Lee is a clinician and specialist in internal medicine, immunopathology, and public health. He is currently professor of infectious disease of The Chinese University of Hong Kong. Between 1991 and 2005, Dr. Lee headed the Hong Kong Government's AIDS program, during which he directed HIV prevention, control, and treatment services. He has, on different occasions, served as consultant to national and international organizations in the assessment of HIV situations, program planning, and evaluations. His major areas of research interests include optimization of HIV treatment,

HIV/AIDS epidemiology, social and spatial contexts of infectious disease transmission.

Dean Lewis is currently the regional coordinator of the ANPUD (The Asian Network of People Who Use Drugs). Dean has been working in the field of drug treatment since 1986 and in the specific field of Harm Reduction since 1993. He has assisted in the implementation of over thirty-five HIV-related projects ranging from home-based and community-based care to palliative care. Since 1994 Lewis was involved with the implementation and administration of the first Buprenorphine pilot study in India, and till 2010 has been involved with the scale-up of harm reduction services in India, including writing the IDU component of four Global Fund country proposals. He also provides technical consultancy to two major research projects: Positive Outcomes for Orphans (POFO)—a longitudinal six-country research project on HIV orphan care—and (AVHI)—Averting HIV Infection among IDUs a two-year project to adapt and evaluate an evidence-based HIV prevention intervention using IDU peer networks as a platform for recruiting IDUs into HIV prevention services. Lewis is also a senior research fellow at the Center for Health Policy, Duke University and is on the advisory board of Lawyers Collective HIV AIDS Unit.

Jih-Heng Li has been devoted to drug policy in Taiwan since the early 1990s. He holds a BS in pharmacy from Kaohsiung Medical University and a PhD in environmental medicine from New York University. Dr. Li was formerly the director general of National Bureau of Controlled Drugs, Department of Health, Taiwan. He is currently professor of toxicology and dean of the College of Pharmacy at Kaohsiung Medical University, Taiwan.

Priya Mannava currently works at the Burnet Institute in Melbourne, Australia, as a fellow in the Women's and Children's Health Team. Prior to this, Mannava worked as a public health consultant for two years, undertaking various tasks including: research on the interrelationships between illicit drugs and socioeconomic development, documenting the response to HIV epidemics in Northeast India, and providing support in the development and review of country proposals to the Global Fund to Fight AIDS, Tuberculosis, and Malaria. Mannava has also worked with the Global Fund to Fight AIDS, Tuberculosis, and Malaria where she undertook research in areas of strategic importance, including an analysis of the organization's funding for harm reduction activities.

Rebecca McKetin is a fellow in mental health research at the Australian National University. Her research interests include the relationship between substance use and mental health, particularly drug-induced psychosis and depression. Much of her research has focused on methamphetamine, for which she received a NSW/ACT Young Tall Poppy Science Award in 2008. Earlier in her career she worked as an epidemiologist for the United Nations Office on Drugs and Crime, and in this context she was involved with the establishment of drug-monitoring systems in Africa and Southeast Asia. McKetin is currently the executive editor for the international journal *Drug and Alcohol Review* and an associate member of the Australian Institute of Policy and Science.

Fifa Rahman has a master's of health law from the University of Sydney and is involved in advocacy and policy recommendations for a wide range of health policy issues, but her primary interests are drug policy, tobacco control, and mental health laws. Formerly with the Malaysian Ministry of Health, she is currently policy manager at the Malaysian AIDS Council. Recently, she was worked for Harm Reduction International, reporting on the death penalty for drug offenses in Southeast Asia. She has spearheaded a national campaign on access to generic medicines, collaborating with numerous patient organizations. She also sits on the panel of reviewers for the journal *Mental Health and Substance Use*. She is currently working on amending urinary testing laws, advocating for human rights-based police practice and introducing police drug diversion in Malaysia. She has worked with the International Drug Policy Consortium (IDPC) on police practice and drug diversion.

Ana Rodas, PhD in criminology, is a research officer at the National Drug and Alcohol Research Centre, UNSW Sydney. Dr. Rodas's work has focused on offender populations and drug use. Her work has included projects such as: an exploration of the relationship between cannabis and crime in a juvenile sample and an examination of supply, demand, and harm reduction strategies in Australian prisoners.

Jennifer Rowe has been working on substance use in compulsory settings for several years. First, from the perspective of national Red Cross and Red Crescent Societies' work in prisons, and then for her PhD in law and public health from the University of Melbourne, focusing on the regulatory framework surrounding substance use in Cambodia. Most recently, Rowe also worked for the UN Office of the High Commissioner for Human Rights in Cambodia, examining the social affairs, drug, and youth rehabilitation centers.

Richard Schottenfeld, MD, is professor of psychiatry at Yale University. His work has focused in the United States and internationally on developing, expanding and disseminating evidence-based drug use treatments, conducting drug use clinical research to improve the efficacy, accessibility, and availability of substance use treatment, and training drug use clinical researchers. The general themes of his research and approaches utilized are evident in the major, interrelated programs of research that he has developed aimed at (1) improving the efficacy of opioid agonist maintenance treatment through investigations of alternatives to methadone for maintenance treatment and investigations of adjunctive behavioral and pharmacological treatments for specific patient subpopulations (e.g., those with co-occurring cocaine dependence or chronic pain), (2) improving the accessibility and effectiveness of opioid dependence treatment by integrating it in office-based and primary care settings, and (3) evaluating and disseminating evidence-based drug use treatment and promoting drug use clinical research in international settings.

Pascal Tanguay worked for the Asian Harm Reduction Network (AHRN) for five years as the communications officer. During this time, Tanguay worked closely with national, regional, and international partners to raise awareness, mobilize funds, and provide technical support to a wide range of stakeholders from the government, civil society, donor, and multilateral sectors. For the past four years, Tanguay has worked closely with the International Drug Policy Consortium (IDPC), first as a focal point for coordination of drug-policy-related activities across Asia, and lately as a fellow with the Consortium to provide guidance and strategic input in the Consortium's operations. Recently, Pascal has joined PSI/Thailand as the program director to oversee the implementation of the Global Fund Round 8 component on injecting drug use. In this latest role, Tanguay works with all relevant national stakeholders to ensure the success of the project.

Nicholas Thomson, MPH PhD, has lived and worked across Southeast Asia over the last twelve years. Initially during that time he worked on HIV prevention research trials with Johns Hopkins School of Public Health and Chiang Mai University's Research Institute for Health Science. Through his work on injecting and non-injecting drug use, he became interested in the intersection of law enforcement, public health, and human rights. This led to further investigation and work into the impacts of compulsory detention. In the last two years, Thomson has embarked on a broad agenda of work around creating and enhancing partnerships between criminal justice systems and public health. He is based at the Nossal Institute for Global Health in Melbourne but maintains Southeast Asian regional projects with the Johns Hopkins and Chiang Mai University collaboration. In addition, Nicholas is a founding director of the Centre for Law Enforcement and Public Health.

Vuong Thi Huong Thu has a master's degree in public health, concentrated on health services management and policy, from Ohio State University in the United States in 2006 on a Fulbright scholarship. From February 2012, with Endeavour scholarship, she pursues her PhD on drug policy research focusing on economic evaluation of drug treatment options. She has had eighteen years of experience in public health work in the areas of HIV and drug policy. She is a key facilitator of dialogue between the international community and the government of Vietnam to achieve a consensus in moving away from the compulsory drug treatment approach toward evidence-based policy and programs for effective drug treatment. The goal of the work is to advance illicit drug policy through improving the evidence base, developing new policy decision-making tools, and understanding the best mix of policy options (law enforcement, prevention, treatment, and harm reduction) and the ways in which these different policy options dynamically interact. Her professional career includes writing for the International Journal of Drug Policy and a considerable career in freelance writing. Her professional efforts have been recognized by the National Assembly of Vietnam and the International Federation of Non-Government Organizations (IFNGO).

Nicole Turner is Australian-based coordinator of the Law Enforcement and HIV Network (LEAHN, www.leahn.org), a bilingual resource jointly hosted by the Nossal Institute for Global Health, Melbourne, Australia, and The Central Asian Centre on Drug Policy, Bishkek, Kyrgyzstan. Turner is a serving police officer with many years' experience in training, education, and mental health. She has worked extensively on police/health partnerships and has recently delivered harm reduction training to police in Vietnam. As the coordinator of the LEAHN project, Turner liaises regularly with law enforcement agencies globally and provides specialist advice and advocacy.

B. Vicknasingam, PhD, is associate professor at the Centre for Drug Research at Universiti Sains Malaysia. His research has focused on conducting epidemiological surveys on the risk behaviors of drug users and how the results from these surveys can be used to improve treatment for drug users. He is currently collaborating with Marek Chawarski and Richard Schottenfeld from Yale University School of Medicine to develop innovative treatment approaches for drug users in Malaysia. He has carried out several consultancy assignments for international agencies to evaluate harm reduction programs in the Asian region. The area of drug policy has also been of interest to him as Malaysia's drug policy continues to evolve.

Alex Wodak, AM, trained as a physician and was director of the Alcohol and Drug Service, St. Vincent's Hospital, Sydney, Australia (1982 to 2012). He worked with others to establish Australia's first needle syringe program and Australia's first medically supervised injecting room (when these were both pre-legal). Dr. Wodak is the president of the Australian Drug Law Reform Foundation and was the President of the International Harm Reduction Association (1996 to 2004). Together with colleagues he helped establish the National Drug and Alcohol Research Centre, the NSW Users AIDS Association (an organization for and run by people who use drugs), and the Australian Society of HIV Medicine. He has often worked in developing countries to help control HIV infection among people who injecting drugs. Dr. Wodak is a Director of Australia21 and was a coauthor of their two reports on drug law reform released in 2012. In 2010 Dr. Wodak was awarded a medal in the Order of Australia (AM).

Mohamad Firdaus Zakaria has been involved in issues related to drug use and harm reduction for over twelve years. His earliest experience in drug policy was as a peer educator at the Malaysian National Anti-Drug Agency (AADK) rehabilitation and service center. From 2004–2005 he became active as a facilitator to issues related to drug use and HIV/AIDS under the Penang Family Health Development Association, Malaysia. From 2005–2010 he served as Program Manager at Alternative Community Centers, an organization which ran the NSEP pilot project in Malaysia. Over the past five years until now, he has been engaged with Asian Network of People who Use Drugs (ANPUD) and currently serves on their board of directors.

Sasha Zegenhagen recently completed a bachelor of arts, bachelor of commerce, and diploma in modern languages (French) at the University of Melbourne, with majors in economics and politics. During this period she undertook an internship at the Nossal Institute for Global Health. She is currently working as an economic analyst at Deloitte Access Economics in Melbourne.

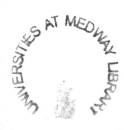